ATTD 2011 Yearbook

ATTD 2011 Yearbook

Advanced Technologies & Treatments for Diabetes

Third Edition

EDITED BY

Moshe Phillip
Tadej Battelino

ASSOCIATE EDITORS

Eran Atlas
Cameron Barr
Jennifer K. Beckerman
Bruce W. Bode
Jan Bolinder
Bruce Buckingham
H. Peter Chase
Thomas Danne
Eyal Dassau
Satish K. Garg
Lutz Heinemann
Irl B. Hirsch
Moshe Hod

Lois Jovanovic
Neal Kaufman
Kelsey Krigstein
Alon Liberman
Christian Lowe
John C. Pickup
Michael C. Riddell
Shlomit Shalitin
Nicole A. Sitkin
Jay S. Skyler
Mark Sueyoshi
Andrei Szigiato
Howard Zisser

WILEY-BLACKWELL

A John Wiley & Sons, Ltd., Publication

This edition first published 2012, © 2012 by John Wiley & Sons Ltd.

Wiley-Blackwell is an imprint of John Wiley & Sons, formed by the merger of Wiley's global Scientific, Technical and Medical business with Blackwell Publishing.

Registered office: John Wiley & Sons, Ltd, The Atrium, Southern Gate, Chichester, West Sussex, PO19 8SQ, UK

Editorial offices: 9600 Garsington Road, Oxford, OX4 2DQ, UK
The Atrium, Southern Gate, Chichester, West Sussex, PO19 8SQ, UK
111 River Street, Hoboken, NJ 07030-5774, USA

For details of our global editorial offices, for customer services and for information about how to apply for permission to reuse the copyright material in this book please see our website at www.wiley.com/wiley-blackwell

Library of Congress Cataloging-in-Publication Data is available for this title

A catalogue record for this book is available from the British Library.

Wiley also publishes its books in a variety of electronic formats. Some content that appears in print may not be available in electronic books.

Set in 10/13 pt Meridien by Aptara® Inc., New Delhi, India

1   2012

Contents

List of Contributors

Editors

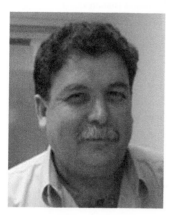

Moshe Phillip
Jesse Z. and Sara Lea Shafer Institute
for Endocrinology and Diabetes
National Center for Childhood Diabetes
Schneider Children's Medical Center of Israel
Petah Tikva
Israel

and

Sackler Faculty of Medicine
Tel-Aviv University, Tel-Aviv
Israel

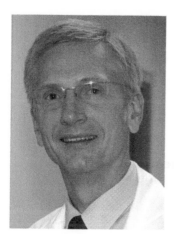

Tadej Battelino
Department of Endocrinology, Diabetes & Metabolism
University Medical Center
University Children's Hospital
Ljubljana
Slovenia

Associate Editors

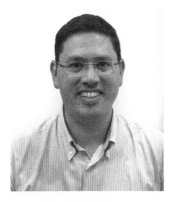

Eran Atlas
Diabetes Technologies Center
Schneider Children's Medical Center of Israel
Jesse Z. and Sara Lea Shafer Institute for
Endocrinology and Diabetes
National Center for Childhood Diabetes
Petah Tikva
Israel

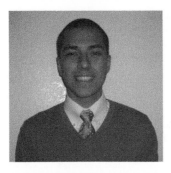

Cameron Barr
University of California at Santa Barbara
Santa Barbara, CA
USA

and

Sansum Diabetes Research Institute
Santa Barbara, CA
USA

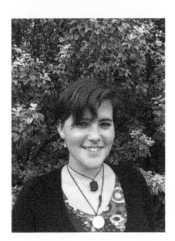

Jennifer K. Beckerman
Sansum Diabetes Research Institute
Santa Barbara, CA
USA

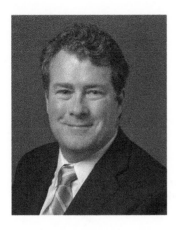

Bruce W. Bode
Atlanta Diabetes Associates
Atlanta, GA
USA

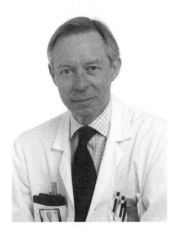

Jan Bolinder
Department of Medicine
Karolinska University Hospital Huddinge
Karolinska Institutet
Stockholm
Sweden

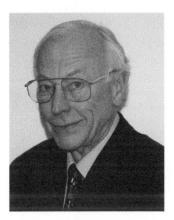

Bruce Buckingham
Stanford University Medical Center
Division of Endocrinology and Diabetes
Stanford, CA
USA

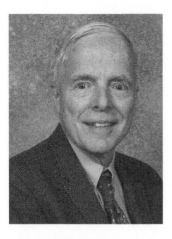

H. Peter Chase
Barbara Davis Center for Childhood Diabetes
University of Colorado
Denver, CO
USA

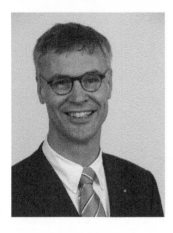

Thomas Danne
Diabetes-Zentrum für Kinder and Jugendliche
Kinderkrankenhaus auf der Bult
Hannover
Germany

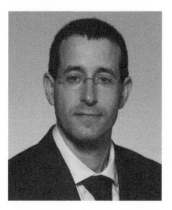

Eyal Dassau
University of California at Santa Barbara
Santa Barbara, CA
USA

and

Sansum Diabetes Research Institute
Santa Barbara, CA
USA

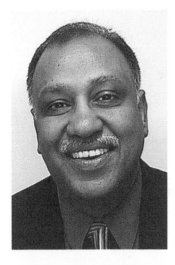

Satish K. Garg
Barbara Davis Center for Childhood Diabetes
University of Colorado Health Sciences Center
Aurora, CO
USA

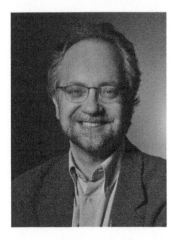

Lutz Heinemann
Science & Co
Düsseldorf, Germany

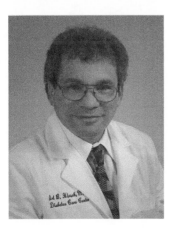

Irl B. Hirsch
University of Washington Medical Center
Seattle, WA
USA

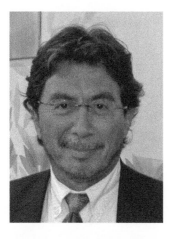

Moshe Hod
Perinatal Division
Helen Schneider Hospital for Women
Rabin Medical Center
Petah Tikva
Israel

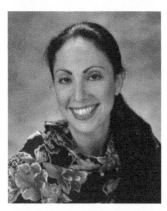

Lois Jovanovic
Sansum Diabetes Research Institute
Santa Barbara, CA
USA

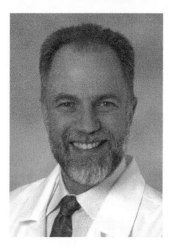

Neal Kaufman
UCLA Schools of Medicine and Public Health
Los Angeles, CA
USA

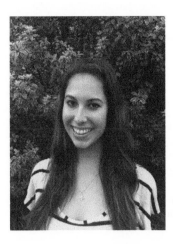

Kelsey Krigstein
Sansum Diabetes Research Institute
Santa Barbara, CA
USA

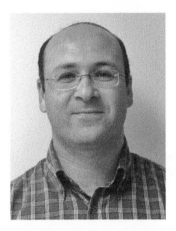

Alon Liberman
Jesse Z. and Sara Lea Shafer Institute for
Endocrinology and Diabetes
National Center for Childhood Diabetes
Schneider Children's Medical Center of Israel
Petah Tikva
Israel

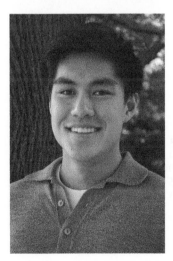

Christian Lowe
University of California at Santa Barbara
Santa Barbara, CA
USA

and

Sansum Diabetes Research Institute
Santa Barbara, CA
USA

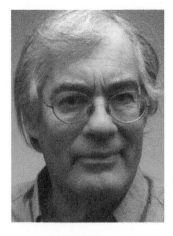

John C. Pickup
King's College London School of Medicine
Guy's Hospital, London
UK

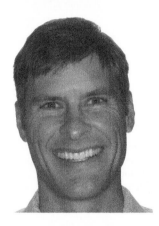

Michael C. Riddell
School of Kinesiology and Health Science
York University
Toronto, ON
Canada

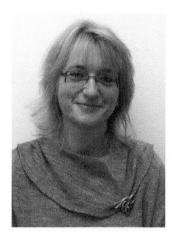

Shlomit Shalitin
Jesse Z. and Sara Lea Shafer Institute
for Endocrinology and Diabetes
National Center for Childhood Diabetes
Schneider Children's Medical Center of Israel
Petah Tikva
Israel

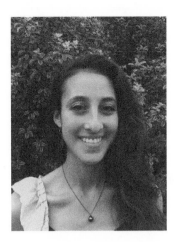

Nicole A. Sitkin
Sansum Diabetes Research Institute
Santa Barbara, CA
USA

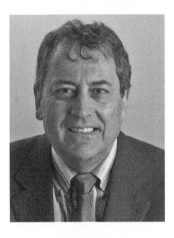

Jay S. Skyler
Division of Endocrinology
Diabetes, and Metabolism, and Diabetes Research
Institute
University of Miami Miller School of Medicine
Miami, FL
USA

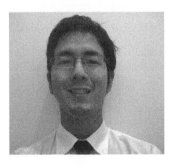

Mark Sueyoshi
Sansum Diabetes Research Institute
Santa Barbara, CA
USA

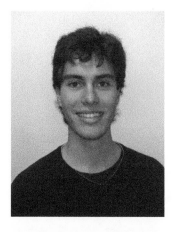

Andrei Szigiato
School of Kinesiology and Health Science
York University
Toronto, ON
Canada

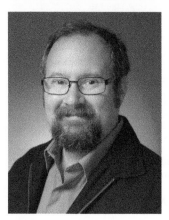

Howard Zisser
Sansum Diabetes Research Institute
Santa Barbara, CA
USA

and

University of California at Santa Barbara
Santa Barbara, CA
USA

Preface

This is the third *ATTD Yearbook* and by now we already know that the book makes its way to the hands of many clinicians, diabetes educators and researchers in academic institutes and to the members of the diabetes industry as well as many others interested in changing the life of people with diabetes all over the world. The availability of the book on the ATTD webpage and in PubMed facilitates access to anybody in the world interested in new technologies and therapies in diabetes. Also this year, the book consists of short summaries of selected papers published in peer-reviewed journals, between July 2010 and June 2011, with comments from the associate editors and editors bringing their expert insight to the reader.

The improvement in quality of life and life expectancy of people with diabetes increasingly depends on the success of innovative people in academia and industry to develop new technologies. This accomplishment is in turn crucially related to the interaction between different disciplines of research collaborating in the endeavour to solve the challenges diabetes presents to patients, caregivers, researchers and the industry. Professional interactive relationships between academia and industry will facilitate progress in the field and will lead not only to great innovations but also to their availability for routine clinical care.

We hope that the ATTD meeting and the present *ATTD Yearbook* will help to raise the attention and facilitate the communication of all interested parties in the field of diabetes for the ultimate benefit of our patients.

Moshe Phillip
Tadej Battelino

CHAPTER 1

Self-Monitoring of Blood Glucose

Satish K. Garg[1] and Irl B. Hirsch[2]

[1] University of Colorado Health Sciences Center, Aurora, CO, USA
[2] University of Washington Medical Center, Seattle, WA, USA

INTRODUCTION

Diabetes prevalence is increasing globally especially in the Asian sub-continent. It is expected that by the year 2030 there may be close to 400 million people with diabetes. All of the research in the past 25 years has clearly documented the effectiveness of improving glucose control in reducing long-term complications of diabetes, both microvascular and macrovascular. The improvement in glucose control usually requires continuous intensive diabetes management, particularly in insulin-requiring patients, which *must* include home self-monitoring of blood glucose (SMBG). Despite the convincing evidence, the role of SMBG in diabetes management is still being debated even though its avail-ability in the past 35 years has revolutionised diabetes care, especially at home.

The International Diabetes Federation (IDF) recently published guidelines for SMBG use in non-insulin-treated diabetic patients, rec-ommending that SMBG should be used only when patients and/or their clinicians possess the ability, willingness and knowledge to incorporate SMBG and therapy adjustment into their diabetes care plan. The IDF also recommends that structured SMBG be performed with the choice of applying different defined blood glucose testing algorithms to patients' individual diabetes care plans. These defined blood glucose testing algorithms give SMBG a medically meaningful structure to collect high quality glucose information and are called structured SMBG. Former SMBG studies have demonstrated SMBG to be beneficial when patients receive feedback regarding the impact of their behaviours on SMBG

Int J Clin Pract 2012; **66** (Suppl. 175): 2–7

results. Other studies which did not link SMBG results to these principal behaviours have shown no SMBG benefit. A new wave of clinical studies performed after the release of the IDF guideline have recently been published and have proved the success of the new application of SMBG.

The reasons for this ongoing debate may in part be due to rising healthcare costs globally, lack of convincing data in non-insulin-requiring patients with type 2 diabetes in randomised controlled clinical trials and multiple controversial meta-analyses performed on several studies. Sometimes the decisions are extended to insulin-requiring patients, even those with type 1 diabetes. For example, last year in the state of Washington in the USA, legislators were going to stop reimbursing glucose test strips for children with type 1 diabetes. After much debate with committee members (who were not diabetologists and or endocrinologists) and law makers, not only SMBG but even in some cases continuous glucose monitoring (CGM) is now reimbursed. The issue was simply educating non-understanding but well-meaning people whose main concern is saving money. In the end, no one, even those not familiar with paediatric type 1 diabetes, can disagree about the need for SMBG in this age group.

It seems to us that we should instead be spending our time and effort in advancing the field and improving diabetes management for patients through newer technologies like CGM and closed-loop systems. As discussed in the section on CGM (Chapter 2) there is ample data from both non-randomised and randomised clinical trials showing the efficacy in reducing time spent in hypoglycaemia and hyperglycaemia along with improvement in glucose control without introducing any additional medication. We hope that the future will be spent in advancing the care rather than useless meta-analyses or going back in time. It is worthwhile to review existing evidence about SMBG to learn, transfer and apply knowledge about the core requirement for good diabetes management, glucose information.

Non-coding glucometers among paediatric patients with diabetes: looking for the target population and an accuracy evaluation of no-coding personal glucometer

Fendler W, Hogendorf A, Szadkowska A, Młynarski W

Department of Pediatrics, Oncology, Hematology and Diabetology, Medical University of Lodz, Poland

*Pediatr Endocrinol Diabetes Metab 2011; **17**: 57–63*

Background

SMBG is one of the major components of diabetes management.

Aims

To evaluate the potential for miscoding of a personal glucometer, to define a target population among paediatric patients with diabetes for a non-coding glucometer and to assess the accuracy of the Contour TS non-coding system.

Methods

Potential for miscoding during SMBG was evaluated by means of an anonymous questionnaire, with worst and best case scenarios evaluated depending on the response pattern. Testing of the Contour TS system was performed according to the national committee for clinical laboratory standards guidelines.

Results

The estimated frequency of individuals prone to non-coding ranged from 68.21% [95% confidence interval (CI) 60.70%–75.72%] to 7.95% (95% CI 3.86%–12.31%) for the worse and best case scenarios, respectively. Factors associated with increased likelihood of non-coding were a smaller number of tests per day, a greater number of individuals involved in testing and self-testing by the patient. The Contour TS device showed intra- and inter-assay accuracy of –95%, a linear association with laboratory measurements ($R^2 = 0.99$, p < 0.0001) and small bias of –1.12% (95% CI –3.27% to 1.02%). Clarke error grid analysis showed 4% of values within the benign error zone (B) with the other measurements yielding an acceptably accurate result (zone A).

Conclusions

The Contour TS system showed sufficient accuracy to be safely used in the monitoring of paediatric patients with diabetes. Patients from families with a high throughput of test-strips or multiple individuals involved in SMBG using the same meter are candidates for clinical use of such devices due to an increased risk of calibration errors.

COMMENT

This study further highlights the role of making SMBG simpler and easier so that patients can monitor the glucose more effectively. The current study used the Contour TS system which does not require coding by the patient and thus removes the barrier of mis-coding of SMBG. We personally think that all meters going forward must be non-coding meters.

Effect of ambient temperature on analytical performance of self-monitoring blood glucose systems

Nerhus K[1], Rustad P[2], Sandberg S[1,3]

[1] *Norwegian Centre for Quality Improvement of Primary Care Laboratories, Department of Public Health and Primary Health Care, University of Bergen, Bergen, Norway,* [2] *Norwegian Clinical Chemistry EQA-Program, Fürst Medical Laboratory, Oslo, Norway,* [3] *Laboratory of Clinical Biochemistry, Haukeland University Hospital, Bergen, Norway*

Diabetes Technol Ther 2011; **13:** *883–92*

Background
Analytical quality of SMBG can be affected by environmental conditions.

Aims
To determine the influence of a shift in the ambient temperature immediately before measurement and taking measurements in the lower and upper part of the operating temperature range.

Methods
Different SMBG systems ($n = 9$) available on the Norwegian market were tested with heparinised venous blood (4.8 and 19.0 mmol/l). To test the effect of a shift in ambient temperature, the glucometer and strips were equilibrated for 1 h at 5 °C or 30 °C before the meter and strips were moved to room temperature, and measurements were performed after 0, 5, 10, 15 and 30 min. To test the lower and upper temperature range, measurements were performed at 10 °C and at 39 °C after 1 h for temperature equilibration of the glucometer and strips. All the measurements were compared with measurements performed simultaneously on a meter and strips kept the whole time at room temperature.

Results
Six of nine SMBG systems overestimated and/or underestimated results by more than 5% after moving meters and strips from 5 °C or 30 °C to room temperature immediately before the measurements. Two systems underestimated the results at 10 °C. One system overestimated and another underestimated the results by more than 5% at 39 °C.

Conclusions
A rapid shift in the ambient temperature affects analytical performance. Therefore patients need to wait at least 15 min for temperature equilibration of affected meters and strips before measuring blood glucose.

COMMENT

This study highlights the importance of ambient temperature on analytical performance of SMBG. The study shows that rapid shift in ambient temperature may affect the accuracy and bias in SMBG measurement and highlights the need for 15 min temperature equilibration. In addition to what has been highlighted in the study, future studies also need to assess the accuracy of existing meters (especially the one using glucose oxidase) at higher altitudes (10,000 feet or higher). It is known that many of these meters do not perform well at high altitudes.

Association between self-monitoring of blood glucose and diet among minority patients with diabetes

McAndrew LM[1,2], Horowitz CR[3], Lancaster KJ[4], Quigley KS[2,5,6], Pogach LM[1,2], Mora PA[7], Leventhal H[8]

[1] *War Related Illness and Injury Study Center and REAP Center for Healthcare Knowledge Management, Department of Veterans Affairs, New Jersey Health Care System, East Orange, NJ, USA,* [2] *University of Medicine and Dentistry of New Jersey, Newark, NJ, USA,* [3] *Department of Health Evidence and Policy, Mount Sinai School of Medicine,New York, NY, USA,* [4] *Department of Nutrition, Food Studies and Public Health, New York University, New York, NY, USA,* [5] *Department of Veterans Affairs, Edith Nourse Rogers Memorial VA Hospital, Bedford, MA, USA,* [6] *Department of Psychology, Northeastern University, Boston, MA, USA,* [7] *Psychology Department, University of Texas at Arlington, Arlington, TX, USA, and* [8] *Institute for Health, Health Care Policy and Research, Rutgers University, New Brunswick, NJ, USA*

J Diabetes 2011; 3: 147–52; Comment in J Diabetes 2011; 3: 93–4

Background

It is unknown whether SMBG can motivate adherence to dietary recommendations.

Aims

To evaluate if patients who used more SMBG would also report lower fat and greater fruit and vegetable consumption.

Methods

This was a cross-sectional study of primarily minority individuals living with diabetes in East Harlem, New York ($n = 401$). Fat intake and fruit and vegetable consumption were measured with the Block Fruit/Vegetable/Fiber and Fat Screeners.

Results

Greater frequency of SMBG was associated with lower fat intake $[r(s) = -0.15; p < 0.01]$, but not fruit and vegetable consumption. The effects of SMBG were not moderated by insulin use. A significant interaction was found between frequency of SMBG and changing one's diet in response to SMBG on total fat intake.

Conclusions

The frequency of SMBG was associated with lower fat intake. The data suggest that participants who use SMBG to guide their diet do not have to monitor multiple times a day to benefit.

COMMENT

This study further highlights the importance of SMBG in daily lifestyle changes. Subjects with higher frequency of SMBG consumed less fat, in part related to overall education and seeing the impact from making dietary changes on SMBG levels.

Accuracy and precision evaluation of seven self-monitoring blood glucose systems

Kuo CY[1,2], Hsu CT[3], Ho CS[3], Su TE[3], Wu MH[4], Wang CJ[2,5]

[1] *Department of Clinical Laboratory, Tai-An Hospital, Taichung, Taiwan,*
[2] *Institute of Biochemistry and Biotechnology, Chung Shan Medical University, Taichung, Taiwan,* [3] *Department of Core Technical Research, Bionime Corporation, Taichung, Taiwan,* [4] *Department of Laboratory Medicine, Min-Sheng General Hospital, Taoyuan, Taiwan,* [5] *Department of Medical Research, Chung Shan Medical University Hospital, Taichung, Taiwan*

Diabetes Technol Ther 2011; 13: 596–600

Background

SMBG systems should at least meet the minimal requirement of the World Health Organization's ISO 15197:2003. For tight glycaemic control, a tighter accuracy requirement is needed.

Methods

Seven SMBG systems were evaluated for accuracy and precision: Bionime Rightest™ GM550 (Bionime Corp., Dali City, Taiwan), Accu-Chek® Performa (Roche Diagnostics, Indianapolis, IN, USA), OneTouch® Ultra®2 (LifeScan Inc., Milpitas, CA, USA), MediSense® Optium™ Xceed

(Abbott Diabetes Care Inc., Alameda, CA, USA), Medisafe (TERUMO Corp., Tokyo, Japan), Fora® TD4227 (Taidac Technology Corp., Wugu Township, Taiwan) and Ascensia Contour® (Bayer HealthCare LLC, Mishawaka, IN, USA). The 107 participants were 23–91 years old. The analytical results of seven SMBG systems were compared with those of plasma analysed with the hexokinase method (Olympus AU640, Olympus America Inc., Center Valley, PA, USA).

Results

The imprecision of the seven blood glucose meters ranged from 1.1% to 4.7%. Three of the seven blood glucose meters (42.9%) fulfilled the minimum accuracy criterion of ISO 15197:2003. The mean absolute relative error value for each blood glucose meter was calculated and ranged from 6.5% to 12.0%.

Conclusions

More than 40% of evaluated SMBG systems meet the minimal accuracy criterion requirement of ISO 15197:2003. However, considering a tighter criterion for accuracy of ±15%, only the Bionime Rightest GM550 meets this requirement. Manufacturers have to try to improve accuracy and precision and to ensure the good quality of blood glucose meters and test strips.

COMMENT

This study further highlights the need for more accurate SMBG systems. Their data concluded that more than 40% of the evaluated SMBG systems meet the minimum ISO criteria. Since patients use blood glucose information for adjusting their insulin dose and/or treating hypoglycaemia, the accuracy of the glucose meters has to be consistent and improved.

Self-monitoring of blood glucose: the use of the first or the second drop of blood

Hortensius J[1], Slingerland RJ[2], Kleefstra N[1,3,4], Logtenberg SJ[1], Groenier KH[5], Houweling ST[3,6], Bilo HJ[1,4]

[1] *Diabetes Centre, Isala Clinics, Zwolle, The Netherlands,* [2] *Department of Clinical Chemistry, Isala Clinics, Zwolle, The Netherlands,* [3] *Medical Research Group, Langerhans, The Netherlands,* [4] *Department of Internal Medicine, University Medical Center, Groningen, The Netherlands,* [5] *Department of General Practice,*

University of Groningen, Groningen, The Netherlands, and [6]*General Practice Sleeuwijk, Sleeuwijk, The Netherlands*

Diabetes Care 2011; **34**: 556–60

Background

There is no agreement regarding the use of the first or second drop of blood for glucose monitoring.

Aims

To investigate whether capillary glucose concentrations, as measured in the first and second drops of blood, differed ≥10% compared with a control glucose concentration in different situations.

Methods

Capillary glucose concentrations were measured in two consecutive drops of blood in 123 patients with diabetes in the following circumstances: without washing hands, after exposing the hands to fruit, after washing the fruit-exposed hands, and during application of different amounts of external pressure around the finger. The results were compared with control measurements.

Results

Not washing hands led to a difference of ≥10% in glucose concentration in the first and in the second drops of blood in 11% and 4% of the participants, respectively. In fruit exposed fingers, these differences were found in 88% and 11% of the participants, respectively. Different external pressures led to ≥10% differences in glucose concentrations in 5%–13% of the participants.

Conclusions

Washing hands with soap and water, drying them, and using the first drop of blood for SMBG is recommended. If washing hands is not possible, it is acceptable to use the second drop of blood after wiping away the first drop. External pressure may lead to unreliable readings.

COMMENT

Over the years we have probably under-emphasised the importance of technique with SMBG. One has to wonder how much iatrogenic hypoglycaemia has occurred due to unintended exposure to glucose on the hands, and how often CGM devices are inaccurate due to poor technique with SMBG use.

Structured self-monitoring of blood glucose significantly reduces A1C levels in poorly controlled, non-insulin-treated type 2 diabetes: results from the Structured Testing Program study

Polonsky WH[1,2], Fisher L[3], Schikman CH[4], Hinnen DA[5], Parkin CG[6], Jelsovsky Z[7], Petersen B[8], Schweitzer M[8], Wagner RS[8]

[1]*University of California, San Diego, CA, USA,* [2]*Behavioral Diabetes Institute, San Diego, CA, USA,* [3]*University of California, San Francisco, CA, USA,* [4]*North Shore University Health System, Skokie, IL, USA,* [5]*Mid America Diabetes Associates, Wichita, KS, USA,* [6]*Health Management Resources, Carmel, IN, USA,* [7]*Biostat International, Tampa, FL, USA, and* [8]*Roche Diagnostics, Indianapolis, IN, USA*

Diabetes Care 2011; 34: 262–7

Aim

To assess the effectiveness of structured blood glucose testing in poorly controlled patients with type 2 diabetes without insulin treatment.

Methods

A 12-month prospective, randomised, multicentre study recruited insulin-naive patients with type 2 diabetes ($n = 483$) and poor glycaemic control (A1C $\geq$ 7.5%) from 34 primary care practices in the USA. Practices were randomised to an active control group (ACG) with enhanced usual care or a structured testing group (STG) with enhanced usual care and at least quarterly use of structured SMBG. STG patients and physicians were trained to use a paper tool to collect/interpret seven-point glucose profiles over three consecutive days. The primary endpoint was HbA1c level measured at 12 months.

Results

The 12-month intent-to-treat analysis (ACG, $n = 227$; STG, $n = 256$) showed significantly greater reductions in mean (SE) HbA1c in the STG compared with the ACG [–1.2% (0.09) vs. –0.9% (0.10); $\Delta = -0.3\%$; $p = 0.04$]. Per-protocol analysis (ACG, $n = 161$; STG, $n = 130$) showed even greater mean (SE) HbA1c reductions in the STG compared with the ACG [–1.3% (0.11) vs. –0.8% (0.11); $\Delta = -0.5\%$; $p < 0.003$]. Significantly more STG patients received a treatment change recommendation at the first month visit compared with ACG patients, regardless of the patient's initial baseline HbA1c level (75.5% vs. 28.0%; $p < 0.0001$). Both STG and ACG patients displayed significant ($p < 0.0001$) improvements in general well-being.

Conclusions

Appropriate use of structured SMBG significantly improves glycaemic control and facilitates more timely/aggressive treatment changes in insulin-naive patients with type 2 diabetes without decreasing general well-being.

COMMENT

It is clear that, with an engaged healthcare team, using a structured glucose testing strategy can improve glucose control in non-insulin-treated patients. Potential benefits are many, including cost of care. Whether this can be repeated in a non-study setting with the more typical time limits encountered in a primary care setting remains to be seen.

Estimates of total analytical error in consumer and hospital glucose meters contributed by haematocrit, maltose and ascorbate

Lyon ME[1,2,3,4], DuBois JA[5], Fick GH[6], Lyon AW[1,4]

[1] *Department of Pathology and Laboratory Medicine, University of Calgary, Calgary, AB, Canada,* [2] *Department of Pharmacology and Physiology, University of Calgary, Calgary, AB, Canada,* [3] *Department of Pediatrics, University of Calgary, Calgary, AB, Canada,* [4] *Calgary Laboratory Services, Calgary, AB, Canada,* [5] *Nova Biomedical Corporation, Waltham, MA, USA, and* [6] *Department of Community Health Sciences, University of Calgary, Calgary, AB, Canada*

J Diabetes Sci Technol 2010; **4**: 1479–94

Aims

To estimate analytical error in consumer and hospital glucose meters contributed by variations in haematocrit, maltose, ascorbate and imprecision.

Methods

The influences of haematocrit (20%–60%), maltose and ascorbate were tested alone and in combination with each glucose meter and with a reference plasma glucose method at three glucose concentrations. Precision was determined by consecutive analysis ($n = 20$) at three glucose levels. Multivariate regression analysis was used to estimate the bias associated with the interferences, alone and in combination.

Results

Three meters demonstrated haematocrit bias that was dependent upon glucose concentration. Maltose had profound concentration-dependent positive bias on the consumer meters, and the extent of maltose bias was dependent on haematocrit. Ascorbate produced small statistically significant biases on three meters. Coincident low haematocrit, presence of maltose and presence of ascorbate increased the observed bias and was summarised by estimation of total analytical error. Among the four glucose meter devices assessed, estimates of total analytical error in glucose measurement ranged from 6% to 68% under the conditions tested.

Conclusions

The susceptibility of glucose meters to clinically significant analytical biases is highly device-dependent. Low haematocrit exacerbated the observed analytical error.

COMMENT

Concerns continue with regard to interferences for SMBG devices, and although the research is consistent, it does not appear that many people appreciate the various problems. This has particular impact on hospitalised patients. Furthermore, as new guidelines for transfusion (allowing greater degrees of anaemia) are implemented, the impact on SMBG accuracy could be profound. Better educational programmes, particularly by the device manufacturers, should be a priority.

Evaluating the cost-effectiveness of self-monitoring of blood glucose in type 2 diabetes patients on oral antidiabetic agents

Pollock RF[1], Valentine WJ[1], Goodall G[2], Brandle M[3]

[1]*Ossian Health Economics and Communications, Basel, Switzerland,* [2]*IMS Health, Basel, Switzerland, and* [3]*Division of Endocrinology and Diabetes, Department of Internal Medicine, Kantonsspital, St Gallen, Switzerland*

Swiss Med Wkly 2010; **140**: *w13103*

Aims

To evaluate the cost-effectiveness of SMBG in patients with type 2 diabetes treated with oral antidiabetic agents (OADs) in Switzerland.

Methods

In a large observational study a validated computer model of diabetes was used to project outcomes reported from a published longitudinal study of SMBG in patients with type 2 diabetes, treated with OADs and with no history of SMBG, over a 30-year time horizon. Cost-effectiveness was assessed from the perspective of a third party healthcare payer. Costs and clinical outcomes were discounted at 3% annually.

Results

Once, twice or three times daily SMBG was associated with improvements in HbA1c which led to increased life expectancy and quality-adjusted life expectancy and reduced incidence of diabetes complications compared with no SMBG in type 2 diabetes patients on OADs. Direct medical costs increased by CHF 528, CHF 1650 and CHF 2899 in patients performing SMBG once, twice or three times daily respectively compared with those not using SMBG. Incremental cost-effectiveness ratios were well below commonly quoted willingness-to-pay thresholds at CHF 9,177, CHF 12,928 and CHF 17,342 per quality-adjusted life year gained, respectively.

Conclusions

SMBG is likely to be cost-effective by generally accepted standards in SMBG-naive patients on OADs in the Swiss setting.

COMMENT

This interesting analysis is based on a 'validated computer model' showing improvements of HbA1c, life expectancy and quality-adjusted life year. The concern of course is that this analysis is not a real randomised controlled trial, and while at best the data are mixed about the efficacy of this population using SMBG, this particular analysis is probably based on controversial assumptions.

Using a cell-phone-based glucose monitoring system for adolescent diabetes management

Carroll AE[1,2], DiMeglio LA[3], Stein S[3], Marrero DG[2,4]

[1]Children's Health Services Research, Indiana University School of Medicine, Indianapolis, IN, USA, [2]Regenstrief Institute for Health Care, Indianapolis, IN, USA, [3]Section of Pediatric Endocrinology, Indiana University School of Medicine, Indianapolis, IN, USA, and [4]Diabetes Prevention and Control Center, Indiana University School of Medicine, Indianapolis, IN, USA

Diabetes Educ 2011; **37**: 59–66

Aim

To assess the feasibility and acceptability of a cell phone glucose monitoring system for adolescents with type 1 diabetes and their parents.

Methods

Patients with type 1 diabetes who had been diagnosed for at least 1 year participated in the study. Each adolescent used the system for 6 months, filling out surveys every 3 months to measure usability and satisfaction with the cell phone glucose monitoring system, as well as how use of the system might affect quality of family functioning and diabetes management.

Results

Adolescents reported positive feelings about the technology, although a large number of them had significant technical issues that affected continued use of the device. Nearly all thought that the clinic involvement in monitoring testing behaviour was acceptable. The use of the Glucophone™ did not change the adolescent's quality of life, their level of conflict with their parents, their reported self-management of diabetes, or their average glycaemic control within the short time frame of the study.

Conclusions

This work demonstrates that cell phone glucose monitoring technology can be used in an adolescent population to track and assist in self-monitoring behaviour.

COMMENT

Mobile technology for both SMBG and CGM is clearly the future for adolescents (and adults) with type 1 diabetes. The real challenge will be to learn how to best use this technology to improve diabetes-related outcomes in this population. To date, the technology is too new to know how best to use it. Many more studies will be required to answer this question.

Accuracy of handheld blood glucose meters at high altitude

de Mol P[1], Krabbe HG[2], de Vries ST[3], Fokkert MJ[2], Dikkeschei BD[2], Rienks R[4], Bilo KM[5], Bilo HJ[5,6]

[1] *Department of Internal Medicine, Canisius Wilhelmina Hospital, Nijmegen, The Netherlands,* [2] *Department of Clinical Chemistry, Isala Clinics, Zwolle, The Netherlands,* [3] *Department of Cardiology, Isala Clinics, Zwolle, The Netherlands,* [4] *Centre for Human Aviation, Dutch Airforce, Soesterberg, The Netherlands,* [5] *Department of Internal Medicine, Isala Clinics, Zwolle, The Netherlands, and* [6] *Department of Internal Medicine, University Medical Centre, Groningen, The Netherlands*

PLoS One 2010; 5: e15485

Background

Patients with diabetes take part in extreme sports (e.g. high-altitude trekking), and thus reliable handheld blood glucose meters (BGMs) are necessary. Prior studies reported bias in blood glucose measurements using different BGMs at high altitude.

Aim

To evaluate if glucose oxidase based BGMs are more influenced by the lower atmospheric oxygen pressure at altitude than glucose dehydrogenase based BGMs.

Methods

Glucose measurements at simulated altitude of nine BGMs (six glucose dehydrogenase, three glucose oxidase BGMs) were compared with glucose measurement on a similar BGM at sea level and with a laboratory glucose reference method. Venous blood samples of four different glucose levels were used. Accuracy criteria were set at a bias <15% from reference glucose (when >6.5 mmol/l) and <1 mmol/l from reference glucose (when <6.5 mmol/l).

Results

No significant difference was observed between measurements at simulated altitude and sea level for either glucose oxidase based BGMs or glucose dehydrogenase based BGMs as a group phenomenon. Two glucose dehydrogenase based BGMs did not meet set performance criteria.

Conclusions

At simulated high altitude all tested BGMs, including glucose oxidase based BGMs, did not show influence of low atmospheric oxygen pressure. All BGMs, except for two glucose dehydrogenase based BGMs, performed within predefined criteria. Most BGMs are generally overestimating true glucose concentration at high altitude. At true high altitude one glucose dehydrogenase based BGM had best precision and accuracy.

COMMENT

Simulated altitude testing for SMBG meters may be problematic. In general, glucose oxidase test strips should be avoided at high altitudes. Although not studied in this analysis, it should be noted that most patients do not take this into consideration when hiking or skiing.

Designing mobile support for glycaemic control in patients with diabetes

Harris LT[1], Tufano J[2], Le T[2], Rees C[1], Lewis GA[3], Evert AB[4], Flowers J[3], Collins C[5], Hoath J[6], Hirsch IB[7], Goldberg HI[7], Ralston JD[8]

[1] *Department of Health Services, University of Washington, Magnuson Health Sciences Center, Seattle, WA, USA,* [2] *Biomedical and Health Informatics, Department of Medical Education and Biomedical Informatics, University of Washington, Seattle, WA, USA,* [3] *Department of Biobehavioral Nursing and Health Systems, University of Washington, Seattle, WA, USA,* [4] *Diabetes Care Center, UW Medical Center-Roosevelt, WA, USA,* [5] *Department of Pharmaceutics, University of Washington, Seattle, WA, USA,* [6] *UW Medicine Information Technology Services, Northgate Executive Center II, Seattle, WA, USA,* [7] *Department of Medicine, University of Washington, Seattle, WA, USA, and* [8] *Group Health Research Institute, Seattle, WA, USA*

J Biomed Inform 2010; **43** *(5 Suppl): S37–40*

Aims

To assess the feasibility and acceptability of using mobile phones as part of an existing web-based system for collaboration between patients with diabetes and a primary care team.

Methods

In design sessions, mobile wireless glucose meter uploads and two approaches to mobile-phone-based feedback on glycaemic control were tested.

Results

Mobile glucose meter uploads combined with graphical and tabular data feedback were the most desirable system features tested. Participants had mixed reactions to an automated and tailored messaging feedback system for self-management support. Participants saw value in the mobile system as an adjunct to the web-based programme and traditional office-based care.

Conclusions

Mobile diabetes management systems may represent one strategy to improve the quality of diabetes care.

> ## COMMENT
>
> How best to integrate mobile technology in a primary care setting for type 2 diabetes is still unclear. It is quite likely that there will be different types of mobile technology that will work better for different patient populations. Still, the growing use of the mobile phone as a primary means of communication makes that device seem like the centre of attention in diabetes management. While the technology now seems to be available, how to get physicians interested is a separate challenge. It may be that separate reimbursements will be the only incentive for many physicians given the burden of time this population already generates.

Immortal time bias and survival in patients who self-monitor blood glucose in the Retrolective Study: Self-monitoring of Blood Glucose and Outcome in Patients with Type 2 Diabetes (ROSSO)

Hoffmann F[1], Andersohn F[2]

[1]*Centre for Social Policy Research, Division of Health Economics, Health Policy and Outcomes Research, University of Bremen, Bremen, Germany, and* [2]*Institute for Social Medicine, Epidemiology, and Health Economics, Charité University Medical Centre Berlin, Berlin, Germany*

*Diabetologia 2011; **54**: 308–11*

Background

Previously the observational Retrolective Study: Self-monitoring of Blood Glucose and Outcome in Patients with Type 2 Diabetes (ROSSO) reported a 51% reduction in the risk of all-cause mortality in patients with type 2 diabetes who performed SMBG.

Aims

To evaluate if these findings are caused by a flawed design that introduced immortal time bias.

Methods

The bias in the ROSSO study was illustrated and demonstrated that it is large enough to explain the apparently protective effect of SMBG on all-cause mortality.

Results

In the ROSSO study, patients were classified as exposed to SMBG for their whole follow-up time if they performed SMBG for at least 1 year during the study period. Thus, the time between cohort entry and

the date after 1 year of self-monitoring was performed is unavoid-
ably 'immortal' for patients with SMBG. Patients had to survive at
least 1 year to be classified as exposed to this intervention and were arti-
ficially 'protected' from death. The total amount of misclassified immortal
person-time in the SMBG group is at least 5082 of 9248 person-years at
risk (55%). After reclassification of immortal person-time as unexposed,
the unadjusted relative risk changed from 0.59 to 1.95.

Conclusions

The apparently protective effect of SMBG on all-cause mortality observed
in the ROSSO study is completely explained by immortal time bias.

COMMENT

The ROSSO study is one of the most-quoted trials in the area of SMBG. Study
design is probably a major reason for non-agreement between the various
studies.

Self-monitoring of blood glucose in tablet-treated type 2 diabetic patients (ZODIAC-17)

*Kleefstra N[1,2], Hortensius J[1], Logtenberg SJ[1], lingerland R[3], Groenier K[4],
Houweling ST[2,5], Gans RO[6], van Ballegooie E[2], Bilo HJ[1,6]*

[1] *Diabetes Centre, Isala Clinics, Zwolle, The Netherlands,* [2] *Medical Research
Group Langerhans, Zwolle, The Netherlands,* [3] *Department of Clinical Chemistry,
Isala Clinics, Zwolle, The Netherlands,* [4] *Department of General Practice,
University of Groningen, Groningen, The Netherlands,* [5] *General Practice
Sleeuwijk, Sleeuwijk, The Netherlands,* [6] *Department of Internal Medicine,
University Medical Center Groningen, Groningen, The Netherlands*

Neth J Med 2010; **68**: *311–6*

Background

It is not clear if SMBG improves glycaemic control in insulin-naive patients with type 2 diabetes.

Aim

To investigate the effects of SMBG in insulin-naive patients with type 2
diabetes who were in persistent moderate glycaemic control.

Methods

Patients aged 18–70 years with an HbA1c level of 7%–8.5%, using one
to two oral blood glucose lowering agents, were included in the study.
Patients ($n = 41$) were randomly assigned to receive either SMBG added

to usual care or to continue with usual care for 1 year. A fasting glucose value and three postprandial glucose values were measured twice weekly. The primary efficacy parameter was HbA1c. Health-related quality of life and treatment satisfaction were assessed using the Short-form 36 Health Survey Questionnaire (SF-36), the T2D Symptom Checklist (DSC-r), the Diabetes Treatment Satisfaction Questionnaire (DTSQ) and the WHO Wellbeing Index (WHO-5).

Results
Change in HbA1c between groups was −0.05% (95% CI −0.51 to 0.41; p = 0.507). There were no significant changes between groups on the DTSQ, DSC type 2, WHO-5 or SF-36, except for the SF-36 dimension 'health change' which was lower in the SBMG group [mean difference −12 (95% CI −20.9 to −3.1)].

Conclusions
Tablet-treated type 2 diabetes patients experienced some worsening of their health perception. Thus, the use of SMBG in these patients is questionable, and its unlimited use should be reconsidered.

COMMENT

This is another negative SMBG study in non-insulin-treated type 2 patients. While the criticism of not adequately teaching patients what to do with the information is quite valid, one has to wonder if this continued signal at some point needs to have some degree of acceptance. At the very least, it is difficult to argue that the average physician in primary care is able to provide more education and time than is done in many of these studies.

The accuracy of home glucose meters in hypoglycaemia

Sonmez A[1], Yilmaz Z[1], Uckaya G[1], Kilic S[2], Tapan S[3], Taslipinar A[1], Aydogdu A[1], YaziciM[1], Yilmaz MI[4], Serdar M[3], Erbil MK[3], Kutlu M[1]

[1] *Department of Endocrinology and Metabolism, Gulhane School of Medicine, Ankara, Turkey,* [2] *Department of Epidemiology, Gulhane School of Medicine, Ankara, Turkey,* [3] *Department of Biochemistry, Gulhane School of Medicine, Ankara, Turkey, and* [4] *Department of Nephrology, Gulhane School of Medicine, Ankara, Turkey*

Diabetes Technol Ther 2010; 12: 619–26

Background

Home glucose meters (HGMs) may not be accurate enough to sense hypoglycaemia.

Aims

Evaluation of the accuracy and the capillary and venous comparability of five different HGMs [Optium Xceed (Abbott Diabetes Care, Alameda, CA, USA), Contour TS (Bayer Diabetes Care, Basel, Switzerland), Accu-Chek Go (Roche Ltd, Basel, Switzerland), OneTouch Select (Lifescan, Milpitas, CA, USA) and EZ Smart (Tyson Bioresearch Inc., Chu-Nan, Taiwan)] in an adult population.

Methods

The insulin hypoglycaemia test was performed for 59 subjects of mean age 23.6 ± 3.2 years. Glucose was measured from venous blood and finger capillary samples before and after injection of regular insulin (0.1 U/kg). Venous samples were analysed in the reference laboratory by the hexokinase method. *In vitro* tests for method comparison and precision analyses were also performed by spiking the glucose-depleted venous blood.

Results

All HGMs failed to sense hypoglycaemia to some extent. EZ Smart was significantly inferior in critical error zone D, and OneTouch Select was significantly inferior in the clinically unimportant error zone B. Accu-Chek Go, Optium Xceed and Contour TS had similar performances and were significantly better than the other two HGMs according to error grid analysis or International Organisation for Standardisation criteria. The *in vitro* tests were consistent with the above clinical data. The capillary and venous consistencies of Accu-Chek Go and OneTouch Select were better than the other HGMs.

Conclusion

Not all HGMs are accurate enough in low blood glucose levels. The patients and the caregivers should be aware of these restrictions of the HGMs and give more credit to the hypoglycaemia symptoms than the values obtained with the HGMs. These results indicate that there is a need for the revision of accuracy standards of HGMs at low blood glucose levels.

COMMENT

We have learned the hard way that today's meters are far from perfect, especially at hypoglycaemic levels. Most patients can state a specific time when they received an inaccurate reading. The implications are obvious, not only for the treatment of hypoglycaemia but also as we move forward with CGM about how this problem impacts calibration. While correspondence about this paper questions the investigators' compliance with the specific manufacturer's recommendations for use of the meters (1), our clinical experience with patient error makes us believe that accuracy remains a tremendous problem for glucose meters at hypoglycaemic levels.

REFERENCE

1. Mahoney JJ, Ellison JM, Cabezudo JI, Cariski AT. Protocol errors may lead to incorrect conclusions. *Diabetes Technol Ther* 2011; **13**: 171

CHAPTER 2

Continuous Glucose Monitoring in 2011

Tadej Battelino[1] and Bruce W. Bode[2]

[1] University Medical Center, University Children's Hospital, Ljubljana, Slovenia
[2] Atlanta Diabetes Associates, Atlanta, GA, USA

INTRODUCTION

Continuous glucose monitoring (CGM) is probably growing from childhood into adolescence, with all the glories and quandaries of this developmental period. The first meta-analysis clearly confirms its benefits on metabolic control in type 1 diabetes, but clinically meaningful improvement in HbA1c and reduction in hypoglycaemia is not readily achievable in all patient populations. First reports from randomised controlled trials in people with type 2 diabetes also suggest its efficacy in this patient population. An unremitting stream of technical improvements and new technologies keeps improving its accuracy and acceptability, slowly spreading its routine use and modifying cautiousness and reluctance of many healthcare professionals. Current patients' satisfaction and quality of life data on the other hand leave ample space for improvement. Successful use of CGM necessitates behavioural adjustments notoriously difficult to achieve and further research of implementation strategies with a focus on sustained use is anticipated.

Glycaemic control in type 1 diabetes during real-time continuous glucose monitoring compared with self-monitoring of blood glucose: meta-analysis of randomised controlled trials using individual patient data

Pickup JC[1], Freeman SC[2,3], Sutton AJ[2]

[1] *Diabetes Research Group, Division of Diabetes and Nutritional Sciences, King's College London School of Medicine, Guy's Hospital, London, UK,* [2] *Department of*

Int J Clin Pract 2012; **66** (Suppl. 175): 8–14

Health Sciences, University of Leicester, Leicester, UK, and [3]MRC Clinical Trials Unit, London, UK

BMJ 2011; **343**: *d3805*

Aim

To assess the impact of real-time continuous glucose monitoring (RT-CGM) on metabolic control in type 1 diabetes compared with self-monitoring of blood glucose (SMBG).

Methods

All randomised controlled trials retrieved through public electronic databases with more than 2 months' duration comparing RT-CGM with SMBG in type 1 diabetes and published until July 2010 were screened. Insulin treatment modality was required to be the same in both arms. Individual patient data were obtained from each trial and analysed with a two-step meta-analysis for HbA1c and in transformed data for area under the curve for hypoglycaemia <3.9 mmol/l (70 mg/dl). A one-step meta-regression analysis on pooled individual patient data was used to assess the effect of the following covariates on main outcomes: baseline HbA1c, sensor use, age, duration of diabetes, and interactions between the covariates and baseline HbA1c. The incidence rate for severe hypoglycaemia (requiring help from another person) was calculated from the summary data in trial reports.

Results

Six randomised controlled trials were eligible with data from 13 to 26 weeks. All trials reached a quality score of 3 out of 6 because of lack of information on concealment and absence of double blinding. Individual data on 892 people with type 1 diabetes (449 randomised to RT-CGM and 443 to SMBG) were available for evaluating the overall reduction in HbA1c with RT-CGM, which was calculated to be 0.30% [95% confidence interval (CI) −0.43% to −0.17%] bigger compared with SMBG. The strongest independent determinant of the final HbA1c was the initial HbA1c, followed by the sensor usage, with every additional day per week of sensor use decreasing HbA1c for a further 0.150% (95% CI −0.194% to −0.106%). Age had a relatively small effect with every year increase in age additionally decreasing HbA1c by 0.002% when RT-CGM was compared with SMBG. With a low level of baseline hypoglycaemia in most individuals, the area under the curve of hypoglycaemia was lower by −0.276 (−0.463 to −0.089) in RT-CGM compared with SMBG, corresponding to a 23% reduction in the median exposure to hypoglycaemia. Higher initial area under the curve of hypoglycaemia and longer duration of diabetes slightly increased the effect of RT-CGM compared with SMBG, but age and sensor usage did not have any effect. The rate of severe hypoglycaemia was not significantly different.

Conclusions

RT-CGM was associated with a significantly greater reduction in HbA1c than SMBG, with a clinically meaningful effect at high baseline HbA1c values and with frequent use. Additionally, hypoglycaemia exposure was lower with RT-CGM.

COMMENT

This first meta-analysis of the efficacy of RT-CGM demonstrates a statistically significant benefit of 0.3% reduction in HbA1c compared with SMBG (1). Overall, this benefit may be of debatable clinical importance. However, at higher baseline HbA1c the benefit is bigger: at baseline HbA1c of 10% the benefit of RT-CGM over SMBG was 0.9% which is clinically relevant and reduces the risk of chronic complications of diabetes. Additionally, this benefit comes with a concomitant reduction in exposure to hypoglycaemia. Another recent meta-analysis included 19 trials in type 1 and type 2 diabetes and also found a benefit of CGM over SMBG with an overall reduction of HbA1c of 0.27% (95% CI −0.44 to −0.10) but higher in adults with type 1 diabetes (0.50%; 95% CI −0.69 to −0.30) and type 2 diabetes (0.70%; 95% CI −1.14 to −0.27) (2). However, the design of this meta-analysis was less stringent and several potential biases are acknowledged. RT-CGM is a multifaceted therapeutic tool involving different patterns of learning, decision-making and behaviour. Compliance with its informed use for frequent intervention is still a considerable barrier, particularly in younger age groups (3).

Effect of continuous glucose monitoring on hypoglycaemia in type 1 diabetes

Battelino T[1], Phillip M[2], Bratina N[1], Nimri R[2], Oskarsson P[3], Bolinder J[3]

[1] *Department of Pediatric Endocrinology, Diabetes and Metabolism, Faculty of Medicine, University Medical Centre University Children's Hospital, University of Ljubljana, Ljubljana, Slovenia,* [2] *The Jesse Z. and Sara Lea Shafer Institute for Endocrinology and Diabetes, National Center for Childhood Diabetes, Schneider Children's Medical Center, Petah Tikva, and Sackler Faculty of Medicine, Tel-Aviv University, Tel-Aviv, Israel, and* [3] *Department of Medicine, Karolinska University Hospital Huddinge, Karolinska Institutet, Stockholm, Sweden*

Diabetes Care 2011; 34: 795–800

Aims

The study was designed to investigate the impact of RT-CGM on hypoglycaemia compared with SMBG in children and adults with type 1 diabetes.

Methods

People with type 1 diabetes diagnosed for more than 1 year, 10–65 years old, HbA1c level <7.5%, and using intensive insulin treatment with either an insulin pump or multiple daily injections (MDI) participated in this multicentre, randomised controlled trial. Participants were randomised after a 1 month run-in period either to SMBG and a masked FreStyle Navigator (Abbott) for 5 days every second week or to continuous RT-CGM with the FreStyle Navigator (Abbott) for 26 weeks. Visits were scheduled at days 1, 60, 120 and 180 for data upload from all devices. HbA1c was determined in a central laboratory at days 1, 60 and 180. The primary outcome was time spent in hypoglycaemia (<3.5 mmol/l, <63 mg/dl) during the entire 6 months' study period, analysed with intent-to-treat approach on all randomised participants. HbA1c was analysed using analysis of covariance (ANCOVA) with the last observation carried forward scheme for all missing data.

Results

The study was completed by 48 participants from 58 randomised to SMBG (83%), and by 53 participants from 62 randomised to RT-CGM (85%). The median sensor wear was 5.6 (paediatric 5.6, adults 4.9) days per week in the SMBG group and 6.1 (paediatric 6.1, adults 6.1) in the RT-CGM group, with a median sensor wear of 5.9 days per week in the last study month. Time spent in hypoglycaemia below 3.5 mmol/l (63 mg/dl) was significantly shorter with RT-CGM (0.48 ± 0.57 h/day) compared with SMBG (0.97 ± 1.55 h/day) [ratio of means 0.49 (95% CI 0.26–0.76), p = 0.03]. Similarly, time spent in hypoglycaemia below 3 mmol/l (55 mg/dl) and 3.9 mmol/l (70 mg/dl) was also significantly shorter with RT-CGM. Additionally, the number of hypoglycaemic excursions below 3 and 3.5 mmol/l (<55 and <63 mg/dl) during the night (00:00–06:00) was significantly lower with RT-CGM compared with SMBG (0.13 ± 0.30 vs. 0.19 ± 0.19, p = 0.01; and 0.21 ± 0.32 vs. 0.30 ± 0.31, p = 0.009). The reduction in time spent in hypoglycaemia with RT-CGM was similar in pump users and participants on MDI (41% vs. 59%), and similar in paediatric and adult participants (48% vs. 54%).

Conclusions

A significant decrease by half in time spent in hypoglycaemia was observed in this trial, with a concomitant significant decrease in HbA1c.

COMMENT

At the end of this study more than 70% of participants achieved the American Diabetes Assocation (ADA) target of HbA1c < 7% without any event of severe hypoglycaemia and with time spent in hypoglycaemia reduced by half (4). The success of RT-CGM was strongly related to sensor use, similar to most trials published so far. Interestingly, in the *post hoc* per-protocol analysis (patients who wore the sensor for >20 days corresponding to one-third of the required time in the SMBG group; 44 of 53 paediatric and 53 of 63 adult patients), the primary outcome was reduced by 64% (p < 0.001) in paediatric and 50% (p = 0.02) in adult patients. With a reasonable compliance with the RT-CGM usage, its effect seems to be comparable in children and adults. A very interesting recent paper described an important benefit of reducing hypoglycaemia with RT-CGM on epinephrine response and hypoglycaemia unawareness in adolescents (5). Eleven adolescents with hypoglycaemia unawareness underwent insulin clamp with 40 min of hypoglycaemia at 2.8 mmol/l and were subsequently randomised to either standard SMBG with a target glucose range of 6–10 mmol/l or RT-CGM with a glucose alarm at 6 mmol/l and target glucose of 8 mmol/l. A second insulin clamp was performed on all participants after 4 weeks. Epinephrine response to hypoglycaemia did not change in the SMBG group but improved in the RT-CGM group with a percentage change of 114 ± 83% vs. 604 ± 234%, SMBG vs. CGM group, respectively; p = 0.048. Perceived adrenergic symptom scores also improved significantly after the intervention in the RT-CGM group compared with SMBG (3.4 ± 0.2 vs. 5.4 ± 0.4; p < 0.001).

Sensor-augmented pump therapy lowers HbA1c in suboptimally controlled type 1 diabetes; a randomised controlled trial

Hermanides J[1], Nørgaard K[2], Bruttomesso D[3], Mathieu C[4], Frid A[5], Dayan CM[6], Diem P[7], Fermon C[8], Wentholt IM[1], Hoekstra JB[1], Devries JH[1]

[1]*Department of Internal Medicine, Academic Medical Centre, Amsterdam, The Netherlands,* [2]*Department of Endocrinology, Hvidovre University Hospital, Hvidovre, Denmark,* [3]*Department of Clinical and Experimental Medicine, Division of Metabolic Diseases, University of Padova, Padova, Italy,* [4]*Department of Endocrinology, Catholic University Leuven, Leuven, Belgium,* [5]*Division of Diabetes and Endocrinology, Malmö University Hospital, Malmö, Sweden,* [6]*Department of Medicine, University of Bristol, Bristol, UK,* [7]*Division of Endocrinology, Diabetes and Clinical Nutrition, University Hospital and University of Bern, Bern, Switzerland, and* [8]*Centre d'éducation pour le traitement de diabète et des maladies de la nutrition, Centre Hospitalier de Roubaix, Roubaix, France*

Diabet Med 2011; 28: 1158–67

Aims

To compare the treatment using a sensor-augmented insulin pump (SAP) with standard MDI therapy in type 1 diabetes with suboptimal control.

Methods

Adult participants with HbA1c above 8.2% were evaluated with a 6-day blinded CGM for initial treatment optimisation and then randomised to either standard MDI with two 6-day blinded CGM (Guardian REAL-Time Clinical, Medtronic) recordings before week 13 and 26, or SAP (Paradigm REAL-Time System, Medtronic) for 26 weeks. HbA1c was the primary outcome, with time spent above 11 or below 4 mol/l recorded during the sensor use in both groups, and patient reported outcomes as secondary endpoints. The analysis was intent-to-treat with the last observation carried forward approach.

Results

Ninety per cent of participants (35/39) completed the study in the MDI group and 98% (43/44) in the SAP group. Baseline HbA1c and centre adjusted treatment effect on HbA1c was −1.21% (95% CI −1.52 to −0.90, $p < 0.001$). A significant proportion of participants (34%) using SAP reached the European Association for the Study of Diabetes/ADA treatment target of HbA1c below 7% compared with those using MDI ($p < 0.001$). Change in percentage of sensor time spent in hyperglycaemia after 26 weeks (the least squares mean difference) was −17.3% (95% CI −25.1 to −9.5, $p < 0.001$) with no significant difference in time spent in hypoglycaemia or number of hyperglycaemic or hypoglycaemic episodes. Several patients reported that outcomes were significantly improved in the SAP group compared with MDI, including the Problem Areas in Diabetes and the Diabetes Treatment Satisfaction Questionnaires scores. The median total contact time during the trial was considerably shorter in the MDI group (240 min; interquartile range 195–353) compared with SAP group (690 min; interquartile range 526–1028) ($p < 0.001$), with a more pronounced difference in the first 13 weeks of the study. The sensor use of more than 60% of total time was achieved in 79% of the patients in the SAP group, and the total mean sensor use was 4.5 (SD 1.0) days per week over the whole trial. The duration of sensor use was not correlated with the decrease in HbA1c. The baseline HbA1c was the only significant predictor for HbA1c decease in a multivariate linear regression model. One episode (6 episodes/100 person-years) of severe hypoglycaemia occurred in the MDI group and four (19 episodes/100 person-years) in the SAP group ($p = 0.21$), all during sensor use.

Conclusions

The use of SAP was associated with a considerable decrease in HbA1c without an increase in hypoglycaemia and with an increase in the quality of life in participants with suboptimally controlled type 1 diabetes. The difference of −1.21% in the HbA1c between the MDI and SAP groups could represent a combined effect of the use of the pump, continuous glucose sensor, bolus calculator and additional education.

COMMENT

The very strong primary outcome of this randomised controlled trial performed in a population with a mean baseline HbA1c around 8.5% is unique (6). Most of the HbA1c decrease in the SAP group (–1.17%) was achieved in the first 13 weeks of the study where most of the contacts between participant and healthcare professional occurred, and plateaued thereafter with only –0.06% additional decrease in the second 13 weeks. The impressive and clinically meaningful difference in the HbA1c is also due to the virtually absent study effect in the MDI group, despite the fact that an average of 4 h of participant–healthcare professional contact in 6 months is likely to be above the average in routine clinical care. This result was achieved with a moderate decrease in time spent in hyperglycaemia > 11 mmol/l (200 mg/dl) of –17.3%, with a probably higher difference in the area under the curve in hyperglycaemia. The time spent in hypoglycaemia was similar in both groups and did not increase with decrease in HbA1c. A non-significantly higher number of severe hypoglycaemia episodes was reported in the SAP group during the study, but this group reported a similarly higher number of severe hypoglycaemia events also in the year before the study. Interestingly, the decrease in HbA1c did not correlate with sensor use, as observed in most other trials (7). This may be related to the relatively high and uniform overall sensor use in the SAP group.

Sensor-augmented pump therapy from the diagnosis of childhood type 1 diabetes: results of the Paediatric Onset Study (ONSET) after 12 months of treatment

Kordonouri O[1], Pankowska E[2], Rami B[3], Kapellen T[4], Coutant R[5], Hartmann R[1], Lange K[6], Knip M[7], Danne T[1]

[1] *Bult Diabetes Centre for Children and Adolescents, Kinderkrankenhaus auf der Bult, Hannover, Germany,* [2] *Department of Paediatric Diabetology and Birth Defects, Medical University of Warsaw, Warsaw, Poland,* [3] *Department of Paediatrics, Medical University of Vienna, Vienna, Austria,* [4] *Universitätsklinik und Poliklinik für Kinder und Jugendliche, Leipzig, Germany,* [5] *Département de Pédiatrie, Centre Hospitalier Universitaire, Angers, France,* [6] *Department of Medical Psychology, Hannover Medical School, Hannover, Germany, and* [7] *Hospital for Children and Adolescents, and Folkhälsan Research Centre, University of Helsinki, Helsinki, Finland*

*Diabetologia 2010; **53**: 2487–95*

Aims

To assess the acceptance, efficacy and safety of SAP used from disease on-set by determining its impact on HbA1c, daily insulin dose, residual β-cell function, incidence of severe hypoglycaemia and quality of life compared with insulin pump with SMBG.

Methods

Children and adolescents with less than 4 weeks from the diagnosis of type 1 diabetes aged 1–16 years were randomised to either an SAP (Paradigm REAL Time, Medtronic) or an insulin pump with SMBG. Gly-caemic targets were the same for both groups with study visits at 6, 26 and 52 weeks and additional routine visits every 6–10 weeks and phone contacts as deemed necessary for individual patients by their healthcare team. A blinded RT-CGM device was used for 6 days before visits at 6 and 52 weeks in the pump with SMBG group. Quality of life questionnaires were given at study entry and at 52 weeks. Fasting C-peptide and all other laboratory measurements were performed centrally and the investigators were blinded for the results. The intent-to-treat approach was used for data analysis.

Results

Out of 295 patients offered the participation 160 (54%) agreed and were randomised at 9.6 ± 6.0 days after the diagnosis. All but six completed the study, 76 in the SAP group and 78 in the pump with SMBG group. No difference was detected in HbA1c at any point of the study with roughly one-third of participants reaching HbA1c $< 7\%$ in both groups. Glycaemic variability assessed with mean amplitude of glucose excursions (MAGE) was significantly lower in the SAP group at the end of the study compared with the pump and SMBG group. Sensor use declined significantly to 1.4 ± 1.0 sensors per week at 26 weeks and 1.1 ± 0.7 sensors per week at the end of the study (one sensor was used for 3 days), with docu-mented sensor use in 55 participants. Participants using at least one sen-sor per week had lower HbA1c than those using less than one sensor per week (7.1% vs. 7.6%, $p = 0.032$). Less SMBG was performed in the SAP group compared with the pump and SMBG group (5.2 ± 2.0 vs.6.5 ± 2.1, $p < 0.001$). The insulin dose was similar in both groups throughout the study, as was the distribution of the dose between the basal and bolus with slightly lower basal dose in the pump with SMBG group. Fasting C-peptide at 52 weeks was slightly higher in the SAP group, but the dif-ference reached significance only in the age 12–16 years subgroup. More frequent sensor use was associated with a reduced decrease in fasting C-peptide at 52 weeks. Not a single episode of severe hypoglycaemia was reported in the SAP group compared with four episodes reported in the pump with SMBG group (p = 0.046). Quality of life scores were similar in both groups throughout the study.

Conclusions

The effectiveness of SAP in children and adolescents from the diagnosis of type 1 diabetes depends on sensor use and may help to preserve fasting C-peptide particularly in the adolescent age group.

COMMENT

This interesting randomised controlled trial seems to raise further questions rather than provide firm answers (8). The lack of an overall reduction in HbA1c with the use of the SAP was probably related to the relatively low sensor use of about half of the required time on average in the second 6 months of the study. Several other studies demonstrated that infrequent sensor use represents the major limitation for its efficacy in children and adolescents. The possible preservation of fasting C-peptide with SAP use in adolescents is of considerable interest and needs further evaluation, possibly with an additional evaluation of the mixed meal stimulated C-peptide. No reported episode of severe hypoglycaemia in the SAP group during the whole year of the study is also of particular interest in this age group and may influence routine clinical care.

Continuous glucose monitoring in youth with type 1 diabetes: 12-month follow-up of the Juvenile Diabetes Research Foundation Continuous Glucose Monitoring randomised trial

Chase HP[1], Beck RW[2], Xing D[2], Tamborlane WV[3], Coffey J[4], Fox LA[5], Ives B[3], Keady J[6], Kollman C[2], Laffel L[6], Ruedy KJ[2]

[1] *Barbara Davis Center, Denver, CO, USA,* [2] *Jaeb Center for Health Research, Tampa, FL, USA,* [3] *Yale University, New Haven, CT, USA,* [4] *University of Iowa, Iowa City, IA, USA,* [5] *Nemours Children's Clinic, Jacksonville, FL, USA, and* [6] *Joslin Diabetes Center, Boston, MA, USA*

*Diabetes Tech Ther 2010; **12**: 507–15*

Aims

A 6 months' extension of the JDRF CGM trial for participants randomised to RT-CGM for description and evaluation of RT-CGM use.

Methods

All participants aged 8 to <18 years with an HbA1c > 7% and < 10% at randomisation were included in this report. A day of sensor use was considered any day with at least one RT-CGM value (one of the following: DexCom SEVEN, CGMS Medtronic or Free Style Navigator, Abbott) recorded. In addition to the central HbA1c measurement, RT-CGM devices upload and monitoring for severe hypoglycaemia, a CGM satisfaction 44-item five-point Likert scale questionnaire was administered at 6 and 12 months to participants and their parents.

Results

The 80 participants with a mean age of 13.0 years, 42 (53%) 8–12 years old and 38 (48%) 13 to <18 years old, had a mean baseline HbA1c level of 8.0 ± 0.7%, 63 (79%) using an insulin pump and the others MDI with insulin including long- and rapid-acting insulin analogues. Seventy-six of the 80 (95%) participants were using RT-CGM for 5.5 days per week (interquartile range 3.6–6.5) at 6 months and 67 (84%) for 4.0 days per week (interquartile range 2.0–6.0) after 12 months, with only 17 (21%) mostly younger children for >6 days per week. These 17 participants had a significantly greater decrease in HbA1c than participants using the sensor <6 days per week (mean change –0.8 ± 0.6% vs. –0.1 ± 0.7%, p < 0.001 adjusted for age), with a markedly higher percentage reaching the ADA glycaemic target (71% vs. 35%, p < 0.01 adjusted for age). These results were paralleled with an increase time spent in the target glucose range without an increase in time spent in hypoglycaemia. The incidence of severe hypoglycaemia was low with 11.2 events per 100 person-years; a total of nine events occurred in seven participants in 12 months, not related to the amount of sensor usage. CGM satisfaction scores were also significantly higher in the 17 participants using the sensor >6 days per week compared with the rest of the group (4.0 vs. 3.3, p < 0.001 for participants; 4.2 vs. 3.7, p < 0.001 for parents).

Conclusions

A considerable reduction of HbA1c levels and a corresponding decrease in frequency of sensor glucose values above the target range was observed in participants 8 to <18 years old when using RT-CGM > 6 days per week, without an increase in time spent in hypoglycaemia. Unfortunately, only 21% were able to sustain such compliance for the 12-month period. The total rate of severe hypoglycaemia was low and not related to sensor use. More sensor use was associated with greater satisfaction in participants and their parents.

COMMENT

This follow-up study clearly demonstrates the close association of sensor use and the efficacy of RT-CGM in the young population (9). The authors conclude that a better, more appealing, less painful and more accurate device is awaited for this population. However, a change in attitude towards diabetes management in this age group may also be pertinent. A separate analysis of 82 children (7–12 years) and 74 adolescents (13–18 years) from the STAR 3 study demonstrated a better compliance with sensor use compared with the JDRF trial, children also being more compliant than adolescents (10). Furthermore, an observational study of 129 children and adolescents (13.5 ± 3.8 years old) using an SAP for an average of 1.4 ± 0.7 years also demonstrated a superior improvement in HbA1c compared with 493 children and adolescents (12.9 ± 3.4 years old) using conventional insulin pump therapy (–0.6% vs. –0.3%; $p = 0.005$) (11). It is therefore possible to improve metabolic control also with currently available RT-CGM devices in most children and adolescents with type 1 diabetes provided that good compliance and motivation is maintained. Further efforts and innovative strategies for overcoming barriers precluding successful use of RT-CGM in this age group are warranted.

Use of continuous glucose monitoring in subjects with type 1 diabetes on multiple daily injections versus continuous subcutaneous insulin infusion therapy: a prospective 6-month study

Garg SK, Voelmle MK, Beatson CR, Miller HA, Crew LB, Freson BJ, Hazenfield RM

Barbara Davis Center for Childhood Diabetes, University of Colorado Denver, School of Medicine, Aurora, CO, USA

Diabetes Care 2011; **34**: 574–9

Aims

To compare the efficacy of CGM in participants with type 1 diabetes using MDI or an insulin pump.

Methods

Sixty adult participants [30 using MDI and 30 continuous subcutaneous insulin infusion (CSII)] with HbA1c between 6.5% and 10%, performing SMBG at least four times a day, agreed to wear an RT-CGM device (DexCom Seven Plus, DexCom) for 24 weeks on a non-randomised basis, with the initial 4 weeks blinded to continuous glucose data. Participants were instructed to wear the CGM device continuously and to capture all insulin administrations, carbohydrate intake and physical activity. Instruction on how to use CGM data as an adjunct to SMBG for diabetes management was provided at the beginning of the study. Study visits were scheduled every 4 weeks. An intent-to-treat analysis for both groups was planned, with a per-protocol analysis of participants wearing the sensor 6 days per week or more.

Results

Fifty-eight participants completed all study visits. The mean change in HbA1c within groups from screening to 24 weeks was 0.16 ± 0.84% in the MDI group and –0.02 ± 0.59% in the CSII group. However, HbA1c was significantly lower at 12 weeks compared with the screening values both in MDI (–0.18%) and CSII (–0.20%). Similar results were obtained in the predefined per-protocol analysis. Time spent within the target range of 3.9–10 mmol/l (70–180 mg/dl) increased on average by 1.4 h in the MDI group and 0.7 h/day in the CSII group compared with the blinded 4 weeks (p = 0.009). The time spent below this range decreased by 30% in the MDI group and by 21% in the CSII group. The total number of glycaemic excursions was also significantly decreased in both groups, with MAGE significantly reduced in the unblinded versus blinded CGM use. Glucose average, time spent in the target range and MAGE were significantly better in the CSII group compared with MDI group in the per-protocol analysis. Compliance with sensor use was similar in both groups. Local skin reactions were recorded, but there was no severe hypoglycaemia or sensor insertion site infection.

Conclusions:

A 24 weeks' use of CGM provides similar benefits to people with type 1 diabetes using MDI or CSII.

COMMENT

This prospective non-randomised study adds to the existing data on RT-CGM efficacy but to some extent surprises with the observation that in most endpoints more sensor use does not improve the outcome (12). Similarly, the amount of sensor use is not correlated with the decrease in HbA1c in a randomised controlled trial comparing SAP with MDI (6). However, many other trials clearly demonstrate the relationship between sensor use and its clinical effectiveness, particularly in the younger population. This apparent discrepancy may be related to differences in motivation for active use of a CGM device, readiness to modify behaviour, and perception of a continuous reminder about the chronic disease. All this may also reflect in disparities in data on quality of life. Despite the substantial satisfaction with the CGM, quality of life did not change very much during the JDRF trial with only marginal although significant differences favouring CGM in some subsets in Hypoglycaemia Fear Score and Social Functioning Health Survey – SF-12 in the adult population (13). The way individual users perceive a CGM device may therefore play a crucial role in compliance with its use and in its effectiveness.

Accuracy and reliability of a subcutaneous continuous glucose-monitoring system in critically ill patients

Brunner R[1], Kitzberger R[1], Miehsler W[1], Herkner H[2], Madl C[1], Holzinger U[1]

[1] *Division of Gastroenterology and Hepatology – ICU 13H1, Department of Medicine III, Medical University of Vienna, Austria, and* [2] *Department of Emergency Medicine, Medical University of Vienna, Austria*

*Crit Care Med 2011; **39**: 659–64*

Aims

To evaluate the accuracy of RT-CGM measurements in critically ill patients.

Methods

Data from two randomised controlled clinical trials conducted in an eight-bed intensive care unit (ICU) at the University Hospital of Vienna, Austria, were polled and analysed for accuracy and reliability. Inclusion criteria incorporated mechanical ventilation, ICU stay of > 48 h and blood glucose above the normal range without insulin. RT-CGM (Guardian, Medtronic) sensor glucose values from 174 different patients were compared with arterial reference blood glucose levels determined by a standard blood gas analyser. An Ellmerer modified error grid analysis was used to analyse the clinical effect of measurement errors on the ICU team decisions about insulin or glucose administration.

Results

A total of 2045 CGM–reference pairs were analysed, excluding outliers [glucose difference > 5.56 mmol/l (> 100 mg/dl) between CGM and reference value]. The CGM mean glucose value of 6.18 mmol/l (CI 6.07– 6.29) [111 mg/dl (CI 109 –113)] was lower than the reference of 6.29 mmol/l (CI 6.19–6.40) [113 mg/dl (CI 111–115)], $p = 0.036$. The mean difference between CGM and reference was –0.10 mmol/l (CI –0.13 to –0.07) [–2 mg/dl (CI –2 to –1)], with the absolute value of the difference 0.44 mmol/l (CI 0.41– 0.47) [8 mg/dl (CI 7–8)], relative difference –0.8% (CI –1.31 to –0.35) and relative absolute difference 7.3% (CI 6.8%–7.8%). Clinical evaluation located 99.1% of the CGM measurements to the acceptable treatment zone, 0.5% to the unacceptable violation zone, and 0.4% to the major violation zone with insulin dosing error grid analysis. No CGM measurements were positioned in the life-threatening zone. The conformity between the two methods assessed by the Pearson correlation coefficient was 0.92. According to the ISO criteria 92.9% of the CGM measurements were accurate, with ± 0.83 mmol/l (± 15 mg/dl) difference for glucose values ≤ 4.20 mmol/l (≤ 75 mg/dl) and ±20% difference for glucose values > 4.20 mmol/l (>75 mg/dl). No malfunction of the CGM was reported during the study periods.

Conclusions

The subcutaneous CGM was reliable and safe for decisions on insulin therapy in critically ill patients with a strong correlation to arterial blood glucose levels, measured by a blood gas analyser.

COMMENT

This analysis of pooled data from two randomised controlled trials presents results for CGM superior to current point of care glucometers in critically ill patients (14). This finding was corroborated in a comparative study of two continuous subcutaneous sensors in a cardiac postoperative ICU, where relative absolute deviation (RAD) between reference and sensor at intervals 0–4 and 5–9 min after the reference glucose was 11% (8–16) and 10% (8–16) compared with 14% (11–18) and 14% (11–17), $p < 0.05$ and $p < 0.001$, for the two investigated sensors (15). Interestingly, the RAD of both sensors was comparable or superior to reported data for routine outpatient use. In a paediatric ICU study with a population of 47 patients aged 6 weeks to 16 years (mean age 4.3 years) a total of 1555 CGM and routine blood glucose measurements were compared using Clarke error grid and Bland–Altman analysis (16). The mean RAD was 15.3% with 97.9% within clinically acceptable agreement (74.6% were in zone A and 23.3% were in zone B). Furthermore, another study performed in children less than 3 years of age admitted to paediatric ICU after cardiac surgery demonstrated the clinical usefulness of RT-CGM for this population (17). Taken together, an increasing amount of evidence supports the safety and efficacy of RT-CGM in critically ill patients of all age groups.

The effect of real-time continuous glucose monitoring on glycaemic control in patients with type 2 diabetes mellitus

Ehrhardt, NM, Chellappa M, Walker MS, Fonda SJ, Vigersky RA

Walter Reed Medical Center, Washington, DC, USA

J Diabetes Sci Technol 2011; 8: 668–75

Aims

To evaluate the utility of RT-CGM in people with type 2 diabetes on a variety of treatment modalities except prandial insulin.

Methods
A prospective, 52-week, two arm, randomised trial comparing RT-CGM ($n = 50$) versus SMBG ($n = 50$) in people with type 2 diabetes not taking prandial insulin was conducted. RT-CGM (DexCom™ SEVEN) was used for four 2-week cycles (2 weeks on/1 week off) for a total of 8 weeks out of the first 3 months. SMBG was asked to be done before meals and bedtime. All patients were managed by their usual healthcare provider with no interventions or recommendations by study staff to either the patient or provider. Primary endpoint was change in A1c.

Results
Mean decline in A1c at 12 weeks was 1.0% ($\pm 1.1\%$) going from 8.4% to 7.4% in the RT-CGM group and 0.5% ($\pm 0.8\%$) going from 8.2% to 7.7% in the SMBG group (p = 0.006). There were no group differences in the net change in the number or dosage of hypoglycaemic medications. Those who used the RT-CGM for ≥ 48 days per protocol reduced their A1c by 1.2% ($\pm 1.1\%$) vs. 0.6% ($\pm 1.1\%$) in those who used it <48 days (p = 0.009). There was no improvement in weight or blood pressure.

Conclusions
Real-time CGM significantly improves A1c compared with SMBG in patients with type 2 diabetes not taking prandial insulin with no significant change in medications, suggesting patients made changes in their behaviour with RT-CGM. The technology using RT-CGM may benefit a larger population of people with diabetes than previously thought.

COMMENT

This is the first randomised controlled study evaluating the potential benefit of RT-CGM vs. frequent SMBG in type 2 diabetes patients not on prandial insulin (18). Neither patients nor healthcare providers were trained or educated on what to do with the real-time readings. Results showed a robust drop in A1c in the RT-CGM group with no major changes in treatment agents, suggesting patients made behaviour changes as a result of seeing the real-time readings. Again, more frequent usage of RT-CGM correlated with a greater decline in A1c. Further studies must validate this finding in type 2 diabetes patients before periodic RT-CGM becomes the standard of care in these patients. One year study results in abstract form have confirmed the durability of this significant drop in A1c at 1 year with no subsequent use of RT-CGM after the eleventh week of the trial.

Continuous glucose monitoring for evaluation of glycaemic excursions after gastric bypass

Halperin F[1,2,3], Patti ME[2,3], Skow M[2], Bajwa M[2], Goldfine AB[1,2,3]

[1]*Brigham and Women's Hospital, Boston, MA, USA,* [2]*Joslin Diabetes Center, Boston, MA, USA, and* [3]*Harvard Medical School, Boston, MA, USA*

J Obes 2011; doi:10.1155/2011/869536. Epub 2011 Feb 7

Aims

To evaluate post gastric bypass hypoglycaemia with either the mixed meal tolerance test (MMTT) or CGM in symptomatic and asymptomatic patients.

Methods

Ten patients treated for symptomatic hypoglycaemia (all with diet advice, eight with α-glucosidase inhibitor, one with octreotide, one with diazoxide) and six patients without any symptoms after Roux-en-Y gastric bypass (RYGB) operation were invited to an MMTT and subsequently to retrospective CGM (iPro, Medtronic) monitoring.

Results

Nine of 10 symptomatic and five of six asymptomatic participants completed the MMTT. No significant differences in mean blood glucose or area under the curve were observed between the two groups, with lower blood glucose in the asymptomatic group after 120 min. Similarly, neither fasting insulin nor insulin area under the curve were significantly different, with a trend to higher insulin secretion in the symptomatic group. During the CGM, the symptomatic group had more total values out of the 3.9–10 mmol/l (70–180 mg/dl) range (8.5 ± 2.1 vs. 3.8 ± 2.3; p = 0.05), with a trend of more frequent hypoglycaemic excursions (1.45 ± 0.42 vs. 0.78 ± 0.44; ns). Minutes per day spent in hypoglycaemia were also higher in the symptomatic group (63 ± 23 vs. 34 ± 22), as was the percentage of time in hypoglycaemia per day (5.5 ± 1.9 vs. 3.1 ± 2.0%), but these did not reach statistical significance. The maximum glucose levels recorded with CGM were significantly higher in the symptomatic group (213 ± 13 vs. 167 ± 13 mg/dl; p = 0.03), with a trend of spending more minutes per day in hyperglycaemia. CGM detected more hypoglycaemia than the MMTT, in three out of six asymptomatic patients.

Conclusions

Asymptomatic hypoglycaemia after RYGB operation is more common than generally thought and is readily detected by CGM.

COMMENT

Symptomatic and asymptomatic hypoglycaemia after RYGB is poorly under-stood but more common than generally believed and potentially associated with a higher incidence of accidents in this patient population (19). CGM was superior to the standard evaluation with MMTT and is potentially a valuable tool to diagnose and possibly prevent hypoglycaemia when used in real time. Another study evaluated glucose excursions in 10 patients after RYGB with CGM and compared them to a group with type 2 diabetes and a healthy con-trol group (20). Early postprandial glucose elevations were present in half of the patients after RYGB and were followed by rapid glucose decrease, some-times causing perceived symptoms of hypoglycaemia, also without reaching hypoglycaemic glucose values. Hypoglycaemia <3.3 mmol/l (<60 mg/dl) was rare in this study. Both studies indicate that further evaluation with CGM of glycaemic fluctuations in patients after RYGB is warranted.

Evaluating the clinical accuracy of GlucoMen®Day: a novel microdialysis-based continuous glucose monitor

Valgimigli F, Lucarelli F, Scuffi C, Morandi S, Sposato I

A. Menarini Diagnostics, Florence, Italy

J Diabetes Sci Technol 2010; 4: 1182–92

Aims

To evaluate the accuracy of a second-generation microdialysis CGM in people with diabetes type 1 and 2.

Methods

Data from two clinical trials involving 12 participants, six with type 1 dia-betes (three females, 30 ± 5 years old, body mass index 25.1 ± 2.5 kg/m^2) and six with type 2 diabetes (two females, 62 ± 11 years old, body mass index 25.6 ± 4.0 kg/m^2) were analysed using the standard and continu-ous glucose error grid analysis (CG-EGA). All participants were inserted with the GlucoMen®Day (A. Menarini) sensor and monitored for up to 100 h. Venous blood sampling was performed at 15 min intervals 2 h after breakfast or after a meal tolerance test for blood glucose measure-ments with a standard analyser. Capillary blood glucose tests (Glucocard G meter, A. Menarini) were used for retrospective calibration of the CGM. Evaluation of the total lag time was done prior to the accuracy analysis as suggested by Kovatchev (Poincaré plot method).

Results

Biofouling and encapsulation usually adding to the sensor 'drift' were minimal. The lag time was calculated to be 11 min. The static accuracy was evaluated from 236 data pairs, with a subset of 120 pairs used for the evaluation of dynamic accuracy. The Clarke error grid analysis showed 90% of points falling within the clinically accurate zone A, 10% of points within zone B, and no data (0%) within zones C, D and E. The Pearson correlation coefficient r was 0.92. The total percentage of values within ±15 mg/dl (<75 mg/dl) and ±20% (≥75 mg/dl) of the reference values was 90%, with a mean absolute error of 11.4 mg/dl, a median absolute error of 9.0 mg/dl, a mean absolute relative error of 10.0% and a median absolute relative error of 7.0%. In dynamic analysis, the percentage of accurate measurements was higher than 95.2% in all glycaemic ranges; no erroneous readings were detected, with some benign errors in the euglycaemic (4.3%) and hyperglycaemic (4.8%) ranges and none (0%) in the hypoglycaemic range.

Conclusions

The GlucoMen®Day microdialysis-based CGM system performs with clinically acceptable accuracy and reliability in people with diabetes for up to 100 h.

COMMENT

The GlucoMen®Day is currently the only microdialysis-based CGM device available for professional use (21). Its accuracy is improved from the previous model and aligns with other commercially available CGM devices, with a particularly strong performance in hypoglycaemia. However, clinical data are rather limited with no data on patient satisfaction available so far. Data on another novel CGM prototype were reported recently from Bayer (22). Its glucose oxidase sensor, composed of platinum and silver/silver chloride with an outer membrane composed of polyurethane, is 0.33 mm (approximately 28 gauge) in diameter and does not require any insertion needle. Fourteen participants (seven type 1 and seven type 2 diabetes) took part in the glucose clamp study composed of four 40 min plateau periods: first hypoglycaemic period (50 mg/dl), hyperglycaemic period (250 mg/dl), second hypoglycaemic period (50 mg/dl) and euglycaemic period (90 mg/dl), with rapidly changing blood glucose between plateaux at an approximate rate of 2 mg/dl/min. Venous plasma samples were collected every 5 min and calibration of the CGM device was done retrospectively using YSI plasma glucose measurements. The accuracy determined from 873 paired data with the Clarke error grid was 79.8% in zone A, 14.9% in zone B and 5.3% in zone D, and the accuracy determined with the Parkes (consensus) error grid was 86.8% in zone A, 12.1% in zone B, 1% in zone C and no results in zones D and E. Rate error grid analysis of the transition period positioned 68.6% of results in zone A, 20.0%

in zone B, 3.8% in zone C, 5.3% in zone D and 2.4% in zone E. No serious adverse events were reported. The development of the above two new CGM devices further demonstrates the strength and importance of CGM in the management of diabetes.

CONCLUSION

Retrospective and real-time CGM is reaching the point of basic consensus (23, 24). However, its successful implementation remains controversial in several aspects, including the proper RT-CGM related education (25), frequency of use (26) and its acceptance in broader social environments such as schools (27). Further search for predictors of clinical benefit (28, 29) and specific target populations will probably improve its routine usefulness and acceptability by users, both professional and patients.

REFERENCES

1. Pickup JC, Freeman SC, Sutton AJ. Glycaemic control in type 1 diabetes during real time continuous glucose monitoring compared with self monitoring of blood glucose: meta-analysis of randomised controlled trials using individual patient data. *BMJ* 2011 Jul 7; 343:d3805 doi:10.1136/bmj.d3805
2. Gandhi GY, Kovalaske M, Kudva Y, Walsh K, Elamin MB, Beers M, Coyle C, Goalen M, Murad MS, Erwin PJ, Corpus J, Montori VM, Murad MH. Efficacy of continuous glucose monitoring in improving glycemic control and reducing hypoglycemia: a systematic review and meta-analysis of randomized trials. *J Diabetes Sci Technol* 2011; **5**: 952–65
3. Battelino T, Phillip M. Real-time continuous glucose monitoring in randomized control trials. *Pediatr Endocrinol Rev* 2010; **7** (Suppl 3): 401–4
4. Battelino T, Phillip M, Bratina N, Nimri R, Oskarsson P, Bolinder J. Effect of continuous glucose monitoring on hypoglycemia in type 1 diabetes. *Diabetes Care* 2011; **34**: 795–800
5. Ly TT, Hewitt J, Davey RJ, Lim EM, Davis EA, Jones TW. Improving epinephrine responses in hypoglycemia unawareness with real-time continuous glucose monitoring in adolescents with type 1 diabetes. *Diabetes Care* 2011; **34**: 50–2
6. Hermanides J, Nørgaard K, Bruttomesso D, Mathieu C, Frid A, Dayan CM, Diem P, Fermon C, Wentholt IM, Hoekstra JB, Devries JH. Sensor-augmented pump therapy lowers HbA(1c) in suboptimally controlled Type 1 diabetes; a randomized controlled trial. *Diabet Med* 2011; **28**: 1158–67
7. Bergenstal RM, Tamborlane WV, Ahmann A, Buse JB, Dailey G, Davis SN, Joyce C, Peoples T, Perkins BA, Welsh JB, Willi SM, Wood MA; STAR 3 Study Group. Effectiveness of sensor-augmented insulin-pump therapy in type 1 diabetes. *N Engl J Med* 2010; **363**: 311–20
8. Kordonouri O, Pankowska E, Rami B, Kapellen T, Coutant R, Hartmann R, Lange K, Knip M, Danne T. Sensor-augmented pump therapy from the diagnosis of childhood type 1 diabetes: results of the Paediatric Onset Study (ONSET) after 12 months of treatment. *Diabetologia* 2010; **53**: 2487–95
9. Chase HP, Beck RW, Xing D, Tamborlane WV, Coffey J, Fox LA, Ives B, Keady J, Kollman C, Laffel L, Ruedy KJ. Continuous glucose monitoring in youth with type 1 diabetes: 12-month follow-up of the Juvenile Diabetes Research Foundation continuous glucose monitoring randomized trial. *Diabetes Technol Ther* 2010; **12**: 507–15

10. Slover RH, Welsh JB, Criego A, Weinzimer SA, Willi SM, Wood MA, Tamborlane WV. Effectiveness of sensor-augmented pump therapy in children and adolescents with type 1 diabetes in the STAR 3 study. *Pediatr Diabetes* 2011 Jul 3; doi:**10**.1111/j.1399-5448.2011.00793.x.

11. Scaramuzza AE, Iafusco D, Rabbone I, Bonfanti R, Lombardo F, Schiaffini R, Buono P, Toni S, Cherubini V, Zuccotti GV; Diabetes Study Group of the Italian Society of Paediatric Endocrinology and Diabetology. Use of integrated real-time continuous glucose monitoring/insulin pump system in children and adolescents with type 1 diabetes: a 3-year follow-up study. *Diabetes Technol Ther* 2011; **13**: 99–103

12. Garg SK, Voelmle MK, Beatson CR, Miller HA, Crew LB, Freson BJ, Hazenfield RM. Use of continuous glucose monitoring in subjects with type 1 diabetes on multiple daily injections versus continuous subcutaneous insulin infusion therapy: a prospective 6-month study. *Diabetes Care* 2011; **34**: 574–9

13. Juvenile Diabetes Research Foundation Continuous Glucose Monitoring Study Group, Beck RW, Lawrence JM, Laffel L, Wysocki T, Xing D, Huang ES, Ives B, Kollman C, Lee J, Ruedy KJ, Tamborlane WV. Quality-of-life measures in children and adults with type 1 diabetes: Juvenile Diabetes Research Foundation Continuous Glucose Monitoring randomized trial. *Diabetes Care* 2010; **33**: 2175–7

14. Brunner R, Kitzberger R, Miehsler W, Herkner H, Madl C, Holzinger U. Accuracy and reliability of a subcutaneous continuous glucose-monitoring system in critically ill patients. *Crit Care Med* 2011; **39**: 659–64

15. Siegelaar SE, Barwari T, Hermanides J, Stooker W, van der Voort PH, DeVries JH. Accuracy and reliability of continuous glucose monitoring in the intensive care unit: a head-to-head comparison of two subcutaneous glucose sensors in cardiac surgery patients. *Diabetes Care* 2011; **34**: e31

16. Bridges BC, Preissig CM, Maher KO, Rigby MR. Continuous glucose monitors prove highly accurate in critically ill children. *Crit Care* 2010; **14**: R176, doi:10.1186/cc9280

17. Steil GM, Langer M, Jaeger K, Alexander J, Gaies M, Agus MS. Value of continuous glucose monitoring for minimizing severe hypoglycemia during tight glycemic control. *Pediatr Crit Care Med* 2011 Apr 14; doi:**10**.1097/PCC.0b013e31821926a5

18. Ehrhardt NM, Chellappa M, Walker MS, Fonda SJ, Vigersky RA. The effect of real-time continuous glucose monitoring on glycemic control in patients with type 2 diabetes mellitus. *J Diabetes Sci Technol* 2011; **5**: 668–75

19. Halperin F, Patti ME, Skow M, Bajwa M, Goldfine AB. Continuous glucose monitoring for evaluation of glycemic excursions after gastric bypass. *J Obes* 2011; **2011**:869536. Epub 2011 Feb 7

20. Hanaire H, Bertrand M, Guerci B, Anduze Y, Guillaume E, Ritz P. High glycemic variability assessed by continuous glucose monitoring after surgical treatment of obesity by gastric bypass. *Diabetes Technol Ther* 2011; **13**: 625–30

21. Valgimigli F, Lucarelli F, Scuffi C, Morandi S, Sposato I. Evaluating the clinical accuracy of GlucoMen®Day: a novel microdialysis-based continuous glucose monitor. *J Diabetes Sci Technol* 2010; **4**: 1182–92

22. Morrow L, Hompesch M, Tideman AM, Matson J, Dunne N, Pardo S, Parkes JL, Schachner HC, Simmons DA. Evaluation of a novel continuous glucose measurement device in patients with diabetes mellitus across the glycemic range. *J Diabetes Sci Technol* 2011; **5**: 853–9

23. Blevins TC, Bode BW, Garg SK, Grunberger G, Hirsch IB, Jovanovič L, Nardacci E, Orzeck EA, Roberts VL, Tamborlane WV; AACE Continuous Glucose Monitoring Task Force, Rothermel C. Statement by the American Association of Clinical Endocrinologists Consensus Panel on continuous glucose monitoring. *Endocr Pract* 2010; **16**: 730–45

24. Hermanides J, Phillip M, DeVries JH. Current application of continuous glucose monitoring in the treatment of diabetes: pros and cons. *Diabetes Care* 2011; **34** (Suppl 2): S197–201

25. Jenkins AJ, Krishnamurthy B, Best JD, Cameron FJ, Colman PG, Hamblin PS, O'Connell MA, Rodda C, Teede H, O'Neal DN. An algorithm guiding patient responses to real-time-continuous glucose monitoring improves quality of life. *Diabetes Technol Ther* 2011; **13**: 105–9

26. Xing D, Kollman C, Beck RW, Tamborlane WV, Laffel L, Buckingham BA, Wilson DM, Weinzimer S, Fiallo-Scharer R, Ruedy KJ; Juvenile Diabetes Research Foundation Continuous Glucose Monitoring Study Group. Optimal sampling intervals to assess long-term glycemic control using continuous glucose monitoring. *Diabetes Technol Ther* 2011; **13**: 351–8

27. Bratina N, Battelino T. Insulin pumps and continuous glucose monitoring (CGM) in preschool and school-age children: how schools can integrate technology. *Pediatr Endocrinol Rev* 2010; **7** (Suppl 3): 417–21

28. Buse JB, Dailey G, Ahmann AA, Bergenstal RM, Green JB, Peoples T, Tanenberg RJ, Yang Q. Baseline predictors of A1C reduction in adults using sensor-augmented pump therapy or multiple daily injection therapy: the STAR 3 experience. *Diabetes Technol Ther* 2011; **13**: 601–6

29. Juvenile Diabetes Research Foundation Continuous Glucose Monitoring Study Group, Fiallo-Scharer R, Cheng J, Beck RW, Buckingham BA, Chase HP, Kollman C, Laffel L, Lawrence JM, Mauras N, Tamborlane WV, Wilson DM, Wolpert H. Factors predictive of severe hypoglycemia in type 1 diabetes: analysis from the Juvenile Diabetes Research Foundation continuous glucose monitoring randomized control trial dataset. *Diabetes Care* 2011; **34**: 586–90

CHAPTER 3

Insulin Pumps

John C. Pickup

King's College London School of Medicine, Guy's Hospital, London, UK

INTRODUCTION

Some identifiable themes for research on continuous subcutaneous insulin infusion (CSII) in the last year are various approaches to further optimising the control in type 1 diabetes (such as by altering the timing of the meal bolus or the type of food eaten), CSII under special circumstances (such as in hospital), the use of CSII from diagnosis rather than after a trial of multiple daily injections (MDI) (particularly in children), and continued interest in whether CSII has a place in the management of type 2 diabetes. These topics form the bulk of the papers reviewed here.

It is interesting that several papers involve continuous glucose monitoring in addition to CSII, either to measure aspects of the control achieved by pumps or in the context of sensor-augmented pump treatment. The latter is likely to be a continued focus of research in the next few years, particularly as low glucose insulin-suspend pumps have been in clinical practice in Europe since 2009 and the first full papers on their efficacy are expected during the coming year.

SYSTEMATIC REVIEWS

Cochrane review: continuous subcutaneous insulin infusion (CSII) versus multiple insulin injections for type 1 diabetes mellitus

Misso ML[1], Egberts KJ[2], Page M[3], O'Connor D[3], Shaw J[4]

[1]Australasian Cochrane Centre, Clayton, Australia, [2]Centre for Obesity Research and Education (CORE), Monash University, Melbourne, Australia,

Int J Clin Pract 2012; **66** (Suppl. 175): 15–19

[3] *Australasian Cochrane Centre, Monash Institute of Health Services Research, Monash University, Clayton, Australia, and* [4] *Baker IDI Heart and Diabetes Institute, Victoria, Australia*

Evidence Based Child Health 2010; 5: 1726–867

Background

The purpose of this study was to perform a meta-analysis of randomised controlled trials comparing glycaemic control in type 1 diabetes during CSII or multiple dose insulin injections (MDI).

Methods

The Cochrane Library, Medline, EMBASE and CINAHL databases were searched for studies meeting the selection criteria, and a random effects meta-analysis was performed using the extracted summary data.

Results

In all, 23 trials were identified, of which 20 reported HbA1c data. CSII was associated with a significant reduction in mean HbA1c vs. MDI: –0.3% (95% confidence interval –0.1% to –0.4%). Severe hypoglycaemia was not suitable for formal meta-analysis, but the authors concluded that 'severe hypoglycaemia appeared to be reduced in those using CSII'. Quality of life measures indicate that CSII is preferred over MDI.

Conclusions

The authors conclude that there is some evidence that glycaemic control may be better on CSII than MDI.

COMMENT

This is the latest of several meta-analyses in recent years that have compared glycaemic control during CSII and MDI. It agrees with previous analyses in that a significant reduction in HbA1c favouring CSII is found, although with a mean of 0.3% the difference in HbA1c reported here is substantially lower than the 0.5%–0.6% found in other reviews (1).

Because of trial selection, this review has reached some conclusions that may mislead some readers. First, many of the 23 studies were from the 1980s, an era when pump technology was less reliable and sophisticated (e.g. no bolus calculators, less programmability of basal rates, no choice of meal bolus profiles) and when monomeric insulin was not used in the pump. Many of the studies were of very short duration and in subjects who had no significant problem with hypoglycaemia at baseline, making it impossible to analyse changes in the frequency of severe hypoglycaemia. Finally, the authors fail to investigate and report on the now well established finding from previous studies that the difference in HbA1c and hypoglycaemia is greatest in those who are worse controlled at baseline. The authors have a rather muted conclusion about a possible beneficial effect of CSII, and if the meta-analysis had included only studies with adequate pump duration and using modern pumps and insulins, the conclusion might have been more positive.

IMPROVING MEALTIME GLYCAEMIC CONTROL DURING CSII

Pre-meal injection of rapid-acting insulin reduces postprandial glycaemic excursions in type 1 diabetes

Luijf YM, Van Bon AC, Hoekstra JB, De Vries JH

Academic Medical Centre, Department of Internal Medicine, Amsterdam, The Netherlands

*Diabetes Care 2010; **33**: 2152–5*

Background

The aim of this study was to test the hypothesis that administration of the meal insulin bolus during CSII lowers postprandial blood glucose levels more when the bolus is given before rather than at the time of eating.

Methods

Ten type 1 diabetic subjects receiving CSII with insulin aspart (or who were switched to aspart) were randomly allocated to give a breakfast insulin bolus −30, −15 or 0 min before the meal. Blood glucose changes were recorded in hospital for 4 h for each test day, and by continuous glucose monitoring which was continued at home over the 3 days of testing.

Results

The maximum glucose concentration and the glucose excursion were lowest when the insulin was given −15 min before the meal. The mean glucose was 2.2 mmol/l lower for −15 min compared to 0 min administration. There was no difference in glycaemic levels <3.5 mmol/l for the different bolus strategies.

Conclusions

Giving the bolus insulin during CSII 15 min before a meal results in lower postprandial blood glucose levels, without an increased risk of hypoglycaemia.

Effects of meals with different glycaemic index on postprandial blood glucose responses in patients with type 1 diabetes treated by continuous subcutaneous insulin infusion

Parillo M[1], Annuzzi G[2], Rivellese AA[2], Bozzetto L[2], Alessandrini R[2], Riccardi G[2], Capaldo B[2]

[1] *AORN S. Anna S. Sebastiano Hospital, Caserta, Italy, and* [2] *Department of Clinical and Experimental Medicine, Federico II University, Napoli, Italy*

Diabet Med 2011; 28: 227–9

Aim

This study aimed to test the effect of the glycaemic index (GI) of foods on the postprandial blood glucose rise in type 1 diabetic subjects treated by CSII.

Methods

Sixteen adult patients with type 1 diabetes who were being treated by CSII were randomly allocated to eat on different days a test breakfast of identical carbohydrate (100 g), fat (28 g), protein (38 g) and fibre (12 g) content but different GI (59 vs. 90). The low GI meal was derived mainly from legumes and pasta, and the high GI meal from bread and rice. The meal insulin bolus was determined according to the total carbohydrate content and insulin sensitivity in the usual way.

Results

Blood glucose levels during the 3 h after eating the low GI meal were significantly lower than during the high GI meal. The blood glucose levels from 60 to 150 min in particular were about 2.0–2.5 mmol/l less during the low GI breakfast.

Conclusions

Meals with identical carbohydrate content but different GI index produce clinically significant differences in postprandial glycaemia.

COMMENT

There is an increasing realisation that the extent of postprandial hypergly-caemia is an important component of the overall control achieved on CSII, and thus lowering meal-related glucose levels may be one approach to im-proving control on pump therapy. These two papers concern different aspects of optimising mealtime glucose increases on CSII: the timing of the insulin bolus and the GI content of the meal. It was common practice before the advent of short-acting monomeric insulins to give the short-acting/regular insulin 15–30 min before the meal, in order to allow for the slow absorption of subcutaneous insulin and better match blood insulin and blood glucose levels. But practitioners were perhaps persuaded by manufacturers that the new insulins were so 'super-fast-acting' that injections could be given at the time of eating or even somewhat after. Although this had little experimental basis, the practice was extended to CSII. A number of studies have appeared recently that have tested the effect of giving the meal bolus at different times before the meal (2) and have consistently reported, as do Luijf et al., that lower levels can be achieved with an approximately 15 min administration. It is slightly puzzling in the Luijf study that the –30 min bolus gave glucose levels similar to that when the bolus is given 0 min before eating, but overall this study provides more evidence that pre-meal rather than at-meal insulin bolusing should be a standard recommendation.

Parillo et al. reflect on the fact that meal insulin on CSII or other intensive insulin programmes is almost always based on total carbohydrate content. Although the GI of foods as a determinant of postprandial glycaemia is a 30-year-old concept, it has not been used much in everyday practice. This study shows a quite marked difference in postprandial blood glucose levels – certainly one that is clinically important. Low GI meals can probably reduce HbA1c by about 10%, so there is scope for further studies examining how easy this will be to put into clinical practice.

CSII IN HOSPITAL

Continuous subcutaneous insulin infusion (CSII) in inpatient setting: unmet needs and the proposal of a CSII unit

Morviducci L[1], Di Flaviani A[2], Luria A[3], Pitocco D[4], Pozzilli P[3], Suraci C[5], Frontoni S[2], for the CSII Study Group of Lazio Region Italy S

[1] Diabetes Unit, San Camillo-Forlanini Hospital, Rome, Italy, [2] Endocrinology, Diabetes and Metabolism, S. Giovanni Calibita Fatebenefratelli Hospital, University of Rome Tor Vergata, Rome, Italy, [3] Department of Endocrinology and Diabetes, University Campus Bio-Medico, Rome, Italy, [4] Diabetes Care Unit, Internal Medicine, Catholic University, Rome, Italy, and [5] Diabetes Unit, Pertini Hospital, Rome, Italy

Diabetes Technol Ther 2011; **13**: 1–4

Background
Information on the role and application of CSII in hospital is limited, although many pump users are keen to continue this therapy when admitted to hospital.

Methods

This report summarises the results of a meeting of the Lazio Region (Italy) CSII Group in December 2010, which considered insulin pump therapy in hospital. The conclusions were based on literature review, personal experience, open discussion and consensus reached by the participants.

Results

It was noted that guidelines have been issued by several authors for the use of CSII in hospital. The meeting proposed that an inpatient 'CSII unit' should be created, consisting of an endocrinologist, diabetes educator, nurse and nutritionist, and that this unit should be responsible for assessing the competence of patients to self-administer CSII, for assisting in deciding the advisability of continued CSII and for helping in adjusting pump rates and maintaining patient independence. When no CSII expertise exists in the hospital, patients should be switched to injection therapy. The experience of CSII in special circumstances in hospital such as before, during and after surgery is limited, but a simple protocol for this is suggested.

Conclusions

A special inpatient CSII unit should be activated in hospital to aid the proper use of CSII, both for new users and for those established pump users who want to continue CSII during their admission.

Outpatient to inpatient transition of insulin pump therapy: successes and continuing challenges

Nassar AA[1], Partlow BJ[2], Boyle ME[2], Castro JC[3], Bourgeois PB[4], Cook CB[2]

[1]*Department of Internal Medicine, Mayo Clinic, Scottsdale, AZ, USA,* [2]*Division of Endocrinology, Mayo Clinic, Scottsdale, AZ, USA,* [3]*Division of Information Technology, Mayo Clinic, Scottsdale, AZ, USA, and* [4]*PBB Associates LLC, Baton Rouge, LA, USA*

J Diab Sci Technol 2010; 4: 863–72

Background

Previous reports on the transition of outpatient-to-inpatient CSII have involved only small groups of patients. The purpose of this study was to review a large group of CSII inpatient users at one institution, with respect to factors such as adherence to procedures, glycaemic control and adverse events.

Methods

Records from 65 patients with insulin pumps undergoing 125 hospitalisations were examined.

Results

The mean age of patients was 55 years, mean diabetes duration 27 years and mean pump duration 6 years. The mean hospital stay was 4.7 days. CSII was continued in 66%. The adherence to guidelines was generally good (endocrinology consultations and nursing assessments in 89%) but bedside flow sheets were found in only 55%. Mean glucose was not different in CSII users vs. those who discontinued (9.7 ± 3.2 vs. 9.7 ± 2.3 mmol/l). Apart from one episode of cannula kinking, no adverse events such as ketoacidosis were observed.

Conclusions

Most CSII users can have their therapy safely continued in hospital. Previously published guidelines for CSII use in hospital can be implemented with good overall compliance. Glycaemic control still needs to be improved.

COMMENT

There is interest in improving the management of CSII in hospital because of the increasing numbers of patients using this therapy worldwide, many of whom will be admitted to hospital either as an emergency or for elective procedures and investigations, and because of the importance that good glycaemic control during the hospital stay has on patient outcomes.

These papers underline the fact that many CSII users prefer to continue this therapy in hospital but that a specific protocol should be in place in hospitals for safe and efficacious pump use. Many healthcare professionals will not be experts in CSII and should therefore call upon specialist help, possibly a dedicated CSII unit, as suggested by Morviducci et al. If procedures are adhered to, CSII is safe to use in hospital, but it is of interest that the quality of glycaemic control, although not different from that achieved with insulin injection therapy, is nevertheless quite poor – a mean blood glucose concentration of 9.7 mmol/l in the survey of Nassar et al. This might be because the relatively short stay in hospital does not allow time to optimise insulin rates. Perhaps attempts should be made to tighten control on CSII before admission, although the mean HbA1c of 7.3% at admission in the Nassar et al. survey suggests that the problem lies in the stress-induced hyperglycaemia in hospital.

CSII AT THE ONSET OF CHILDHOOD DIABETES

Sensor-augmented pump therapy from the diagnosis of childhood type 1 diabetes: results from the Paediatric Onset Study (ONSET) after 12 months' treatment

Kordonouri O[1], Pankowska E[2], Rami B[3], Kapellen T[4], Coutant R[5], Hartmann R[1], Lange K[6], Knip M[7,8], Danne T[1]

[1] *Bult Diabetes Centre for Children and Adolescents, Kinderkrankenhaus auf der Bult, Hannover, Germany,* [2] *Department of Paediatric Diabetology and Birth Defects, Medical University of Warsaw, Warsaw, Poland,* [3] *Department of Paediatrics, Medical University of Vienna, Vienna, Austria,* [4] *Universitätsklinik und Poliklinik für Kinder und Jugendliche, Leipzig, Germany,* [5] *Département de Pédiatrie, Centre Hospitalier Universitaire, Angers, France,* [6] *Department of Medical Psychology, Hannover Medical School, Hannover, Germany,* [7] *Hospital for Children and Adolescents and Folkhälsan Research Centre, University of Helsinki, Helsinki, Finland, and* [8] *Department of Paediatrics, Tampere University Hospital, Tampere, Finland*

*Diabetologia 2010; **53**: 2487–95*

Background

The purpose of this study was to examine the value of managing type 1 diabetes in children and adolescents from diagnosis using CSII and continuous glucose monitoring. In particular, the authors tested whether sensor-augmented insulin pump therapy led to better glycaemic control and preserved β-cell function, with lower insulin requirements, lower rates of hypoglycaemia and better quality of life, compared with conventional CSII with self-monitoring of blood glucose.

Methods

Children aged 1–16 years, within 4 weeks of the diagnosis of type 1 diabetes, were randomised to CSII with continuous glucose monitoring or CSII with self-monitoring of blood glucose for 12 months.

Results

HbA1c, quality of life and insulin requirements did not differ between the groups during the study. Glycaemic variability was lower in the sensor group. Those who used the sensor more regularly had lower HbA1c levels: 7.1 vs. 7.6% (p = 0.032). Higher C-peptide levels were observed in 12–16 year olds in the sensor-augmented pump group at 12 months. Severe hypoglycaemia only occurred in those who did not use a sensor.

Conclusions

Sensor-augmented pump therapy used from diagnosis in type 1 diabetes may lead to less decline in C-peptide than conventional CSII, particularly in older children, but regular sensor use is necessary.

Metabolic control in children with diabetes mellitus who are younger than 6 years at diagnosis: continuous subcutaneous insulin infusion as a first-line treatment?

Sulmont V, Souchon P-F, Gouillard-Darnaud C, Fartura A, Salmon-Musial AS, Lambrecht E, Mauran P, Abely M

Department of Pediatrics, American Memorial Hospital, University Hospital of Reims, Reims, France

J Pediatr 2010; **157**: *103–7*

Background

The aim of this study was to compare metabolic outcomes in young children who were either treated from diagnosis by CSII or treated initially by multiple daily insulin injections (MDI) and then switched to CSII.

Methods

From a cohort of children with type 1 diabetes who were diagnosed before the age of 6 years, 34 were selected who received initial treatment with MDI, and all but three of these switched to CSII after a mean of 3.9 years, mostly because of elevated HbA1c. Thirty-two children were also selected who were treated by CSII from diagnosis. The groups did not differ at baseline in HbA1c or age.

Results

The mean annual HbA1c was lower in those on CSII from diagnosis compared with those on MDI [6.9 vs. 7.6% (p = 0.011) at year 1; 7.4 vs. 8.1% (p = 0.006) at year 4]. The pump group was associated with lower rates of severe hypoglycaemia (9.8 vs. 22.3 episodes per 100 patient-years, p = 0.016). In those who switched from MDI to CSII, the rate of severe hypoglycaemia reduced from 22.3 to 12 episodes per 100 patient-years. Ketoacidosis did not differ between groups. Only 5% of families expressed difficulties learning to use CSII; 10% reported technical difficulties at school time and physical activities; 9.1% of patients abandoned CSII.

Conclusions

Better glycaemic control and reduced hypoglycaemia can be achieved with CSII, especially when used from diagnosis.

COMMENT

The usual pattern of CSII use in adults with type 1 diabetes has been as a 'last resort' in those who have failed to achieve target levels of control on MDI because of continued elevated HbA1c or disabling hypoglycaemia, and this practice has been followed in children until quite recently. However, because of practical difficulties in implementing MDI in young children, especially at school, there is increasing exploration of CSII from diagnosis in children, as a first-line therapy. Sulmont *et al.* show that not only is this feasible and acceptable for at least 90% of patients and parents, but metabolic control is also significantly better than on MDI. The additional importance of this study is that it is one of the first to supply long-term information on CSII use from diagnosis in children, here up to 8 years.

The issue of whether good control obtained by CSII from diagnosis can better preserve β-cell function than conventional therapy has been discussed for decades but never conclusively settled. The study of Kordonouri *et al.* partly addresses this problem but compares CSII not with MDI but with CSII plus continuous glucose monitoring. Perhaps not surprisingly, there was little difference in HbA1c in the two treatment arms, although there was less glycaemic variability with sensor-augmented pump users compared with conventional CSII. The hint of a higher C-peptide level in one age group of sensor-augmented pump users suggests that pump-related good control might have real benefits in preserving β-cell function. It would have been interesting to know C-peptide levels in the study of Sulmont *et al.* (though that study was not randomised). Clearly, more work is needed in this area.

PUMP INSULIN

Insulin glulisine compared to insulin aspart and to insulin lispro administered by continuous subcutaneous insulin infusion in patients with type 1 diabetes: a randomised controlled trial

Van Bon AC[1], Bode BW[2], Seri-Langeron C[3], DeVries JH[1], Charpentier G[4]

[1] *Department of Internal Medicine, Academic Medical Center, Amsterdam, The Netherlands,* [2] *Atlanta Diabetes Associates, Emory University School of Medicine, Atlanta, GA, USA,* [3] *Sanofi-aventis, Paris, France, and* [4] *Department of Internal Medicine, Endocrinology and Diabetology, Centre Hospitalier Sud Francilien, Corbeil, France*

Diabetes Technol Ther 2011; 6: 607–14

Background

The aim of this study was to compare the performance of glulisine (glu) compared with aspart (asp) and lispro (lis) as pump insulins during CSII, particularly with respect to unexplained hyperglycaemia and perceived infusion set occlusions.

Methods

In this multicentre study involving 12 countries and 44 centres, 256 adult subjects with type 1 diabetes who were being treated by CSII were randomised to one of three treatment orders, glu-asp-lis, asp-lis-glu or lis-glu-asp, with each insulin for 13 weeks of treatment.

Results

The percentage of subjects with at least one episode of unexplained hyperglycaemia (>300 mg/dl, 16.7 mmol/l) and/or perceived infusion set occlusion was not significantly different between insulins, although there was a non-significant trend towards more hyperglycaemia or occlusions with glu. There was no difference in HbA1c, severe hypoglycaemia or ketoacidosis at endpoint between the treatments. Glu was associated with a higher frequency of symptomatic hypoglycaemia, possibly because of slight overdosing.

Conclusions

Glu, asp and lis were found to have similar performance when used as pump insulins, with no difference in metabolic outcome or infusion set occlusion. The authors conclude that any of the insulins can be used for CSII.

COMMENT

Papers continue to appear with rather conflicting conclusions on whether one pump insulin is more suitable for CSII than another. This study finds no strong evidence for the outcome of most importance (HbA1c) being any different when glulisine, aspart or lispro insulin was used – nor in fact for pump occlusions or ketoacidosis. If there were subtle differences in the pharmacokinetics or stability of these short-acting insulins it would be difficult to show that effect on HbA1c, given the large day-to-day variations in control in individuals using any one insulin, due to a huge number of variables such as meal size, insulin sensitivity, errors in estimated carbohydrate content, insulin absorption etc.

CSII IN TYPE 2 DIABETES

Efficacy of continuous subcutaneous insulin infusion in type 2 diabetes mellitus: a survey on a cohort of 102 patients with prolonged follow-up

Reznik Y, Morera J, Rod A, Coffin C, Rousseau E, Lireux B, Joubert M

Department of Medicine, Department of Endocrinology, Caen University Hospital, Caen, France

*Diabetes Technol Ther 2010; **12**: 931–6*

Background

Most reported trials of CSII in type 2 diabetes have been short term, but this retrospective study reports on the long-term efficacy of CSII in this group of patients at a single centre in France.

Methods

All 102 type 2 diabetic subjects who started CSII at the centre were included in a retrospective analysis, with follow-up for 6 months to 6 years (mean pump duration 2 years). Prior to CSII, 80% were treated by MDI. CSII was initiated because of various factors including elevated HbA1c on insulin injection therapy (77%), diabetes complications (6%), patient's desire to use CSII (6%), frequent hypoglycaemia (1%) and pregnancy (1%).

Results

Most patients were obese (mean body mass index 35 kg/m^2) with poor control at baseline. HbA1c improved from 9.3 ± 1.8% to 7.8 ± 1.4% at the 1-year evaluation (p < 0.001), and the decrease was maintained until 6 years. The best HbA1c reduction was in those with highest pre-treatment HbA1c. There was no significant change in insulin dose. There was a mean bodyweight increase of 3.9 kg at 1 year which remained stable for the follow-up period.

Conclusions

CSII is safe and effective in type 2 diabetes, and improves control in those with an HbA1c > 8%. The benefit is sustained for at least 6 years in this population.

Associations between improved glucose control and patient-reported outcomes after initiation of insulin pump therapy in patients with type 2 diabetes mellitus

Peyrot M[1,2], Rubin RR[2], Chen X[3], Frias JP[3]

[1] *Loyola University Maryland, Baltimore, MD, USA,* [2] *Johns Hopkins University School of Medicine, Baltimore, MD, USA, and* [3] *LifeScan Inc., Milpitas, CA, USA*

Diabetes Technol Ther 2011; 13: 471–6

Background

The purpose of this study was to examine the relationship between changes in glycaemic control in type 2 diabetic patients who started CSII and patient-reported outcomes (PRO) such as quality of life and treatment satisfaction.

Methods

Type 2 diabetic patients ($n = 54$) who initiated CSII were studied over 16 weeks. Pre-CSII treatments were 17 on oral agents, 17 on basal insulin $\pm$ oral agents, and 20 on MDI $\pm$ oral agents. Control was measured by self-monitoring of blood glucose, patient-blinded continuous glucose monitoring and HbA1c. Multiple validated measures of PRO were used including health related quality of life and EQ-5D and treatment satisfaction.

Results

All measures of glycaemia (except for standard deviation of continuous glucose monitoring-measured night-time glucose values) and PRO improved with CSII. HbA1c reduced by a mean of 0.94%. Decreased HbA1c was associated only with perceived clinical efficacy. Continuous glucose monitoring and self-monitoring of blood glucose reductions were associated with improved EQ-5D, symptom score, perceived clinical utility and treatment satisfaction.

Conclusions

HbA1c as a measure of average control may not capture aspects of glycaemia which have the greatest impact on health-related quality of life. Reduced glycaemic variability was strongly associated with improved health-related quality of life.

COMMENT

The evidence from observational studies that HbA1c in type 2 diabetes can be improved by switching to CSII continues to appear, and both these reports support that. Unfortunately, only 30 of the 102 patients in Reznik and colleagues' study were treated by MDI before the switch to CSII, which is probably regarded as the insulin injection regimen most likely to achieve good control in type 2 diabetic patients who have failed other measures. No large-scale randomised controlled trials of CSII in type 2 diabetes have appeared in the last few years, and arguably what is of most interest is a trial in those who have not reached target control with MDI.

The study of Peyrot *et al.* underlines the fact that many of the measures of quality of life and patient perceived outcomes are insensitive to the improvements in glycaemic control achieved by technologies such as CSII, at least when control is assessed by HbA1c. Interestingly, they show that PRO can be correlated with measures of glycaemic variability. Glycaemic variability seems to set the HbA1c that can achieved on MDI, perhaps because patients with a high variability are concerned about lowering the HbA1c in case hypoglycaemia is induced. In any case, it is valuable to see that quality of life and treatment satisfaction is improved by CSII in type 2 diabetes.

REFERENCES

1. Pickup JC, Sutton AJ. Severe hypoglycaemia and glycaemic control in type 1 diabetes: meta-analysis of multiple daily insulin injections compared with continuous subcutaneous insulin infusion. *Diabet Med* 2008; **25**: 765–74
2. Cobry E, McFann K, Messer L, Gage V, VanderWel B, Horton L, Chase HP. Timing of meal insulin boluses to achieve optimal postprandial glycemic control in patients with type 1 diabetes. *Diabetes Technol Ther* 2010; **12**: 173–7

CHAPTER 4

Closing the Loop

Eyal Dassau[1,2], Christian Lowe[2], Cameron Barr[1,2], Eran Atlas[3] and Moshe Phillip[3,4]

[1] University of California at Santa Barbara, Santa Barbara, CA, USA,
[2] Sansum Diabetes Research Institute, Santa Barbara, CA, USA,
[3] Diabetes Technolgies Center, Jesse Z and Sara Lea Shafer Institute for Endocrinology and Diabetes, Schneider Children's Medical Center of Israel, Petah Tikva, Israel
[4] Sackler Faculty of Medicine, Tel-Aviv University, Tel-Aviv, Israel

INTRODUCTION

Closed-loop systems have become necessary components of our technologically dependent world. Algorithms are responsible for implementing control in a variety of settings ranging from the temperature of your home to the altitude and speed at which you fly on an airplane. The closed-loop algorithms eliminate the need for constant monitoring and adjustment by an individual. Diabetes mellitus is a disease where the human body's innate ability to control blood glucose levels fails, making glycaemic control extrinsic and up to the conscious efforts of that individual. However, the ever-increasing amount of variation and unpredictability in people's lives have led to difficulties with manual 'open-loop' control and have ushered in the need to develop a system that can more effectively control blood glucose. An artificial pancreas aims to greatly reduce the difficulty of maintaining euglycaemia and improve the individual's quality of life in the process. Although the idea of an artificial pancreas has existed for decades, the feasibility of such a device has only recently come into focus with the combination of user friendly continual glucose monitors and insulin infusion devices. The degree of control that the algorithm possesses as well as the method of administration of one or two hormones are the variables that researchers are currently adjusting. This past year has seen dramatic advances in clinical trials of closed-loop systems ranging from a multinational study of subcutaneous model predictive closed-loop control to a study of closed-loop insulin delivery during pregnancy complicated by type 1 diabetes (T1D). Trials with overnight control in adults and bi-hormonal infusion have also provided further evidence for the feasibility of a closed-loop system.

Int J Clin Pract 2012; **66** (Suppl. 175): 20–29

Advances in controller technology have led to the use of euglycaemic zones in place of discrete set-points and the development of adaptive model predictive controllers based on the utilisation of past behaviour profiles. The inclusion of new safety precautions aims to further reduce the amount of time spent outside the euglycaemic range. Further refinement of controllers *in silico* brings researchers closer to achieving the ultimate goal of fully automated artificial pancreases. Our goal was to select the most influential and ground-breaking publications that focus on the quest to make an artificial pancreas available to people afflicted with diabetes mellitus around the world.

REVIEW AND EDITORIAL PAPERS

Closed-loop insulin delivery: from bench to clinical practice

Hovorka R

Institute of Metabolic Science, University of Cambridge, Cambridge, UK

Nat Rev Endocrinol 2011; 7: 385–95

The artificial pancreas consists of a continuous glucose monitoring (CGM) device, an insulin pump, and a control algorithm that mediates the delivery of insulin to achieve glycaemic control. Two algorithmic approaches, a model predictive control and a proportional-integral-derivative control, have emerged as the top choices for the controller of the closed-loop method. These algorithms are implemented in a number of different systems that vary in complexity from the more simple suspended insulin delivery to the intricate dual-hormone closed-loop system using both insulin and glucagon. The introduction of artificial pancreas prototypes into clinical practice has already begun with the use of a low-glucose suspend pump in 2009 in parts of Europe. The more complex systems, however, are still being tested either *in silico* or *in vivo* and will not see clinical use for at least several years. These closed-loop therapy systems are targeted for use in patients who struggle with hypoglycaemia and children who have difficulties managing their diabetes; however, it is hoped that all patients suffering from T1D will be able to use a fully closed-loop artificial pancreas in the near future.

COMMENT

Hovorka provides a synopsis of the current status of closed-loop artificial pancreas technology as well as a brief yet effective analysis of the controllers that have undergone clinical studies. The inclusion of the suspended insulin delivery system in the review reflects the increasing utilisation and research of semi-closed-loop delivery methods as a stepping stone in the development of a fully automated closed-loop artificial pancreas. The different physiological and lifestyle factors, such as subcutaneous insulin delivery and exercise, serve as the biggest hurdles for closed-loop glycaemic control. Hovorka rightly points out that the future success of an artificial pancreas does not rest merely on the effectiveness of the control algorithm, but also on the establishment of an appropriate infrastructure to educate both healthcare professionals and patients; user-friendliness and portability will factor greatly into the wide acceptance of the artificial pancreas. However, there is also a stress not to delay clinical use of such a medical device because of its phased process of improvement. Small future updates, as with any other software, should be expected. Although hybrid insulin delivery systems are probably the next step, fully automated closed-loop control will hopefully reach clinical use in the next one to two decades.

Semi-closed-loop insulin delivery systems: early experience with low-glucose insulin suspend pumps

Pickup JC

Diabetes Research Group, Division of Diabetes and Nutritional Sciences, King's College London School of Medicine, Guy's Hospital, London, UK

*Diabetes Technol Ther 2011; **13**: 695–8*

Although much of the current research involving the artificial pancreas involves closed-loop insulin delivery, the concept of using a hybrid or semi-closed-loop delivery system has existed for over 30 years. Current subcutaneous glucose measurement and insulin infusion in the mealtime setting present large hurdles for the closed-loop method; therefore, the simplicity of the semi-closed-loop system has regained attention. Although many attempts at hybrid insulin delivery have involved long periods of closed loop with short pre-meal boluses, 'control-to-target' or 'control-to-range' stress the exact opposite approach. The majority of the time is spent in an open-loop setting with short periods of closed-loop management when blood glucose levels become too high or low. An insulin pump with an automatic low-glucose suspend (LGS) (Paradigm® Veo™, Medtronic Inc., Northridge, CA, USA) has been used clinically in parts of Europe since 2009. The LGS functions by stopping basal insulin delivery when the blood glucose levels fall below a certain set-point. Studies have shown that the LGS pump has effectively reduced the frequency of hypoglycaemic events, especially nocturnal incidences, in both adult and paediatric diabetic patients (1, 2). There is still much to be studied about the LGS pump including the personal thresholds and the best response to an LGS alarm. Future research is aimed at using insulin boosters to eliminate hyperglycaemic events and the use of an algorithm that can predict the trend towards a hyperglycaemic or hypoglycaemic event rather than a reaction once the event has already occurred.

COMMENT

The challenges of a fully automated closed-loop insulin delivery system have made the semi-closed-loop system a likely first step in the development of an artificial pancreas. Pickup explains that the hybrid control offers overall better glycaemic control than current insulin management with minimal user intervention. LGS pumps are already being used in Europe and it seems likely that pumps that both suspend and boost insulin delivery are the next steps. Other semi-closed-loop systems have been developed that focus on a long period of closed-loop management with short open-loop periods. Research is on its way with different strategies to address meal disturbance and to find ways to minimise postprandial hyperglycaemic events. However, the semi-closed-loop model should be seen as an intermediate step in the development process, not the end-product. Even though the hybrid model is currently the most effective controller, insulin infusion without any user intervention is the ultimate goal.

CLINICAL STUDIES – UNI-HORMONE (INSULIN ONLY)

Multinational study of subcutaneous model predictive closed-loop control in type 1 diabetes mellitus: summary of the results

Kovatchev B[1,2], Cobelli C[3], Renard E[4], Anderson S[5], Breton M[1], Patek S[2], Clarke W[6], Bruttomesso D[7], Maran A[7], Costa S[7], Avogaro A[7], Mann CD[3], Facchinetti A[3], Magni L[8], Nicolao GD[8], Place J[4], Farre A[4]

[1]*Department of Psychiatry and Neurobehavioral Sciences, University of Virginia, Charlottesville, VA, USA,* [2]*Department of Systems and Information Engineering, University of Virginia, Charlottesville, VA, USA,* [3]*Department of Information Engineering, University of Padova, Padova, Italy,* [4]*Department of Endocrinology and UMR CNRS, CHU and University of Montpellier, Montpellier, France,* [5]*Department of Medicine, Section Endocrinology, University of Virginia, Charlottesville, VA, USA,* [6]*Department of Pediatrics, University of Virginia, Charlottesville, VA, USA,* [7]*Department of Clinical and Experimental Medicine, University of Padova, Padova, Italy, and* [8]*Department of System and Informatics, University of Pavia, Pavia, Italy*

J Diabetes Sci Technol 2010; 4: 1374–81

Background

Increasing effort has been focused on the development of subcutaneous–subcutaneous (SC-SC) closed-loop glucose control, using CGM coupled with an insulin pump and a control algorithm. This paper summarised data found in a previous publication.

Methods

The design of the control algorithm was done entirely *in silico*. Adults ($n = 20$) were recruited for the clinical experiments from the USA, Italy and France. All subjects participated in both open-loop and closed-loop sessions, which were scheduled 3–4 weeks apart lasting 22 h each. A CGM and an insulin pump were used. During open-loop control the patient performed insulin dosing under physician supervision, whereas a control algorithm performed insulin dosing during closed-loop control.

Results

The *in silico* design resulted in quick and cost-effective system development, testing and regulatory approvals (which took less than 6 months compared with the years it would have taken with animal trials). Closed-loop control reduced nocturnal hypoglycaemia from 23 to five episodes ($p < 0.01$). There was a mean of 1.15 hypoglycaemic episodes per subject overnight on open-loop control, which was reduced to 0.25 episodes per subject on closed-loop control. Closed-loop control also increased the amount of time spent overnight within the target range from 64% to 78% ($p = 0.03$). However, the percentage of time within the blood glucose target range of 3.9–10 mmol/l during postprandial breakfast control decreased from 61% in open-loop control to 52% in closed-loop control. This equates to 9% less time spent below 10 mmol/l on closed-loop after breakfast with 0.4 mmol/l higher average blood glucose. During closed-loop control, an attending physician decided to override the insulin suggested by the closed-loop algorithm on four occasions, resulting in 2.5 h (2%) loss of closed-loop control time in all 20 patients.

Conclusions

A system using personalised model predictive control (MPC) to control blood glucose in T1D was developed *in silico* and then tested in a clinical setting. Subsequent studies have adopted such technology in their clinical approaches.

COMMENT

The practicality of an 'artificial pancreas' has been contested by the feasibility of its outpatient use due mainly to the cumbersome technology it requires and the difficulties of creating a closed-loop system that is fully automated.

Applications such as minimally invasive subcutaneous CGM, which samples glucose through a minimally invasive sensor implanted in the subcutaneous tissue, have risen to the forefront of artificial pancreas research. This paper by Kovatchev and co-workers made two significant contributions: (1) *in silico* designs for control algorithms; and (2) multinational testing of SC-SC closed-loop glucose control using fully automated CGM data transfer.

The study was a pilot study designed to evaluate a hybrid control methodology. Hence, all subjects participated in both open-loop and closed-loop control under identical conditions in a tightly controlled hospital setting; however, the order of open-loop vs. closed-loop control was not randomised. Typically, randomisation is necessary to avoid learning effects. In this study, data from the open-loop control were used to supply the algorithm with information regarding meals during the closed-loop control. Furthermore, the control cannot be considered fully automated because the algorithm did not automatically control the insulin pump. Future studies should include randomisation, real-life meals as well as full automation as a step toward ambulatory evaluation of the proposed technology.

Overall, the study provided strong evidence for the use of closed-loop insulin delivery as it did reduce the number of hypoglycaemic events nearly fivefold and increased the time spent in the target glucose range. But, despite the overall success of CGM performance, there were 15 instances across all subjects when the CGM devices suffered from a transient loss of sensitivity and the sensor readings did not correspond to the reference blood glucose. This highlights the challenge of CGM accuracy in the context of a closed-loop system. While the need for more accurate sensors may solve the problem, CGM technology may still face some inaccuracies that could raise a safety issue to a closed-loop system. Therefore, other solutions need to be developed such as algorithms to detect sensor inaccuracy or drift and combining glucometer data as additional input to the closed-loop system.

Overnight closed-loop insulin delivery (artificial pancreas) in adults with type 1 diabetes: crossover randomised controlled studies

Hovorka R[1,2], Kumareswaran K[1,3], Harris J[1], Allen JM[1,2], Elleri D[1,2], Xing D[4], Kollman C[4], Nodale M[1], Murphy HR[1], Dunger DB[1,2], Amiel SA[5], Heller SR[6], Wilinska ME[1,2], Evans ML[1,3]

[1] *Institute of Metabolic Science, University of Cambridge, UK,* [2] *Department of Paediatrics, University of Cambridge, UK,* [3] *Department of Medicine, University of Cambridge, UK,* [4] *Jaeb Center for Health Research, Tampa, FL, USA,* [5] *Diabetes Research, Weston Education Centre, King's College London, London, UK, and* [6] *Diabetes Centre, Clinical Sciences Centre, Northern General Hospital, Sheffield, UK*

*BMJ 2011; **342**: d1855*

Background

Overnight closed-loop control can reduce the risk of hypoglycaemia in children and adolescents. This study was done to extend these findings to adults.

Methods

This study carried out two sequential, open-label, randomised controlled crossover studies comparing overnight closed-loop delivery of insulin with conventional insulin pump therapy after two meal scenarios: 'eating in' and 'eating out'. Thirteen adults participated in the 'eating in' scenario 60 g carbohydrate (CHO) meal and were randomly assigned overnight treatment with either closed-loop delivery of insulin or conventional insulin pump therapy during two separate study nights, separated by an interval of 1 to 3 weeks. Twelve adults were recruited for the 'eating out' scenario and followed the same protocol except that their meals were larger (100 g CHO) and accompanied by alcohol. The primary outcome was the time plasma glucose concentrations were in target (3.91–8.0 mmol/l) during closed-loop control.

Results

In the "eating in scenario," overnight closed-loop insulin delivery increased the time plasma glucose concentrations were in target by a median 15% (interquartile range 3%–35%), p = 0.002. In the "eating out" scenario, closed-loop insulin delivery increased the time plasma glucose concentrations were in target by a median 28% (2%–39%), p = 0.01. Analysis of the data showed that with closed-loop delivery the overall time plasma glucose was in target increased by a median 22% (3%–37%), p = 0.001. In conclusion, closed-loop delivery reduced overnight time spent hypoglycaemic (plasma glucose ≤3.9 mmol/l) by a median 3% (0%–20%), p = 0.04, and eliminated plasma glucose concentrations below 3.0 mmol/l after midnight.

Conclusions

These two crossover trials provided evidence that in adults with T1D, closed-loop delivery of insulin may improve overnight control of glucose concentrations and reduce the risk of nocturnal hypoglycaemia.

COMMENT

According to Hovorka and co-workers, no evidence prior to this study had been shown to support that overnight closed-loop insulin delivery in adults could reduce the number of glucose excursions. Thus, this study was designed to test overnight closed-loop systems in adults with T1D and made two significant contributions to the field: (1) overnight closed-loop delivery of insulin in adults with T1D improves nocturnal glucose control; and (2) overnight closed-loop delivery of insulin can operate safely and effectively across a range of age groups and lifestyles, including scenarios with large meals and alcohol consumption. The success of this study can be attributed to its use of a robust and computationally efficient algorithm, which resulted in a complete avoidance of hypoglycaemia, and the controller's ability to discriminate between both slowly and rapidly absorbed meals, thus coping with the considerable variability in gut absorption. In addition, the study's incorporation of 'eating in' and 'eating out' scenarios enhanced the real-world applicability of the control system and brings the artificial pancreas one step closer to outpatient use. One main downside of the study was its need for manual inputting of sensor glucose concentrations into the algorithm and manual adjustment of the insulin pump, which rendered the control semi-automated as opposed to fully automated. In addition, the study team delivered the meal bolus at mealtime based on exact estimation of the meal CHO content. While this study presented its limitations with closed-loop control, the research community should strive to refine their algorithms, miniaturise their devices, include real-life challenges as well as variation in meal content and time and then follow up with more advanced solutions for glucose control during both day and night.

Closed-loop insulin delivery during pregnancy complicated by type 1 diabetes

Murphy HR[1], Elleri D[1,2], Allen JM[1], Harris J[1], Simmons D[3], Rayman G[4], Temple R[5], Dunger DB[2], Haidar A[1], Nodale M[1], Wilinska ME[1,2], Hovorka R[1,2]

[1] *Institute of Metabolic Science, Metabolic Research Laboratories, University of Cambridge, Cambridge, UK,* [2] *Department of Paediatrics, University of Cambridge, Cambridge, UK,* [3] *Institute of Metabolic Science, Cambridge University Hospitals NHS Foundation Trust, Cambridge, UK,* [4] *Diabetes Centre, Ipswich Hospital NHS Trust, Ipswich, UK, and* [5] *Elsie Bertram Diabetes Centre, Norfolk and Norwich University Hospital NHS Trust, Norwich, UK*

*Diabetes Care 2011; **34**: 406–11*

Background

There has been evidence to support the use of insulin pump therapy, continuous glucose measurements (CGM) and sensor-augmented pump (SAP) therapy in pregnancy; however, the benefits have not been well established, particularly during late pregnancy. This study aimed to evaluate closed-loop insulin delivery with an MPC algorithm during early (12–16 weeks) and late (28–32 weeks) gestation in pregnant women with T1D.

Methods

Ten women with T1D were studied over 24 h during early and late gestation. Basal insulin infusion rates were calculated using CGM sensor glucose values and the MPC algorithm every 15 min. A nurse adjusted the basal insulin infusion rate before each insulin delivery as a safety precaution. At 18:00 h, women ate a standardised evening meal. At 07:00 h, they ate a standardised morning meal. Prandial insulin boluses were calculated according to the women's insulin–carbohydrate ratio and capillary fingerstick glucose concentrations. The study ended at 12:00 h. Mean glucose and time spent in target (63–140 mg/dl), hyperglycaemic (>140 to ≥180 mg/dl) and hypoglycaemic (<63 to ≤ 50 mg/dl) ranges were calculated using plasma and sensor glucose measurements. At the end of the study, models were used to compare glucose control during early and late gestation.

Results

Throughout closed-loop insulin delivery, median plasma glucose concentrations were 117 mg/dl in early gestation and 126 mg/dl in late gestation (p = 0.72). The overnight mean plasma glucose time in target was 84% and 100% in early and late pregnancy, respectively (p = 0.09). Overnight mean time spent hyperglycaemic (>140 mg/dl) was 7% in early and 0% in late pregnancy (p = 0.25) and hypoglycaemic (<63 mg/dl) was 0% and 0%, respectively (p = 0.18). Postprandial glucose control, glucose variability, insulin infusion rates and CGM sensor accuracy were no different in early or late pregnancy. However, it must be noted that time spent with plasma glucose within the target range after breakfast was 59% in early and 47% in late pregnancy, and time spent hyperglycaemic after breakfast was 28% in early and 44% in late pregnancy. Sensor accuracy was reported as the mean absolute relative difference between sensor glucose and paired plasma glucose divided by plasma glucose and was 13.3% (14.7% in early vs. 11.9% in late pregnancy; p = 0.15).

Conclusions

This study demonstrates that closed-loop control could be performed in women with T1D during pregnancy; however, much more work is needed to achieve optimal glycaemic control.

COMMENT

Pregnant women suffering from T1D are faced with physiological and hormonal changes during pregnancy, which can contribute to poor glycaemic control and progressive insulin resistance in late gestation. Prior to this study, the effectiveness of a closed-loop system in pregnant women with T1D had not been reported. The study was unique in that it was the first to use plasma glucose measurements during pregnancy, which allowed for the evaluation of sensor accuracy. Unfortunately, the ability of the glucose sensors and algorithm to achieve tight glycaemic control was less than optimal. In this proof of concept study, the algorithm was not modified to distinguish between preprandial and postprandial glucose targets, and postprandial glycaemia was shown to be a major challenge in the closed-loop system. In addition, the closed-loop system was not fully automated. During closed-loop insulin delivery, a nurse had to manually adjust the insulin rate based on the values given by the CGM, which were fed into the MPC algorithm.

By way of current CGM technology and tighter glycaemic targets to treat pregnant women with T1D, it can be inferred that the risk for hypoglycaemic events increases because of lower glycaemic setpoint. To confirm clinical effectiveness of closed-loop insulin delivery in women with T1D, a larger randomised study comparing closed-loop with SAP therapy will be needed.

The effect of insulin feedback on closed-loop glucose control

Steil GM[1], Palerm CC[2], Kurtz N[2], Voskanyan G[2], Roy A[2], Paz S[3], Kandeel FR[3]

[1]Children's Hospital Boston, Boston, MA, USA, [2]Medtronic MiniMed, Northridge, CA, USA, and [3]City of Hope National Medical Center, Duarte, CA, USA

J Clin Endocrinol Metab 2011; **96**: 1402–8

Background

Initial studies of closed-loop proportional integral derivative (PID) control in individuals with T1D have shown good overnight performance; however, breakfast meals are routinely more difficult to control and require supplemental carbohydrates to prevent hypoglycaemia. This study assessed the ability of insulin feedback (IFB) to improve the breakfast meal profile.

Methods

Subjects with previously diagnosed with T1D ($n = 8$) were recruited for participation with closed-loop control over approximately 30 h at an inpatient clinical research facility. Participants completed both an open-loop CGM procedure and a closed-loop PID-with-IFB procedure. During open-loop monitoring, adjustments were made to normalise blood glucose to between 90 and 120. An intravenous catheter was inserted for collecting blood samples. Meals were served at 07:00 (44.5 g) [breakfast on day 1 (B1)], 12:00 (62.5 g) [lunch (L)] and 18:00 h (59.5 g) [dinner

(D)], with a snack given at 21:00 h and breakfast the next day (B2) at 07:00 h (45 g). A manual 2-U meal bolus was delivered before every meal. If plasma glucose fell below 50 mg/dl, 15 g of supplemental carbohydrate was provided. Outcome measures were plasma insulin concentration, model-predicted plasma insulin concentration, 2-h postprandial and 3- to 4-h glucose rate of change following breakfast after 1 day of closed-loop control. There was also a measure of the need for supplemental carbohydrate in response to nadir hypoglycaemia.

Results

Plasma concentrations during closed-loop were well correlated with model predictions. Two-hour postprandial glucose concentration values were 138 ± 24, 158 ± 17, 138 ± 9 and 132 ± 16 mg/dl (B1 L, D and B2, respectively). No hypoglycaemia was observed overnight. Sensors tracked plasma glucose with a mean absolute relative difference of 11.9% (7.3%–20.6%). Glucose concentration during the 3–4 h period after B2 was stable (rate of change of glucose, -0.03792 ± 0.0884 mg/dl/min, not different from zero; $p = 0.68$) and at daytime target (97 ± 6 mg/dl, not different from 90; $p = 0.28$). During the 30-h closed-loop period, supplemental carbohydrate was given on eight occasions and three subjects received supplemental carbohydrate during B2. Overall, six instances of hypoglycaemia requiring supplemental carbohydrate were observed, and two subjects did not require any interventions with closed-loop insulin delivery.

Conclusions

PID control with insulin feedback can achieve a desired breakfast response but more studies will be necessary to achieve optimal control.

COMMENT

Steil and co-workers have been conducting research and clinical trials on the closed-loop system for years, but this study was the most successful in obtaining optimal results. A previous study in 2006 showed peak breakfast glucose concentrations on day 2 reported as 231 ± 12 mg/dl, which were reduced in a study done in 2008 to 204 ± 17 mg/dl, and in this study to 175 ± 8 mg/dl with the use of insulin feedback (3, 4).

The overall results of the study are good with excellent glucose control. However, the tuning of the PID algorithm remains a problem with what seems like excessive delivery due to integral error for some of the subjects.

Although this study highlights the need for an improved system, the effect of insulin feedback on closed-loop glucose control was shown to improve overnight control. This study reported that it was unclear whether the need for supplemental carbohydrate, eight times during a nine-patient study, could be eliminated by changes in the PID algorithm parameters or whether the algorithm needed further modification. During this trial, pre-meal boluses were also administered, which renders the system semi-automated. Future IFB and PID closed-loop algorithms for the artificial pancreas will require better control tuning as well as additional algorithms to alert against sensor errors and impending hypoglycaemia.

Preliminary study on glucose control with an artificial pancreas in postoperative sepsis patients

Takahashi G[1], Sato N[1], Matsumoto N[1], Shozushima T[1], Hoshikawa K[1], Akitomi S[1], Kikkawa T[1], Onodera C[1], Kojika M[1], Inoue Y[1], Suzuki K[2], Wakabayashi G[3], Endo S[1]

[1] *Department of Critical Care Medicine,* [2] *Department of Anesthesiology, and* [3] *Department of Surgery, Keio University School of Medicine, Tokyo, Japan*

*Eur Surg Res 2011; **47**: 32–8*

Background

Glucose control has been a topic of serious debate within the Surviving Sepsis Campaign Guidelines (SSCG) over the past years due to arguments both for and against its use in postoperative sepsis patients. Current SSCG state that following initial stabilisation of patients with severe sepsis, blood glucose should be maintained <150 mg/dl. This study sought to evaluate the feasibility of an artificial pancreas in such patients.

Methods

Patients who had surgery for sepsis caused by infections ($n = 8$) underwent tight glucose control using an artificial pancreas continuously for 7 days after surgery. Patients were sedated and mechanically ventilated. Primary outcomes included blood glucose concentrations over time, insulin dose received, and occurrence of hypoglycaemia. At the end of the study, the patients were divided into two groups (HG, higher insulin requirement; LG, lower insulin requirement) and analysed on the basis of total insulin dose they received over the 7 days.

Results

The blood glucose concentration before glucose control was 203.3 ± 9.9 mg/dl, but was successfully brought down to < 150 mg/dl with the use of the artificial pancreas with no events of hypoglycaemia. Patients in the HG group required a mean of $21,824 \pm 6,030.4$ mU/kg of insulin, and patients in the LG group required $6,254.5 \pm 3,402.3$ mU/kg.

Conclusions

Targeted glucose concentrations could be achieved safely and feasibly with the use of an artificial pancreas in postoperative sepsis patients.

COMMENT

Notwithstanding studies in the past which present data both for and against glucose control in postoperative patients, Takahashi's study is unique in that it demonstrates the feasibility of a closed-loop control system in postoperative sepsis patients. While it is understood that this was a preliminary study, more research is needed to present the need for tight glucose control in postoperative patients. This study did not have a control group where patients did not undergo glucose control with the artificial pancreas. Takahashi *et al.* mention, however, that they do plan to assess a larger number of patients and conduct a randomised controlled trial to make their results more conclusive.

There seems to be uncertainty on how much insulin requirement is actually necessary for postoperative patients in intensive care in order to avoid the complications that can potentially arise from hypoglycaemia due to the glucose control and hyperglycaemia due to no glucose control. This study purports that, because their artificial pancreas achieved glucose concentrations within a target range of 80–150 mg/dl, the artificial pancreas is capable of acute control; however, if the study were designed to measure glucose concentrations within a narrower target range, more insulin may have been administered and the results might differ. As a preliminary study evaluating the feasibility of an artificial pancreas, it presents an innovative solution for controlling glucose concentrations in postoperative patients with a method that reduces human intervention while optimising control.

CLINICAL STUDIES – DUAL-HORMONE (INSULIN–GLUCAGON SYSTEMS)

Novel use of glucagon in a closed-loop system for prevention of hypoglycaemia in type 1 diabetes

Castle JR[1], Engle JM[2], Youssef J[1], Massoud RG[2], Yuen K[1], Kagan R[2], Ward WK[1,2]

[1] *Oregon Health and Science University, Department of Medicine, Division of Endocrinology, Portland, OR, USA, and* [2] *Legacy Health, Division of Research, Portland, OR, USA*

*Diabetes Care 2010; **33**: 1282–7*

Background

In 1963, Kadish proposed the concept of incorporating glucagon delivery into a bi-hormonal closed-loop glycaemic control system (5). Studies such as this have outlined the limitations of a traditional uni-hormonal insulin delivery system as follows: (1) analogue insulin is slow to take effect; (2) it can have a prolonged effect when delivered subcutaneously; and (3) inaccuracy of current glucose sensors presents a risk for the development of hypoglycaemia, which can lead to seizures, coma and death. This study reports on a novel, automated, sensor-controlled method of insulin delivery accompanied by glucagon delivery in order to minimise hypoglycaemia in subjects with T1D.

Methods

Thirteen patients with T1D participated in a total of 21 closed-loop studies of insulin plus placebo and insulin plus glucagon over both 7- and 28-h study periods. Seven subjects received glucagon delivered in a brisk fashion (high-gain) and six in a slower fashion (low-gain). All subjects were monitored for glucose levels every 10 min, and manually adjusted for glucose and insulin infusions every 5 min based on the output given by the Fading Memory Proportional Derivative (FMPD) algorithm. Insulin rates were increased for high or rising glucose levels and glucagon was given for low or falling glucose levels at times of impending hypoglycaemia. An open-loop bolus was given before every meal.

Results

The six subjects who underwent a high-gain glucagon and a placebo study exhibited a 56% reduction of time spent in the hypoglycaemic range (18 ± 11 vs. 41 ± 13 min/day, $p = 0.01$). The amount of insulin delivered was nearly identical in both series (48.9 ± 6.2 vs. 48.3 ± 5.5 units/day, $p = $ ns). In the six subjects who received low-gain glucagon compared with the placebo, there was no significant reduction in time spent in the hypoglycaemic range (15 ± 8 vs. 40 ± 10 min/day, $p = $ ns) and no significant difference in the amount of insulin delivered (60.1 ± 14.1 vs. 46.9 ± 5.5 units/day). Combining both high- and low-gain results, glucagon led to a 63% reduction of time spent in the hypoglycaemic range compared with placebo (15 ± 6 vs. 40 ± 10 min/day, $p = 0.04$). Although it did not reach statistical significance, the mean dose of glucagon delivered during the low-gain glucagon studies was higher than the high-gain glucagon studies (746 ± 134 vs. 516 ± 108 g/day, $p = $ ns).

Conclusions

During closed-loop treatment in subjects with T1D, high-gain glucagon can be used to decrease the time spent in the hypoglycaemic range, the number of hypoglycaemic events and the number of treatments needed for hypoglycaemia.

COMMENT

Advances in the field of artificial pancreas systems have led groups such as Castle and collaborators to test the feasibility of bi-hormonal closed-loop gly-caemic control systems that deliver both insulin and glucagon in the event of impending hypoglycaemia. Although most diabetes-related complications are caused by hyperglycaemia, most patients with diabetes are fearful of hy-poglycaemia, which can cause acute complications such as seizure, loss of consciousness and even death. However, closed-loop control systems have not been able to prevent severe hyperglycaemia without running the risk of hypoglycaemic events because of two main factors: sensor inaccuracy and slow onset and offset of insulin. In this study, hypoglycaemia occurred in 87.5% of cases when the venous blood glucose was less than 90 mg/dl at the start of glucagon delivery due to overestimation of glucose, and it was estimated that insulin on board at the start of glucagon delivery was significantly higher in the failures compared with successes (5.8 ± 0.5 vs. 2.9 ± 0.5 U, $p < 0.001$). It can be concluded that glucagon may fail to prevent hypoglycaemia if neither of these two factors can be prevented. Thus, further improvement in sensor accuracy and more robust glucagon deliverance will be vital to the future of bi-hormonal closed-loop control systems.

Furthermore, Castle *et al.* (6) reported in a follow-up paper that 'repeated doses of glucagon could become increasingly less effective if multiple doses resulted in depletion of liver glycogen', which prompts us to question the prac-ticality of glucagon deliverance if 'cumulative glucagon dose was examined for each episode of glucagon delivery'. If a bi-hormonal control system were to be adopted by diabetics, glucagon deliverance would be considered foremost a safety precaution rather than the primary method for hypoglycaemic avoid-ance. Current treatment utilises oral CHO as a first line of defence against hypoglycaemic events and glucagon should be kept for the second line of defence and not be used as part of the nominal control design. Moreover, the side effects of frequent use of glucagon should be assessed as part of the design question.

Efficacy determinants of subcutaneous microdose glucagon during closed-loop control

Russell SJ[1], El-Khatib FH[2], Nathan DM[1], Damiano ER[2]

[1] *Diabetes Unit and Department of Medicine, Massachusetts General Hospital and Harvard Medical School, Boston, MA, USA, and* [2] *Department of Biomedical Engineering, Boston University, Boston, MA, USA*

J Diabetes Sci Technol 2010; 4: 1288–304

Background

In a previous study by the same group of researchers, it was found that glucagon was not uniformly effective in preventing hypoglycaemia in a bi-hormonal closed-loop system. This paper presented the various factors that contributed to the success or failure of microdose glucagon administration.

Methods

Thirty-six episodes in which glucagon was delivered by a closed-loop system in an attempt to prevent hypoglycaemia were taken from the previous study and analysed for a number of factors including the rate of blood glucose (BG) descent toward hypoglycaemia, $\Delta BG/\Delta t$, the mean plasma insulin levels, the error in the controller's online estimate of mean plasma insulin, the mean and peak plasma glucagon levels, and the ratio of glucagon to insulin levels. Hypoglycaemia was defined as a BG less than 70 mg/dl. 'Glucose episodes' were defined as beginning when BG fell below 120 mg/dl or when BG began a descent from a plateau between 70 and 120 mg/dl.

Results

In 20 of the 36 'glucose episodes', BG did not fall below 70 mg/dl and these were thus considered 'glucagon successes'. In the other 16 episodes, BG did fall below 70 mg/dl and these were considered 'glucagon failures'. There was a statistically significant difference between the success and failure groups in the rate of BG decrease (1.03 ± 0.45 vs. 1.50 ± 0.62 mg/dl/min, $p = 0.02$). The levels of plasma insulin were significantly higher in failures (5.2 vs. 3.7 times the baseline insulin level, $p = 0.01$). A significant difference was found between the success and failure groups in error in the controller's online estimate of the mean plasma insulin level relative to the measured mean plasma insulin level for each episode ($30 \pm 17\%$ vs. $50 \pm 21\%$, $p = 0.003$). The peak plasma glucagon levels were higher in episodes ending in hypoglycaemia (183 vs. 116 pg/ml, $p = 0.007$), as were the mean plasma glucagon levels (142 vs. 75 pg/ml, $p = 0.02$). Although it was not statistically significant ($p = 0.14$), the ratio of glucagon to insulin levels tended to be 59% higher during episodes ending in hypoglycaemia.

Conclusions

Glucagon successfully prevents hypoglycaemia when the control algorithm estimates plasma insulin levels within an average error of 30% but not greater than 60% at the time of impending hypoglycaemia.

COMMENT

Unless a closed-loop system takes into account the insulin already delivered but not yet in the blood stream, excess delivery of insulin is inevitable and the need for glucagon made apparent as the risk of impending hypoglycaemia increases. This study showed that by adjusting the algorithm's PK parameters such that slower insulin absorption was assumed, insulin dosing was conserved and microdose glucagon administered was more effective in reducing hypoglycaemia while maintaining normal plasma glucagon levels. The main question remains, do we need glucagon as part of the closed-loop system or just as a secondary safety layer? The goals for bi-hormonal closed-loop systems are to regulate BG safely while maintaining normal plasma glucagon concentrations, and thus it will be necessary for future controllers to operate as precisely and appropriately as possible in the deliverance of insulin to ensure only the most economically conservative deliverance of glucagon. As such, it is important that studies testing the feasibility of glucagon present data on the side effects due to the relatively large doses of glucagon administered during closed-loop control. This paper showed that glucagon can prevent hypoglycaemia, but only with a consideration of the side effects of glucagon injections will we be able to determine its practicality in outpatient use.

This study was successful in showing that for all successful glucagon episodes the mean plasma glucagon concentrations remained within normal range (50–150 pg/ml). Future research in the physiological variables that control glucose absorption in terms of its relation to fluctuating insulin levels may be appropriate for the development of more advanced control systems. The stability of glucagon in solution has also been a concern for the use of glucagon in a bi-hormonal closed-loop system. This study reported, 'in order for glucagon to be approved as part of an artificial endocrine pancreas, a formulation that is stable in pump reservoirs without fibrillation for at least 3 days must become available'.

Hypoglycaemia may be unavoidable, especially in the hybrid configuration when the patient is allowed to deliver pre-meal boluses. Since the artificial pancreas is a high risk device, several layers of prevention and protection against extreme events such as hypoglycaemia should be embedded as an integral part of the overall design. In this study, the efficacy determinants of microdose glucagon is a promising look into the future of artificial pancreas systems and supports the use of bi-hormonal closed-loop control; however, the combination of insulin and glucagon as a dual hormone artificial pancreas system should be further studied and incorporated with other methods to mitigate hypoglycaemia.

ADVANCES IN CLOSED-LOOP ALGORITHMS/CONTROL STRATEGIES

Zone model predictive control: a strategy to minimise hyperglycaemic and hypoglycaemic events

Grosman B[1,2,3], Dassau E[1,2,3], Zisser HC[1,3], Jovanovič L[1,3], Doyle FJ III[1,2,3]

[1]*Department of Chemical Engineering, University of California, Santa Barbara, Santa Barbara, CA, USA,* [2]*Biomolecular Science and Engineering Program,*

*University of California, Santa Barbara, Santa Barbara, CA, USA, and [3] Sansum
Diabetes Research Institute, Santa Barbara, CA, USA*

J Diabetes Sci Technol 2010; 4: 961–7

Background

The usage of MPC algorithms in the development of the artificial pancreas has grown due to their ability to deal with the large time delays and constraints encountered in the subcutaneous delivery of insulin. The authors of this paper aimed to mimic the physiology of the pancreatic β-cell by utilising zone model predictive control (zone-MPC) which defines euglycaemia as a range of values rather than a discrete point.

Methods

Zone-MPC incorporates different MPC algorithms that can be classified into four approaches to specify future process response: fixed setpoint, zone, reference trajectory, and funnel. The ultimate goal is to maintain the controlled variable in the desired range and in the process become more efficient because of the fewer calculations and processes that the controller must execute in the pursuit of a discrete point. The zone-MPC also integrates second-order input transfer functions to generate an artificial input memory to account for insulin-on-board. The zone-MPC was tested on 10 adult *in silico* subjects from the UVa/Padova Metabolic Simulator that consumed mixed meals with 75, 75 and 50 g of carbohydrates consumed at 7 am, 1 pm and 8 pm, respectively. Three different modes were tested: announced meals at their nominal value, announced meals with 40% uncertainty, and unannounced values. Data from the zone-MPC closed-loop trials were compared with those of patient-direct, open-loop control.

Results

When the meals were unannounced, the zone-MPC was found to perform better than the open-loop treatment with more time spent in the euglycaemic range and no bouts of hypoglycaemia. The zone-MPC with the tighter control range, 100–120 mg/dl, had a mean glucose value of 160 mg/dl compared with the mean of the open-loop control which was 180 mg/dl. It was also found that the narrower the range of the zone-MPC, the more variable the control signal becomes. The zone-MPC led to much better glycaemic control when meals were unannounced or when the meals were announced with a 40% uncertainty. In the unannounced meal scenario, the zone-MPC with the tighter control range had a mean glucose value of 141 mg/dl; the open-loop control had a mean of 180 mg/dl.

Conclusion

Zone-MPC displayed the ability to deal with announced and unannounced meals with meal uncertainties with a distinct advantage over the patient-direct open-loop treatment. A reduction in control move variability was not accompanied with a loss of performance compared with the setpoint control.

COMMENT

Grosman and collaborators utilised a range of euglycaemia rather than a discrete setpoint in their zone-MPC, and in the process they were able to more closely mimic the physiological behaviour of the pancreatic β-cell. The controller attempts to keep or move the expected outputs into a zone defined by upper and lower bands rather than driving the output to a specific point. It is impressive that the zone-MPC controller prevented all hypoglycaemic events whilst also minimising the total time spent with a blood glucose greater than 180 mg/dl. The algorithm's ability to handle announced and unannounced meals with similar effectiveness is important because it is crucial for a closed-loop delivery system to deal with unexpected changes in the user's eating behaviour.

The concept of zone-MPC not only produced much better results than the patient-direct open-loop control, but also reduced the number of processes that the controller must perform. This translates to improved battery life, an important factor if the artificial pancreas is going to be small and portable. Although the results are promising, the algorithm will still need further adjustment to decrease the number of hyperglycaemic events. Further research will be needed to elucidate the personalisation capabilities of zone-MPC in human patients.

Hypoglycaemia prevention via pump attenuation and red-yellow-green 'traffic' lights using continuous glucose monitoring and insulin pump data

Hughes CS[1], Patek SD[1], Breton MD[2], Kovatchev BP[2]

[1] *Department of Systems and Information Engineering, University of Virginia, Charlottesville, VA, USA, and* [2] *Department of Psychiatry and Neurobehavioral Sciences, University of Virginia, Charlottesville, VA, USA*

J Diabetes Sci Technol 2010; 4: 1146–55

Background

One of the main risks in a closed-loop, open-loop or advisory-mode system is the threat of hypoglycaemia. Therefore, safety measures must be incorporated into the system to curb this risk as well as maintain overall system stability. The authors of this paper proposed two algorithms for hypoglycaemia prevention and detection as well as a signalling system to alert the user of three possible 'levels' of hypoglycaemic risk.

Methods

The two algorithms proposed, Brakes and Power Brakes, were formulated as a component of the independent safety system module proposed in the modular control-to-range architecture. Both algorithms alter the insulin injection rate of the pump to avoid hypoglycaemia; however, Brakes is an insulin pump attenuation function that factors in only CGM information while Power Brakes utilises both CGM information and a metabolic state observer with insulin input. In addition to smoothly attenuating the insulin pump, the two algorithms are designed to provide a signal to the user of their current hypoglycaemic risk in the form of a traffic light. The algorithms were tested in two different simulated scenarios using the UVa/Padova Metabolic Simulator. One was an elevated basal rate scenario and one was a scenario in which a bolus is delivered for a meal that is skipped.

Results

With hypoglycaemia defined at 70 mg/dl based on the American Diabetes Association, Power Brakes was shown to reduce the total time of hypoglycaemia by 88% in the elevated basal rate scenario compared with no intervention; the reduction was 94% in the missed meal scenario. The red light alarm was also triggered in about 94% of both scenarios with a false alarm being triggered in 6.77% and 3.3% of the elevated basal rate trials and the missed meal trials, respectively. In both scenarios, the alert occurred at least 17 min prior to the hypoglycaemic event allowing the administration of carbohydrates to avoid the hypoglycaemic event in 98% of the cases.

Conclusion

The two algorithms provide a method for smoothly reducing insulin delivery to prevent hypoglycaemia in individuals with T1D whilst avoiding hyperglycaemic rebound that exceeded 180 mg/dl. The alert system also provides a secondary measure to avoid hypoglycaemia by triggering further intervention.

COMMENT

Hughes and collaborators have proposed two algorithms that have been shown to reduce the number and duration of hypoglycaemic events, with the Power Brakes algorithm being much more effective. The superiority of the

Power Brakes algorithm over its less complex counterpart should make it the focus of further research. Also, the two scenarios that were simulated *in silico* are common, real-world situations that frequently affect patients with T1D; therefore, the effectiveness of the Power Brakes is more *relevant*. However, the effectiveness of the safety algorithm may be slightly inflated due to the method with which it was compared, i.e. no intervention. A comparison to a current, accepted treatment method for T1D would have provided more meaningful data.

The most impressive aspect of the study may in fact be the red light alarm that is triggered in anticipation of the hypoglycaemic event; the alarm would be displayed on the CGM device display together with an alert sound or vibration. Its ability to anticipate the event more than 17 min in advance in the elevated basal rate scenario and more than 28 min in advance in the missed meal scenario provides ample time for a patient to supplement their blood glucose with carbohydrates. Further clinical studies are needed to measure the effectiveness of the algorithm *in vivo* as well as to assess user compliance.

Anticipating the next meal using meal behavioral profiles

Hughes CS[1], Patek SD[1], Breton M[2], Kovatchev BP[1,2]

[1]*Department of Systems and Information Engineering, University of Virginia, VA, USA, and* [2]*Diabetes Technology Program, University of Virginia, Charlottesville, VA, USA*

*Comput Methods Programs Biomed 2011; **102**: 138–48*

Background

MPC is thought to be a solution to the time delay associated with subcutaneously administered insulin in the closed-loop artificial pancreas. However, there still exists the need for adaptation of the controller to the patient's time-varying physiological behaviour and parameters. The authors of the paper attempt to address this by developing an MPC controller that can anticipate meals given a probabilistic history of the patient's eating behaviour.

Methods

The control law is based upon a shock-anticipating linear quadratic regulator (SA-LQR) methodology that uses a random meal profile that predicts the likelihood, timing and carbohydrate content of the next meal. The SA-LQR algorithm is then combined with an open-loop strategy where the patient delivers a meal bolus which takes into account insulin-on-board delivered by the controller resulting in a hybridised controller.

This hybrid was tested on a population of 100 *in silico* adult patients with T1D. The scenario ran from midnight to 12:30 pm and included one meal at 7 am; if the meal arrived at all, it would include 55 g of carbohydrates. The meal behaviour profile allotted a time interval, from 4 am to 8:45 am, in which the meal would most likely occur. The controller was then tested multiple times with different probabilities of the meal being skipped, p(skip), and then compared against normal open-loop control; the controller was set to hold the patient at a blood glucose level of 112.5 mg/dl.

Results

It is seen that the lower the value of p(skip), the larger the dose of insulin delivered in anticipation of the meal. When a p(skip) value of 0.0001 is used, the open-loop meal bolus is 8.51 U, while a p(skip) of .5 value has a corresponding dose of 9.71 U; the larger dose compensates for the smaller, less aggressive anticipatory insulin dose. A p(skip) value of 0.1 had the best results with values of 73.56 mg/dl and 144.86 mg/dl for the mean pre-breakfast minimum and the mean post-breakfast maximum respectively. Smaller p(skip) values had a much greater risk of hypoglycaemia. The increase in insulin delivery in anticipation of the meal drove down blood glucose levels prior to meal consumption resulting in a lower postprandial blood glucose than with open-loop treatment.

Conclusion

The integration of past meal profiles with an MPC controller yielded better glycaemic control than basic open-loop therapy with a greater amount of time spent below 180 mg/dl when the meal was eaten and above 80 mg/dl when the meal was skipped (88% vs. 75%). The results also suggest the existence of an optimal p(skip) value that balances hypoglycaemia avoidance and hyperglycaemia management.

COMMENT

Meals are one of the biggest challenges of people with T1D. The questions of how many carbohydrates are in this dish, how much insulin should be injected for this meal, and/or do I need to use a dual wave/extended bolus are being asked on a daily basis. An artificial pancreas that is required to regulate glucose control will face similar questions. Currently two main approaches are being evaluated in clinical settings; the first is to announce the meal to the controller with an estimated meal size, whilst the other is to allow the controller the freedom and flexibility to overcome the meal challenge on its own. The presented paper suggests an interesting method to anticipate a future meal which allows insulin to be delivered at the anticipated mealtime and as such minimises hyperglycaemia excursion. Simulation results seem promising; however, the use of a probability approach in dosing insulin seems on the dangerous side. Detecting a meal or adjustment of the controller setting based on learning effect seems a more prudent method that will not rely on a probability function. Future clinical studies will be needed to effectively evaluate this method.

Model predictive control with learning-type setpoint: application to artificial pancreatic β-cell

Wang Y[1,2,3], Zisser H[1,2], Dassau E[1,2], Jovanovic L[1,2], Doyle FJ III[1,2]

[1] *Department of Chemical Engineering, University of California, Santa Barbara, CA, USA,* [2] *Sansum Diabetes Research Institute, Santa Barbara, CA, USA, and* [3] *Beijing University of Chemical Technology, Beijing, China*

AIChE J 2010; **56***: 1510–18*

Background

Iterative learning control (ILC) is often used when the process displays a repetitive behaviour; therefore, the cyclic profile of glycaemic control makes ILC a suitable candidate for an artificial pancreatic β-cell. The authors of this paper propose a novel controller for the artificial pancreas that combines ILC and MPC to create a learning-type MPC (L-MPC).

Methods

The ILC used in this experiment is an indirect ILC because it updates the setpoint of another controller that is used in conjunction; the MPC controls the signal directly. The tracking error from the previous day is used by the ILC to adjust the setpoint of the MPC for the current day. Eleven adult *in silico* subjects, adults 1–10 and the adult average, were used from the UVa/Padova diabetes simulator in the study. Five different scenarios were tested: repetitive diets, meal size variations, meal timing variations, timing and meal size variations, and subject variations. Each scenario was run for 20 days. In the repetitive diet scenario the L-MPC was compared with a normal MPC controller as well as a constrained L-MPC that utilised some limitations to avoid potential risks of an excessive setpoint range.

Results

For the repetitive diets scenario, the L-MPC performed better than the MPC with more time spent in the acceptable glycaemic range, 60–180 mg/dl. On the final day, the range of blood glucose concentrations for the MPC was 68–201 mg/dl while the range for the continually improving L-MPC was 68–145 mg/dl. It was found that the large variation in setpoints on a day-to-day basis would decrease the L-MPC's robustness;

therefore, the constrained L-MPC was developed for testing in the rest of the scenarios. When the carbohydrate content of the meal was varied ±75% or the mealtime was varied within ±60 min, the constrained L-MPC was robust and displayed good glycaemic control. The same result was seen in the scenario where there were both meal size variations within ±50% and mealtime variations within ±40 min. When tested in a variety of subjects, there was one subject that was consistently hyperglycaemic and many had a large number of hyperglycaemic events; however, most had no hypoglycaemic events.

Conclusion

The constrained L-MPC was able to effectively improve glycaemic control as time progressed, utilising the ILC to make adjustments to the setpoint of the MPC. The controller showed better glycaemic control than the MPC alone and was shown to adequately deal with variations in the timing, the carbohydrate composition of the meal, and the subjects.

COMMENT

The constrained L-MPC developed by Wang and collaborators is a novel technique that shows great robustness and overall glycaemic control in a variety of scenarios mimicking the everyday life of individuals with T1D. However, it was shown that the constraints on the L-MPC caused a decrease in performance suggesting an improvement in the limitations imposed on the ILC-based setpoint should be considered; it must be noted that the constrained L-MPC still performed better than the MPC on its own. It is impressive to see the level of glycaemic control achieved by a fully closed-loop artificial pancreas, a system requiring no intervention from the subject. The authors also noted that the ILC is independent of the local controller and may be implemented on other controllers to create new combinations. Further research should be aimed at not only refining overall glycaemic control in different subjects but dealing with the possibility of meals that are skipped entirely, another real-life variation in diet.

Development of a multi-parametric model predictive control algorithm for insulin delivery in type 1 diabetes mellitus using clinical parameters

Percival MW[1,2], Wang Y[1,2,3], Grosman B[1,2], Dassau E[1,2], Zisser H[1,2], Jovanovic L[1,2], Doyle FJ III[1,2]

[1] *Department of Chemical Engineering, University of California, Santa Barbara, CA, USA,* [2] *Sansum Diabetes Research Institute, Santa Barbara, CA, USA, and* [3] *Beijing University of Chemical Technology, Beijing, China*

*J Process Control 2011; **21**: 391–404*

Background

The development of an effective controller that can account for the lag time associated with subcutaneous insulin infusion is one of the main challenges to the artificial pancreas. The authors of this paper aimed to develop a multi-parametric model predictive control (mpMPC) algorithm that is computationally efficient, robust to insulin variations, and involves minimal burden for the user.

Methods

The study aimed to show the feasibility of using simple models, clinical parameters and mpMPC for control of glycaemia via the subcutaneous route; parameters derived from physicians were incorporated into the safety constraint of the controller. Closed-loop simulations using the mpMPC algorithm were conducted on two virtual subject cohorts: four patients were based on the model of Hovorka *et al.* and 10 patients were based on the UVa/Padova model. The algorithm was developed and tested using three different modelling scenarios: an unannounced meal, a measured meal, and an announced meal. The simulations were performed assuming a daily meal plan of 200 g of carbohydrates, divided into three meals of 50, 85 and 65 g ingested at 7 am, noon and 7 pm, respectively. Two constraint cases, one being only physical constraints and the other being a combination of both physical constraints and insulin-on-board safety constraints, were also considered in the closed-loop simulations.

Results

Initial model development led to the selection of two algorithm variations, models D and F, to use in further experimentation. It was found that when testing model D in the Hovorka cohort, unannounced meals resulted in low postprandial blood glucose. Although announced meals also reduced peak blood glucose, it was at the cost of further decreasing the postprandial blood glucose. In the UVa/Padova cohort, tests with model D showed that 30% of the trials had satisfactory results when meals were unannounced; 30% needed announced meals to avoid hypoglycaemia, 30% needed insulin-on-board safety constraints to avoid hypoglycaemia, and 10% suffered hypoglycaemia due to a failed safety constraint. In the trials with model F as the controller in the UVa/Padova cohort, 70% achieved glycaemic control that were identical with or without safety constraints and the other 30% avoided hypoglycaemia with some sort of safety constraint, whether it was physical or insulin-on-board dependent. The authors found that controller F performed better than controller D in closed-loop scenarios.

Conclusion

The robustness of the mpMPC controller was demonstrated, and the safety constraints that were implemented successfully improved performance by reducing the number of hypoglycaemic events. The low order functions with clinically meaningful parameters were relatively able to control glycaemia and remain compact enough to be implemented on a simple electronic device.

COMMENT

Percival and co-workers were able to use simple models and several clinical parameters to almost completely eliminate hypoglycaemic episodes in the *in silico* patients. The combination of the physical constraints with the insulin-on-board safety constraints proved to be the most effective at preventing hypoglycaemic events. However, it is difficult to say that the controller achieved glycaemic control. Both controllers tested, D and F, were unable to stop blood glucose levels from reaching the upper end of the glycaemic index after meals; 40% of the patients in the UVa/Padova cohort had measured postprandial blood glucose levels greater than or equal to 300 mg/dl in both controllers while another 20% had measured postprandial blood glucose levels greater than or equal to 400 mg/dl. The lack of some type of control in the experiment also makes it difficult to critically evaluate the overall effectiveness of the mpMPC. The incorporation of another closed-loop or an open-loop administration of insulin as a comparison would have provided more relevant data as well as a basis to make adjustments to the algorithm.

The controller for the closed-loop administration must be able to control both ends of the blood glucose spectrum. The mpMPC has been shown to reduce the number of hypoglycaemic events but now the research should focus on limiting postprandial blood glucose. It is important to note that future personalisation of the controller could be accomplished by a non-specialist due to the reduced complexity of the mpMPC. Also, the use of an mpMPC reduced the size of the controller such that it can be implemented on a reasonably simple computational device, an important factor in the development of a user-friendly artificial pancreas.

SUMMARY

The artificial pancreas system has been the hope of both people with diabetes and caregivers around the world for the last four decades. Its great potential is 'freeing' the patients from the day-to-day burden of the treatment while safely controlling the patient's blood glucose concentration. An artificial pancreas will integrate two currently available technologies: (a) continuous glucose monitors and (b) insulin pumps with control and safety algorithms that adjust insulin delivery when needed or based on some level of user interaction. The papers in this chapter have been selected because they successfully illustrated the feasibility of several types of algorithms and artificial pancreas systems as well as promising advanced algorithms that should be tested in future clinical studies. Pilot clinical studies results are extremely encouraging; however, in most studies the systems were tested in ideal conditions and more work is needed to allow the translation of this amazing technology to the home setting. The dream of the artificial pancreas is around the corner but the following challenges need to be addressed as part of the path forward to a commercial system: (a) system integration, that is communication standards between CGM, continuous subcutaneous insulin infusion and the algorithms; (b) safety and monitoring algorithms that can provide early alert in the event of sensor drifts, infusion site failure, as well as hypoglycaemia/hyperglycaemia prevention algorithms; (c) user interactions and human factor studies to evaluate the interaction of the end user with the different artificial pancreas designs.

The papers in this chapter clearly suggest that we are moving in the right direction and are gradually bringing the idea of an artificial pancreas to a reality.

REFERENCES

1. Choudhary P, Shin J, Wang Y, Evans ML, Hammond PJ, Kerr D, Shaw JA, Pickup JC, Amiel SA. Insulin pump therapy with automated insulin suspension in response to hypoglycemia. *Diabetes Care* 2011; **34**: 2023–5
2. Danne T, Kordonouri O, Holder M, Haberland H, Golembowski S, Remus K, Bläsig S, Wadien T, Zierow S, Hartmann R, Thomas A. Prevention of hypoglycemia by using low glucose suspend function in sensor-augmented pump therapy. *Diabetes Technol Ther* 2011 Aug 9 [Epub ahead of print]
3. Steil GM, Rebrin K, Darwin C, Hariri F, Saad MF. Feasibility of automating insulin delivery for the treatment of type 1 diabetes. *Diabetes* 2006; **55**: 3344–50
4. Weinzimer SA, Steil GM, Swan KL, Dziura J, Kurtz N, Tamborlane WV. Fully automated closed-loop insulin delivery versus semiautomated hybrid control in pediatric patients with type 1 diabetes using an artificial pancreas. *Diabetes Care* 2008; **31**: 934–9
5. Kadish AH. Automation control of blood sugar a servomechanism for glucose monitoring and control. *Trans Am Soc Artif Intern Organs* 1963; **9**: 363–7
6. Castle JR, Engle JM, El Youssef J, Massoud RG, Ward WK. Factors influencing the effectiveness of glucagon for preventing hypoglycemia. *J Diabetes Sci Technol* 2010; **4**: 1305–10

CHAPTER 5

New Insulins and Insulin Therapy

Thomas Danne[1] and Jan Bolinder[2]

[1]Diabetes-Zentrum für Kinder and Jugendliche, Kinderkrankenhaus auf der Bult, Hannover, Germany

[2]Department of Medicine, Karolinska University Hospital Huddinge, Karolinska Institutet, Stockholm, Sweden

INTRODUCTION

While the pharmacokinetic properties of the long-acting insulin analogues, insulin glargine and insulin detemir, clearly demonstrate clinical benefits over NPH insulin in terms of reduced frequency of overall and nocturnal hypoglycaemic events and lowered glycaemic variability, several new insulin analogues with even longer and smoother time-action profiles are being developed and explored. Among these, insulin degludec is the first to enter the market. The ultra-long action profile of this insulin analogue is mainly the result of a slow and stable release of insulin degludec monomers from soluble multihexamers that form after subcutaneous administration. In the last year, the results of the first phase II trials with insulin degludec have been published, where the efficacy and safety of this basal insulin analogue have been compared with insulin glargine in patients with type 1 (T1D) and type 2 (T2D) diabetes.

With regard to short-acting insulins for mealtime insulin supplementation, there is also a search for new insulins with a more rapid onset of action, and hence improved postprandial glucose control. Linjeta™ (formerly named VIAject) is a human insulin formulation with faster insulin absorption and action than insulin lispro and regular human insulin. A new drug application to market Linjeta™ as a treatment for diabetes was submitted to the US Food and Drug Administration (FDA) by the manufacturer at the beginning of 2010. However, the FDA's review cycle, which was announced late in 2010, concluded that the application could not be approved in its present form. The FDA's complete response

Int J Clin Pract 2012; **66** (Suppl. 175): 30–32

letter included comments related to clinical trials, statistical analysis and chemistry, manufacturing and controls. The FDA requested that the company should conduct two new phase III clinical trials using the commercial formulation, one in patients with T1D and the other in patients with T2D, to establish efficacy and safety with regard to hypo-glycaemia and toleration. Co-administration of hyaluronidase together with insulin is another novel concept which has been proven to accel-erate the absorption of both insulin lispro and regular human insulin in healthy subjects. In this review, we comment on two recent publications in which the pharmacokinetic and pharmacodynamic characteristics of Linjeta™ and co-formulations of prandial insulins with recombinant hu-man hyaluronidase were investigated in patients with T1D. Lastly, a re-cent review on the ongoing discussion regarding insulin treatment and cancer risk is included.

NOVEL LONG-ACTING INSULIN ANALOGUES

Insulin degludec in type 1 diabetes. A randomised controlled trial of a new-generation ultra-long-acting insulin compared with insulin glargine

Birkeland KI[1], Home PD[2], Wendisch U[3], Ratner RE[4], Johansen T[5], Endahl LA[5], Lyby K[5], Jendle JH[6], Roberts AP[7], DeVries JH[8], Meneghini LF[9]

[1] *Oslo University Hospital and Faculty of Medicine, Oslo, Norway,* [2] *Newcastle University, Newcastle upon Tyne, UK,* [3] *Group Practice in Internal Medicine and Diabetology, Hamburg, Germany,* [4] *Medstar Research Institute, Washington, DC, USA,* [5] *NovoNordisk A/S, Soeborg, Denmark,* [6] *Örebro University Hospital, Örebro, Sweden,* [7] *Royal Adelaide Hospital, Adelaide, SA, Australia,* [8] *University of Amsterdam, The Netherlands, and* [9] *University of Miami Miller School of Medicine, Miami, FL, USA*

*Diabetes Care 2011; **34**: 661–5*

Background
To investigate the efficacy and safety of two formulations of insulin degludec (IDeg), administered once daily together with mealtime insulin aspart in patients with T1D. Comparison was made with a similar basal-bolus regimen consisting of insulin glargine (IGlar) and aspart.

Methods
Adult patients with T1D (mean A1c 8.4%) were randomised (open-label) to be treated for 16 weeks with once-daily (evening) subcutaneous

injections of either of two different insulin degludec formulations, IDeg(A) (600 μmol/l; $n = 59$), IDeg(B) (900 μmol/l; $n = 60$), or with IGlar ($n = 59$). All patients received insulin aspart at mealtimes.

Results

At 16 weeks, mean A1c was comparable for all three basal insulin therapies: IDeg(A) $7.8 \pm 0.8\%$, IDeg(B) $8.0 \pm 1.0\%$ and IGlar $7.6 \pm 0.8\%$. Similarly, there was no difference in mean fasting plasma glucose across treatment groups (8.3 ± 4.0, 8.3 ± 2.8 and 8.9 ± 3.5 mmol/l, respectively). In comparison with IGlar, the estimated mean rate of confirmed hypoglycaemia (<3.1 mmol/l) was 28% lower for IDeg(A) [rate ratio (RR) 0.72, 95% confidence interval (CI) 0.52–1.00] and 10% lower for IDeg(B) [RR 0.90 (0.65–1.24)], and rates of nocturnal hypoglycaemia were reduced by 58% with IDeg(A) [RR 0.42 (0.25–0.69)] and by 29% with IDeg(B) [RR 0.71 (0.44–1.16)]. Mean total daily insulin doses remained essentially unchanged from baseline values in all treatment arms. The overall rates and nature of adverse events were comparable between groups.

Conclusions

IDeg is a safe and well tolerated basal insulin in patients with T1D, providing comparable glycaemic control to IGlar at similar doses but with lower frequency of hypoglycaemia.

Insulin degludec, an ultra-long-acting basal insulin, once a day or three times a week versus insulin glargine once a day in patients with type 2 diabetes: a 16-week, randomised, open-label, phase 2 trial

Zinman B[1], Fulcher G[2], Rao PV[3], Thomas N[4], Endahl LA[5], Johansen T[5], Lindh R[5], Lewin A[6], Rosenstock J[7], Pinget M[8], Mathieu C[9]

[1] *Samuel Lunenfeld Research Institute, Mount Sinai Hospital, University of Toronto, Toronto, ON, Canada,* [2] *Royal North Shore Hospital and University of Sydney, Sydney, NSW, Australia,* [3] *Nizam's Institute of Medical Sciences University, Hyderabad, India,* [4] *Christian Medical College, Vellore, India,* [5] *Novo Nordisk, Soeborg, Denmark,* [6] *National Research Institute, Los Angeles, CA, USA,* [7] *Dallas Diabetes and Endocrine Center at Medical City, Dallas, TX, USA,* [8] *University Hospital Strasbourg, France, and* [9] *UZ Gasthuisberg Katholieke Universiteit Leuven, Leuven, Belgium*

*Lancet 2011; **377**: 924–31*

Background

To assess the efficacy and safety of insulin degludec administered once daily or three times a week in patients with T2D. Comparison was made with insulin glargine injected once daily.

Methods

Insulin-naive patients with T2D (age 18–75 years), inadequately controlled with oral antidiabetic drugs (A1c 7%–11%), were eligible in this 16-week, multicentre, open-label trial. Sixty-two patients were randomised to administer insulin degludec (900 μmol/l) three times a week (starting dose 20 U per injection; 1 U = 9 nmol), 60 patients to receive insulin degludec (600 μmol/l) once daily (starting dose 10 U; 1 U = 6 nmol), 61 patients to receive insulin degludec (900 μmol/l) once daily (starting dose 10 U; 1 U = 9 nmol) and 62 to administer insulin glargine once daily (starting dose 10 U; 1 U = 6 nmol). All patients were on combination therapy with metformin. The primary outcome was HbA1c following 16 weeks of treatment.

Results

At 16 weeks, the mean HbA1c values were comparable in the four treatment groups: 7.3% (SD 1.1), 7.4% (1.0), 7.5% (1.1) and 7.2% (0.9), respectively. The estimated mean HbA1c difference in comparison with insulin glargine was 0.08% (95% CI –0.23 to 0.40) for insulin degludec administered three times a week, and 0.17% (–0.15 to 0.48) and 0.28% (–0.04 to 0.59), respectively, for the 600 μmol/l and 900 μmol/l insulin degludec formulations given once daily. The overall rate of hypoglycaemic events was low, and the frequency and pattern of adverse events were similar across the treatment groups.

Conclusions

Insulin degludec provides comparable glycaemic control and safety profile to insulin glargine in patients with T2D, and – according to its ultra-long action profile – it might allow prolonged dosing intervals.

A new-generation ultra-long-acting basal insulin with a bolus boost compared with insulin glargine in insulin-naive people with type 2 diabetes

Heise T[1], Tack CJ[2], Cuddihy R[3], Davidson J[4], Gouet D[5], Liebl A[6], Romero E[7], Mersebach H[8], Dykiel P[8], Jorde R[9]

[1] *Profil Institut für Stoffwechselforschung, Neuss, Germany,* [2] *Radboud University Nijmegen Medical Centre, Nijmegen, The Netherlands,* [3] *International Diabetes Center, Park Nicollet, Minneapolis, MA, USA,* [4] *Department of Medicine,*

Division of Endocrinology, University of Texas, Southwestern Medical School, Dallas, TX, USA, [5]Hopital Saint Louis, Centre Hospitalier de La Rochelle, La Rochelle, France, [6]Center for Diabetes and Meabolism, Fachklinik, Bad Heilbrunn, Germany, [7]University of Valladolid, Instituto de Endocrinologia y Nutricion, Valladolid, Spain, [8]Novo Nordisk A/S, Soeborg, Denmark, and [9]Institute of Clinical Medicine, University of Tromsoe, Tromsoe, Norway

*Diabetes Care 2011; **34**: 669–74*

Background

To compare the safety and efficacy of two formulations of a soluble co-formulation of insulin degludec and insulin aspart (70%/30% v/v and 55%/45% v/v, respectively) and insulin glargine in insulin-naive patients with T2D inadequately controlled with oral antidiabetic drugs.

Methods

Patients with T2D (mean age 59.1 years, A1c 8.5%, body mass index 30.3 kg/m^2) were randomly allocated (open-label) to 16 weeks of treatment with once-daily injection (before evening meal) of insulin degludec/aspart 70/30 ($n = 59$), insulin/aspart 55/45 ($n = 59$), or insulin glargine ($n = 60$). All patients received combination therapy with metformin. Insulin doses were titrated to a fasting plasma glucose target of 4–6 mmol/l.

Results

At 16 weeks, mean A1c had decreased to comparable levels across the treatment groups: insulin degludec/aspart 70/30 7.0%, insulin degludec/aspart 55/45 7.2% and insulin glargine 7.1%. There was a similar relative proportion of patients who improved their A1c below 7.0% without experiencing confirmed hypoglycaemia (plasma glucose <3.1 mmol/l) over the last 4-week period of the trial (51%, 47% and 50% in the three treatment groups, respectively). Mean 2-h post-dinner plasma glucose increase was less prominent for insulin degludec/aspart 70/30 (0.13 mmol/l) and insulin degludec/aspart 55/45 (0.24 mmol/l) than for insulin glargine (1.63 mmol/l), whereas fasting plasma glucose was similar (6.8 mmol/l, 7.4 mmol/l and 7.0 mmol/l, respectively). Estimated rates of confirmed hypoglycaemic events were lower for insulin degludec/aspart 70/30 (1.2 events per patient-year) and insulin glargine (0.7 events per patient-year) than for insulin degludec/aspart 55/45 (2.4 events per patient year). Likewise, nocturnal hypoglycaemia occurred more frequently with insulin degludec/aspart 55/45 (27 events) than with insulin degludec/aspart 70/30 (1 event) and insulin glargine (3 events).

Conclusions

The 70%/30% (v/v) co-formulation of insulin degludec and insulin as-part administered once daily provided comparable overall glycaemic control and hypoglycaemia rates compared with insulin glargine but better postprandial glucose control after dinner.

COMMENT

Insulin degludec is a soluble, basal insulin analogue with a smooth and stable pharmacokinetic profile, with a duration of action exceeding 24 h (1) and with low within-subject variability (2). In the referenced reports, the safety and efficacy of different formulations of insulin degludec were compared with insulin glargine in short-term, proof-of-concept trials. In patients with T1D, once-daily injection of insulin degludec together with insulin aspart at mealtimes resulted in essentially the same glycaemic control as that observed when insulin glargine was used for basal insulin supplementation. The rates of confirmed hypoglycaemic episodes were lower for insulin degludec; this was most readily observed during night-time, and in those patients who were allocated to use the 600 μmol/l formulation of insulin degludec [according to the authors, the higher strength insulin degludec formulation (900 μmol/l) has therefore been discontinued from further clinical development]. Similarly, in patients with T2D, insulin degludec administered once daily as add-on to metformin did not differ from insulin glargine in terms of glycaemic control or risk of hypo-glycaemia or other adverse events. Interestingly, demonstrating its prolonged duration of action, insulin degludec (900 μmol/l) also provided comparable glycaemic outcomes when given only three times a week, although with a tendency to more frequent hypoglycaemic episodes. The latter finding may have been due to the fact that approximately twice as much insulin was ad-ministered per injection when insulin degludec was given three times a week in comparison with the once-daily insulin regimens. Another intriguing feature of insulin degludec is that it can be co-formulated with a rapid-acting insulin analogue (pre-mixed insulin). In the study by Heise *et al.*, the two tested for-mulations of insulin degludec and insulin aspart (relative proportions 70/30 and 55/45, respectively) injected once daily provided comparable overall gly-caemic control to insulin glargine. The postprandial glucose excursion after dinner was less pronounced with the two insulin degludec formulations than with glargine. This was perhaps an expected finding, given the prandial, rapid-acting component of insulin aspart in these formulations. Notably, the rate of hypoglycaemic events, and especially the frequency of nocturnal hypogly-caemia, was considerably higher with the 55/45 degludec/aspart formulation. Based on this finding, the clinical development of this co-formulation has been stopped. In summary, the results of these phase 2 trials are promising and in-dicate that insulin degludec may allow more flexible insulin regimens with less frequent insulin injections in patients with T2D. Moreover, the findings suggest that insulin degludec may have the potential to further reduce the risk of hypoglycaemia, in particular in patients with T1D as well as in patients with T2D necessitating more complex insulin regimens. Additional data from longer term studies are much awaited to clarify in more detail the efficacy and safety characteristics and the potential clinical benefits of this novel basal insulin analogue.

RAPID-ACTING INSULIN FORMULATIONS

Comparable efficacy and safety of insulin glulisine and insulin lispro when given as part of a basal-bolus insulin regimen in a 26-week trial in paediatric patients with type 1 diabetes

Philotheou A[1], Arslanian S[2], Blatniczky L[3], Peterkova V[4], Souhami E[5], Danne T[6]

[1]University of Cape Town Diabetes Clinical Trials Unit, New Groote Schuur Hospital, Cape Town, South Africa, [2]Divisions of Pediatric Endocrinology, Metabolism and Diabetes Mellitus, and Weight Management and Wellness, Children's Hospital of Pittsburgh, University of Pittsburgh Medical Center, Pittsburgh, PA, USA, [3]Buda Children's Hospital, Budapest, Hungary, [4]Endocrinological Scientific Centre, Russian Academy of Science, Moscow, Russia, [5]Sanofi-aventis, Antony, France, and [6]Children's Hospital auf der Bult, Hannover, Germany

*Diabetes Technol Ther 2011; **13**: 327–34*

Background

To evaluate the efficacy and safety of insulin glulisine compared with insulin lispro as part of a basal-bolus regimen in children and adolescents with T1D.

Methods

Children and adolescents aged 4–17 years ($n = 572$) using insulin glargine or NPH insulin as basal insulin were enrolled in a 26-week, multicentre, open, centrally randomised, parallel-group study. Subjects were randomised to receive glulisine ($n = 277$) or lispro ($n = 295$) 0–15 min before a meal.

Results

Both groups exhibited similar A1c levels at baseline. The adjusted mean change in A1c from baseline to endpoint was $+0.10 \pm 0.08\%$ in the glulisine group and $+0.16 \pm 0.07\%$ in the lispro group. The difference in the adjusted means for the change from baseline in A1c between the treatments was equal to −0.06% (95% CI −0.24 to 0.12), confirming non-inferiority of glulisine vs. lispro. Similar effects on A1c levels were reported in both groups after 12 and 26 weeks. For all age groups, the percentage of subjects achieving the American Diabetes Association recommended A1c target was significantly higher (p = 0.039) with glulisine (38.4%) than with lispro (32.0%). This difference was most pronounced in adolescents (13–17 years). At baseline, the mean blood glucose profiles were comparable for all three time points in both groups. At endpoint, only the mean pre-breakfast blood glucose was significantly lower in the glulisine group. Most subjects had three to four bolus insulin injections at baseline, which remained stable throughout the study. No significant differences between the two treatment arms were reported for the monthly events rate per patient of all, severe, nocturnal, or severe nocturnal symptomatic hypoglycaemia from month 4 to treatment to endpoint for glulisine and lispro, respectively. Frequency and type of adverse events, serious adverse events, or hypoglycaemia reported as serious adverse events were similar between the groups.

Conclusions
In children and adolescents withT1D, glulisine is non-inferior to lispro in terms of A1c change, and is similarly well tolerated to lispro.

Reduction of postprandial glycaemic excursions in patients with type 1 diabetes: a novel human insulin formulation versus a rapid-acting insulin analogue and regular human insulin

Heinemann L[1,2], Hompesch M[2], Flacke F[3], Simms P[3], Pohl R[3], Albus K[3], Pfützner A[4], Steiner S[3]

[1] *Profil Institut für Stoffwechselforschung, Neuss, Germany,* [2] *Profil Institute for Clinical Research Inc., San Diego, CA, USA,* [3] *Biodel Inc., Danbury, CT, USA, and* [4] *IKFE, Institute for Clinical Research and Development, Mainz, Germany*

J Diabetes Sci Technol 2011; 5: 681–6

Background
To compare postprandial glucose control in patients with T1D following administration of VIAject™ (Linjeta™), insulin lispro and regular human insulin.

Methods
On three occasions, and with normalised preprandial glucose control, patients (*n* = 18) received an individually tailored dose of each insulin immediately before a standardised mixed meal.

Results

Insulin absorption was faster following injection of VIAject™ than after administration of insulin lispro and human regular insulin, the time to half-maximum serum insulin being 13.1 ± 5.2 min, 25.4 ± 7.6 min and 38.4 ± 19.5 min, respectively (VIAject™ vs. insulin lispro p $= 0.001$; VIAject™ vs. regular human insulin p < 0.001; and insulin lispro vs. regular human insulin p < 0.001). Peak postprandial blood glucose (0–180 min) was lower with VIAject™ (157 ± 30 mg/dl, p $= 0.002$) and insulin lispro (170 ± 42 mg/dl; p $= 0.008$) compared with regular human insulin (191 ± 46 mg/dl). The difference between maximum and minimum glucose levels was smaller after administration of VIAject™ (70 ± 17 mg/dl) than after injection of either insulin lispro (89 ± 18; p $= 0.011$) or regular human insulin (91 ± 33 mg/dl; p $= 0.007$), and the area under the blood glucose curve was 23% smaller with VIAject™ than with regular human insulin (p < 0.001).

Conclusions

The more rapid absorption of VIAject™ results in less pronounced postprandial glucose excursions.

Accelerated insulin pharmacokinetics and improved postprandial glycaemic control in patients with type 1 diabetes after coadministration of prandial insulins with hyaluronidase

Hompesch M[1], Muchmore DB[2], Morrow L[1], Vaughn DE[2]

[1]*Profil Institute for Clinical Research, Chula Vista, CA, USA, and* [2]*Halozyme Therapeutics, San Diego, CA, USA*

Diabetes Care 2011; **34**: *666–8*

Background

To assess the effect of co-administration of recombinant human hyaluronidase (rHuPH20) on safety, pharmacokinetics and pharmacodynamics of insulin lispro and human regular insulin in patients with T1D.

Methods

Patients ($n = 22$) were given individually titrated optimum doses of insulin lispro or human regular insulin with or without co-administration of rHuPH20 before a standardised liquid test meal.

Results

With co-administration of rHuPH20, the early (0–60 min) insulin uptake increased by 54% (p $= 0.0011$) for insulin lispro and by 206%

(p < 0.0001) for human regular insulin, compared with administration of the respective insulin without rHuPH20. Mean peak blood glucose decreased 26 mg/dl for insulin lispro (p = 0.002) and 24 mg/dl for human regular insulin, and the total postprandial glycaemic excursions (area under the curve for blood glucose above 140 mg/dl) were reduced by 79% (p = 0.09) and 85% (p = 0.049) for insulin lispro and human regular insulin, respectively. Frequency of hypoglycaemia was similar for insulin lispro with or without co-administration of rHuPH20, whereas it was reduced when human regular insulin was administered together with rHuPH20.

Conclusions

Co-administration of rHuPH20 with insulin lispro and human regular insulin resulted in accelerated insulin absorption and improved postprandial blood glucose control.

COMMENT

The largest paediatric T1D study with rapid-acting insulin analogues to date showed comparable efficacy in a head-to-head comparison between lispro and glulisine. However, it raised the question whether all currently available fast acting insulin analogues are clinically equivalent, or if certain patient populations may benefit using one over the other. Notably, despite the introduction of the fast acting insulin analogues, many patients remain unable to achieve effective control of postprandial glucose excursions. Thus, there is a clinical need for insulin formulations that are absorbed even more rapidly from the subcutaneous injection site, and mimic the normal meal-induced insulin response. Linjeta™ is a special formulation of human insulin which promotes monomerisation of insulin. Previous studies in healthy subjects have demonstrated that Linjeta™ has a faster onset of action compared with regular human insulin and insulin lispro (3, 4). The study by Heinemann *et al.* confirms similar findings in patients with T1D, and also that the faster rate of absorption of Linjeta™ is mirrored by a less pronounced increase in postprandial glucose levels. Nevertheless, the FDA request additional studies prior to approval, as mentioned above. The report by Hompesch and co-workers describes another interesting approach to accelerate the absorption of insulin, namely by co-administration of prandial insulins with hyaluronidase. For more than six decades, hyaluronidase has been utilised as an adjuvant to enhance the absorption and dispersion of other injected molecules. This enzyme catalyses the breakdown of hyaluronan polymers in the subcutaneous space, leading to facilitated permeation of co-administered compounds (5, 6). In the case of insulin, the depolymerisation of hyaluronan mediates a dilution effect that favours dissociation of insulin hexamers and hence enhances the rate of insulin absorption (7). In addition, the insulin molecules are dispersed over a larger capillary bed, which facilitates their absorption. In the current experimental study in patients with T1D, co-administration of rHuPH20 enhanced the absorption of both regular human insulin and insulin lispro, leading to a faster and greater maximum insulin exposure and a corresponding lowering of the postprandial glucose excursions. While the findings are encouraging, larger long-term trials are warranted to clarify the potential clinical benefit of this approach of constructing ultra-fast insulins.

INSULIN THERAPY AND CANCER

Insulin therapy in diabetes and cancer risk: current understanding and implications for future study: Proceedings of a meeting of a European Insulin Safety Consensus Panel, convened and sponsored by Novo Nordisk, held Tuesday 5 October 2010 at the Radisson Edwardian Heathrow Hotel, Hayes, Middlesex, UK

Gough SC[1], Belda-Iniesta C[2], Poole C[3], Weber M[4], Russell-Jones D[5], Hansen BF[6], Mannucci E[7], Tuomilehto J[8]

[1] Oxford Centre for Diabetes Endocrinology and Metabolism and Oxford (NIHR) Biomedical Research Centre, Churchill Hospital, Oxford, UK, [2] IdiPAZ, University Hospital La Paz, Madrid, Spain, [3] Department of Epidemiology, Pharmatelligence, Pharma Research Centre, Cardiff Medicentre, University Hospital of Wales, Heath Park, Cardiff, UK, [4] I Medical Department, University Hospital Mainz, Mainz, Germany, [5] Royal Surrey County Hospital and University of Surrey, Guildford, UK, [6] Diabetes Biology, Novo Nordisk A/S, Novo Nordisk Park, Måløv, Denmark, [7] Diabetes Agency, Department of Emergency, Medicine and Surgery, Careggi Teaching Hospital, Florence, Italy, and [8] Department of Public Health, University of Helsinki, Helsinki, Finland

Adv Ther 2011; **28** (Suppl 5): 1–18

Background

The possibility of certain insulin treatments having the potential to modify cancer development and prognosis was raised again in 2009, following publication of several epidemiological studies addressing this issue. Together with the possibility that diabetes itself might be linked to cancer, an exchange of expert views and knowledge was essential in order to enhance understanding on this subject among those treating diabetes and cancer, and those developing diabetes therapies.

Methods

A European meeting was convened with participants who are experts in the fields of endocrinology, oncology, epidemiology and insulin analogue design and investigation. The experts were invited to present on relevant topics, with open discussions held after each presentation.

Results

Some epidemiological studies have raised concern over the potential mitogenic properties of certain insulin analogues, although confounding factors render interpretation controversial. Meanwhile, pharmacological studies, and a consideration of cancer pathophysiology, implicate increased insulin-like growth factor 1 receptor affinity and/or deranged insulin receptor interaction/signalling properties as possible causes for concern with some insulin analogues. However, interpretation of the pharmacological evidence is confounded by the array of test systems and methodologies used, and by studies frequently succumbing to methodological pitfalls. Most available insulin analogues do not differ in their receptor interaction response profile to human insulin, and for those that do there are reasons to question any potential clinical relevance. Yet, it is preferred that new experimental models are devised that can better determine the likely clinical consequences of any variance in receptor response profile vs. human insulin.

Conclusions

We need more data to increase our understanding of this issue, with close cooperation and communication between diabetologists, epidemiologists, oncologists and insulin engineers.

COMMENT

This review summarises the most recent papers on the insulin treatment and cancer debate. Although the proceedings have to be interpreted with caution as the panel was convened by a single pharmaceutical company (Novo Nordisk) it allows a quick update. Despite the growing knowledge base the authors conclude that current gaps in our understanding do not allow clear recommendations on how to discuss this issue adequately with patients to reach an 'informed choice'.

REFERENCES

1. Jonassen I, Havelund S, Ribel U, Hoeg-Jensen T, Steensgaard DB, Johansen T, Haar H, Nishimura E, Kurtzhals P. Insulin degludec is a new generation ultra-long acting basal insulin with a unique mechanism of protraction based on multi-hexamer formation. *Diabetes* 2010; **59** (Suppl 1): A11 (Abstract)
2. Heise T, Hermaniski L, Nosek L, Feldmann A, Rasmussen S, Stryhn TK, Haahr H. Insulin degludec: less pharmacodynamics variability than insulin glargine under steady-state conditions. *Diabetologia* 2010; **53** (Suppl 1): S387 (Abstract)

3. Steiner S, Hompesch M, Pohl R, Simms P, Flacke F, Mohr T, Pfützner A, Heinemann L. A novel insulin formulation with a more rapid onset of action. *Diabetologia* 2008; **51**: 1602–6

4. Hompesch M, McManus L, Pohl R, Simms P, Pfützner A, Bülow E, Flacke F, Heinemann L, Steiner SS. Intra-individual variability of the metabolic effect of a novel rapid-acting insulin (VIAject™) in comparison to regular human insulin. *J Diabetes Sci Technol* 2008; **2**: 568–71

5. Chain E, Duthie ES. Identity of hyaluronidase and spreading factor. *Br J Exp Pathol* 1940; **21**: 324–38

6. Frost GI. Recombinant human hyaluronidase (rHuPH20): an enabling platform for subcutaneous drug and fluid administration. *Expert Opin Drug Deliv* 2007; **4**: 427–40

7. Vaughn DE, Yocum RC, Muchmore DB, Sugarman BJ, Vick AM, Bilinsky IP, Frost GI. Accelerated pharmacokinetics and glucodynamics of prandial insulins injected with recombinant human hyaluronidase. *Diabetes Technol Ther* 2009; **11**: 345–52

CHAPTER 6

New Ways of Insulin Delivery

Lutz Heinemann

Science & Co, Kehler Str. 24, 40468 Düsseldorf, Germany

INTRODUCTION

The last year was not a good year for new ways of insulin delivery, at least when you regard the number of publications about this topic as a reflection about the scientific and commercial interest in this area of research. Not only has the number of papers published from the middle of 2010 to the middle of 2011 about inhaled insulin decreased in comparison with the years before, but also in general there were a limited number of publications about alternative routes of insulin administration (ARIA). Thus the number of clinical studies published in leading peer-reviewed journals that can be presented here is small. Simply no data from a clinical study were published about nasal insulin, dermal insulin or transdermal insulin developments; it appears as if there is a standstill with these approaches. It would be quite helpful for this area of research if at least one product came to the market in 2012 (e.g. inhaled insulin/Technosphere insulin). It might be that an oral insulin formulation will come to the market in the next few years, but most probably in less regulated markets. The story is clearly different when it comes to insulin pens; there is an increasing number of publications about these widely used devices.

INHALED INSULIN

Clearly the failure of Exubera (combined with the stop of the clinical development of most other inhaled insulin programmes) is the major reason for the drastic decline in the number of publications about clinical trials with inhaled insulin. Currently there is only one company active in the clinical development of an inhaled insulin formulation: MannKind has

Int J Clin Pract 2012; **66** (Suppl. 175): 33–35

submitted a New Drug Application to the US Food and Drug Administration (FDA) and received a certain setback from this regulatory authority, but is still in a good mood that they will get market approval sometime in the near future. However, as we have learned from the Exubera story, market approval is not all, without appropriate acceptance by the market (=sales); also an inhaled insulin with demonstrated and unique advantages when it comes to insulin absorption and insulin action might fail in the long run.

Market approval for Afrezza would be good news also for another company that has a profound scientific background in the inhalation of peptides (www.dancepharma.com) and that is interested in starting over with the clinical development of inhaled insulin formulations (1). Also a good review was published that argues for keeping inhaled insulin as a valid option for insulin application in mind (2).

It appears as if the submission of the necessary documents to the FDA and performance of additional clinical studies has required a lot of focus inside this company; there were no publications by MannKind about clinical studies in the last year that can be presented here. However, they published a number of other interesting studies, some more methodological, that will be presented here in brief only, e.g. one human study about lung deposition of Technosphere particles (3). Two good reviews were published by the same authors about Technosphere insulin (4,5).

MannKind also tried to support the position of inhaled insulin in general by performing surveys at the physician (6) and patient level (7). Also some pharmacokinetic/pharmacodynamic modelling papers about inhaled insulin were published that highlight the advantages of this route of insulin administration when it comes to insulin absorption, also in subjects with diabetic nephropathy, chronic liver disease and chronic obstructive pulmonary disease (8–11). There might be special paediatric cases in which treatment with inhaled insulin is helpful to overcome massive subcutaneous insulin resistance, but a number of aspects have to be considered (12,13).

One animal study was published that declares to have identified a potentially serious side effect of inhalation based insulin delivery, the formation of aggregates of inhaled insulin at the interface presented in the lungs through an amyloid formation mechanism (14). The authors state that their data highlight the need for caution when considering other novel methods of insulin delivery due to the amyloidogenic nature of this protein.

ORAL INSULIN

Oral insulin (OI) has also seen some setbacks, resulting in the fact that only one paper presenting data from a clinical trial was published in the last year. The negative outcome of Biocon's phase 2 trial with their OI candidate IN-105 led to a recent offer by this large Indian company that produce a lot of insulin to sell this development, i.e. they are looking for another company that is interested in pursuing this development further. Novo Nordisk reported in a press release that they have stopped the development of one of their OI candidates (NN-1952), which was a co-development with the Irish company Merrion Pharmaceuticals. Somewhat in contrast to previous years the publication activities of the Israel based company Oramed were reduced. Access Pharmaceuticals – which has an OI in which the insulin is bound to cobalamin (vitamin B12) – announced plans to initiate clinical trials; however, again no data have been presented so far. Nevertheless, a considerable number of papers about OI were published in pharmaceutical journals in the last year. We shall have to see how many, if any, of these approaches make it to clinical development.

Rather different is the story of buccal insulin. For a number of years one company was quite prominent in the world of ARIA – the Canadian company Generex with their buccal insulin development. The company was present at many scientific congresses with a relatively large booth and has hired a number of renowned diabetologists. For a while the company also sent out press releases at weekly intervals that gave the impression that the product is highly successfully in a number of markets such as Ecuador and India. Also the start of a phase 3 study some time ago signals that this company was quite confident in the success of their development. Nevertheless, after a period of silence (accompanied by the lack of any publications and press releases . . .) it has become obvious that the fate of the development is uncertain. A new management is trying to sort out what the true level of development is and whether there is chance to develop this to a product also for highly regulated markets. It will be interesting to see how the story continues in the next few years.

A dose range finding study of novel oral insulin (IN-105) under fed conditions in type 2 diabetes mellitus subjects

Khedkar A[1], Iyer H[1], Anand A[1], Verma M[1], Krishnamurthy S[1], Savale S[2], Atignal A[2]

[1] Research and Development, Biocon Limited, Bangalore, India, and
[2] Clinigene International Limited, Bangalore, India

Diabetes, Obesity Metab 2010; 12: 659–64

Background

To evaluate the dose–response of an OI formulation (IN-105 tablets) and explore a possible therapeutic window in patients with type 2 diabetes (T2D) poorly controlled on oral antidiabetic agents.

Methods

Primary endpoints were evaluation of the effect of sequential ascending doses of IN-105 on the plasma glucose levels under fed conditions. All participants received, sequentially, matching placebo or 10, 15, 20 and 30 mg IN-105 tablets in five consecutive periods 20 min prior to a meal in all periods. Plasma insulin, C-peptide and glucose levels were measured up to 180 min from the time of dosing. Comparison between the IN-105 tablets and placebo in the changes in postprandial glycaemic excursions at 120 min was done.

Results

Decreases in plasma glucose from baseline (mean $\pm$ SD) at 140 min (2 h postprandial) were 94.8 ± 22.3, 79.5 ± 43.0, 70.7 ± 35.7, 63.5 ± 42.8 and 53.1 ± 47.3 mg/dl, respectively, and exhibited a linear dose–response. The maximal plasma insulin levels were observed to be 51 ± 26 mU/l for placebo, 100 ± 67 with 10 mg IN-105, 178 ± 150 with 15 mg IN-105, 246 ± 245 with 20 mg IN-105 and 353 ± 279 mU/l with 30 mg of IN-105.

Conclusions

This OI formulation is absorbed in a dose-proportional relationship and circulating C-peptide levels were suppressed in proportion to the IN-105 exposure. The 2-h postprandial glycaemic excursion was in a dose-proportional reduction in the relationship. The OI formulation seems to have a wide therapeutic window as no clinical hypoglycaemia was observed at any of the doses studied.

COMMENT

This clinical-experimental study investigated in 18 subjects with T2D the pharmacokinetic and pharmacodynamic properties of the only OI formulation that is in a later stage of clinical development. A rapidly absorbable OI formulation that allows a good coverage of prandial insulin requirements in such patients would be of high clinical relevance. Not only might it enable a good control of postprandial glycaemic excursions, due to a reduced entering barrier, such a pain-free insulin therapeutic option might allow insulin therapy to be started at an earlier stage in many patients. This well performed study showed that tablet administration 20 min before a carbohydrate-rich meal led to a clear dose-dependent change in PK properties and also in postprandial glycaemic excursions. However, the drop in glycaemia was not much different with the three highest of four OI doses tested. Also the observed considerable inter-subject variability in insulin levels after OI application is of note. Adequately designed and performed studies addressing intra-individual variability are needed to evaluate the therapeutic relevance of OI.

INSULIN PENS

The first insulin pen was introduced into the marketplace by Novo Nordisk in 1985 (Novo Pen I). After more than 25 years we have to acknowledge that not many devices have revolutionised diabetes therapy as insulin pens did, probably with the exception of blood glucose monitors (15). In some countries/continents >75% of patients are using insulin pens nowadays. However, in other countries, like the USA, the market share is much lower, but with a clear increase also in recent years.

Reflecting their widespread usage today, insulin pens are the only way of insulin administration which has gained more attraction in the last few years when it comes to publications. Practically all of these publications were sponsored by one of the companies which have insulin pens in their portfolio. There is a certain feature war about pens (each company is promoting which property of their pen is better than that of the competitor, using scientific publications as ammunition); however, some people do believe that we are close to having the ideal insulin pen in the near future.

Randomised trial on the influence of the length of two insulin pen needles on glycaemic control and patient preference in obese patients with diabetes

Kreugel G, Keers JC, Kerstens MN, Wolffenbutte BHR

University Medical Center Groningen, University of Groningen, Groningen, The Netherlands

*Diabetes Technol Ther 2011; **13**: 737–41*

Background
To evaluate the influence of two different needle lengths on metabolic control and patient preference in obese patients with type 1 (T1D) and type 2 (T2D) diabetes.

Methods
This is a comparison of a multicentre, open-label crossover study of insulin pen needles with 5- and 8-mm lengths. Insulin-treated obese

patients ($n = 130$; body mass index 30 kg/m^2) with T1D and T2D were randomised, and 126 patients completed the study. Patients started using the 5-mm needle for 3 months and thereafter they switched to injecting insulin with the 8-mm needle for another 3 months, or vice versa. The endpoints were HbA1c, fructosamine and 1,5-anhydroglucitol, and self-reported side effects and patient preference.

Results

With respect to HbA1c, serum fructosamine, 1,5-anhydroglucitol, hypoglycaemic events, bruising and pain no within-group differences were observed. There was a small difference between needle lengths (5 mm, HbA1c 7.5 ± 0.9%; 8 mm, 7.6 ± 1.0%; p = 0.02). Patients reported less bleeding with the 5-mm needle (p = 0.04) and less insulin leakage from the skin with the 8-mm needle (p = 0.01). There were no significant differences in patient preference.

Conclusions

Use of a 5-mm needle led to a similar outcome as use of an 8-mm needle in obese patients with diabetes with respect to metabolic control, injection-related complaints or patient preference, and shorter needles can be used safely in this population.

COMMENT

Different lengths of pen needles are a hot topic (at least for some companies). Currently in Europe, 92% of adult patients on insulin treatment were using an insulin pen with a disposable needle, and 63% were using an 8-mm needle or longer. There were concerns that in overweight people shorter needles do not result in proper subcutaneous administration. However, recent studies have shown that the body mass index has only a small impact on skin thickness, but clearly a large impact on the thickness of the subcutaneous tissue layer. In this clinical study with a considerable sample size and an adequate study design a small but significant benefit of a shorter needle length on insulin action (measured by HbA1c when data of all subjects were pooled) could be shown in obese subjects. This means that also in obese subjects shorter needles can be used safely.

Performance of a new reusable insulin pen

Penfornis A

Department of Endocrinology – Metabolism and Diabetology – Nutrition, University of Franche-Comté, Besançon, France

*Diabetes Technol Ther 2011; **13**: 373–9*

Background

This was a multinational study that compared the simplicity of use and performance of the ClikSTAR insulin pen with other commonly used reusable pens based on participant and interviewer assessments.

Methods

In total 654 patients with diabetes were asked to demonstrate four pens consecutively – ClikSTAR, Lilly Luxura and NovoPen 3 and 4 – according to the instruction manuals. Assessment was performed by a rating from the participants and the interviewer. While the patients focused on the pen's ease of use, the interviewer considered the patients' difficulty in preparing and delivering a 40 U dose.

Results

Up to 24% of participants had T1D. Approximately 50% of participants had prior insulin pen experience. A higher proportion of patients, including those with dexterity or visual impairments, reported ClikSTAR as easier to use than other pens ($p < 0.05$). Patients assessed the ClikSTAR and NovoPen 4 as the most highly rated pens. The number of patients not requiring help in completing the tasks with ClikSTAR was rated as higher than, or similar to, that with the other pens.

Conclusions

One of the reusable insulin pens, the ClikSTAR was significantly easier to use, which, taken together with overall performance, meets the need of people with diabetes.

COMMENT

Comparison of widely used reusable insulin pens is of high importance. Clearly the question is which factors/features are regarded as important and which not. A stated above, each company clearly has an interest in having the most 'attractive' pen (see below). For different patient groups (depending on age, visual impairment etc.) pens might differ in their usability; most probably there is no pen 'that fits all patients'. Such an assessment is based on the assumption that all pens deliver the selected dose precisely, that no handling errors can take place etc. As with glucose meters where people tend to forget that the precision of glucose measurement is of higher importance than the colour of the cover or the size of the display, with each evaluation of an insulin pen the technical performance and safety should remain the most important criteria. The results of the evaluation of many of the parameters studied in this performance study differ only marginally between the pens studied, even if these differences are significant in some cases.

Correct use of a new reusable insulin injection pen by patients with diabetes: a design validation study

Schwartz S

Diabetes and Glandular Disease Research Associates, San Antonio, TX, USA

J Diabetes Science Technol 2010; **4***: 1229–35*

Aim

To evaluate whether individuals with diabetes can use the ClikSTAR pen, a novel reusable insulin pen for injecting long-acting insulin glargine or short-acting insulin glulisine, correctly.

Methods

This was an open-label, single-centre study in which patients with diabetes delivered three 40 U insulin doses after receiving training from a diabetes specialist (group A, $n = 256$; 68% females, 93% Hispanic ethnicity, 97% T2D, age 52 ± 11 years, diabetes duration 11 ± 7 years) or after self-training (group B, $n = 47$; demographic/baseline characteristics similar to group A but 70% had not previously used an injection pen). Administration of a dose of 75%–115% of the intended dose was considered successful. Adverse events and product technical complaints were recorded.

Results

Half of the patients in group A had prior experience in using insulin pen devices. All except one participant (99.6%) in group A successfully delivered three insulin doses. The lower one-tailed 95% confidence limit for the success rate (98.2%) was higher than the predefined target of 90%. Group B also showed success; 93.6% of participants successfully completed three dose deliveries.

Conclusions

This study successfully validated the ClikSTAR pen for use by patients with diabetes.

COMMENT

It is of interest to read the analysis paper for this publication (16). The authors of this comment highlight that the sample of patients studied should have covered a wider range of diabetes patients, particularly users who are visually impaired. For such patients, who are a large portion of all patients with diabetes, selecting the right dose and applying it correctly is a big hurdle. More such patients should be involved in the development of these medical devices at an early stage. This would generate a win–win situation: better products to meet the needs of a specific group of patients and a new market for the manufacturers. From my point of view (and in view of the small therapeutic window of insulin) it is obvious that each and every patient should participate in a good teaching and training programme prior to use of any insulin application device/start of insulin therapy. In the group of patients without adequate training 6.4% of the patients did not apply the correct dose (with a tendency to under-dosing). In view of the many insulin doses patients with diabetes have to apply, this is surely a much too high portion. It is also of note that 26% of the patients enrolled in this group were excluded due to extreme difficulty in using the ClikSTAR device. In addition, comparison of the two groups in the study was hampered by the massively different size of the two patient groups. It would have been of interest to see whether patients using a different pen (from a different manufacturer) would perform better or worse under the same conditions.

Do different body colours and labels of insulin pens enhance a patient's ability to correctly identify pens for injecting long-acting versus short-acting insulins?

Lefkowitz M

Lieberman Research Group, Great Neck, NY, USA

J Diabetes Science Technol 2011; 5: 136–49

Aim
To evaluate how successfully patients with diabetes are able to distinguish between pens of the same pen type containing rapid- and long-acting insulin formulations.

Methods
In all, 400 patients with diabetes in the USA were interviewed about using either a differentiated ($n = 100$) or undifferentiated ($n = 100$) SoloSTAR® (insulin glargine vs. insulin glulisine) or ($n = 200$) FlexPen® (insulin detemir vs. insulin aspart). A pair of each pen type was presented simultaneously, and participants were asked to identify the pen that they would use (1) to inject at lunch, (2) to inject once daily and (3) to inject at breakfast, and how they differentiate between pens. The pen containing the rapid-acting insulin analogue was then presented, and the patients were asked whether this was the correct pen to administer insulin once or thrice daily.

Results
More patients successfully identified the correct SoloSTAR pen across the tests vs. FlexPen, and the error rate was significantly lower. The most common reason for correct responses among all patients was colour (of the label/pen, according to pen type).

Conclusions

This handling study suggests that the insulin pen with full body colour enhances the patient's ability to differentiate between the pens for rapid- and long-acting insulin. This appears to be a notable improvement compared with the standard approach of differing label colour.

COMMENT

On first glance this paper reports an evaluation that might appear as being not relevant for a scientific journal. However, from a practical and safety point of view, it is crucial that patients with diabetes do not falsely select the insulin pen for prandial or basal insulin coverage. In reality many patients do not understand the differences between the insulin formulations and cannot memorise the names of the different insulin products they use correctly (this is the case with many of the pills patients take). We are lacking a good survey about the understanding and knowledge of patients with diabetes about insulin formulations, details of insulin therapy etc. One can assume that there will be considerable differences in the outcome of such a survey depending on the patient group considered (T1D vs. T2D, younger vs. elderly etc.). Therefore something that helps the patient to select the right insulin pen on first glance (it might be something simple like the colour or other elements of the pen) can be of significant importance for practical insulin therapy. Clearly confirmation of this statement requires larger studies under daily life conditions. Nevertheless, publication of this relatively small study by a well known author provides relevant hints also for the pen manufacturers for the design of future pens that enable unanimous detection of the right pen by patients with diabetes for a given therapeutic situation.

MISCELLANEOUS

The following two papers do not refer to new ways to deliver insulin in the strict sense; however, they report interesting results relevant for a successful insulin therapy.

A quantitative assessment of patient barriers to insulin

Casciano R[1], Malangone E[1], Ramachandran A[2], Gagliardino JJ[3]

[1] *Analytica International, New York, NY, USA,* [2] *India Diabetes Research Foundation, Dr A. Ramachandran's Diabetes Hospitals, Chennai, India, and* [3] *CENEXA (UNLP-CONICET), PAHO/WHO Collaborating Centre for Diabetes, National University of La Plata, La Plata, Buenos Aires, Argentina*

*Int J Clin Pract 2011; **65**: 408–14*

Aim

To assess diabetes treatment preferences with a focus on patient barriers to insulin treatment.

Methods

As part of the International Diabetes Management Practices Study (IDMPS) a questionnaire using indirect and direct methods was administered. Discrete choice modelling was used to assess how product attributes influence patients' preferences for diabetes treatment.

Results

The IDMPS questionnaire was administered to patients with diabetes in 18 countries ($n = 14{,}033$, 53% women, 85% with T2D). Administration (i.e. oral vs. injection) was a driver of preference across subgroups; patient preferences varied according to diabetes type; individuals with T2D assigned much higher relative importance to administration than those with T1D (30.9% vs. 5.0%; $p < 0.0001$). Patients with T2D treated with insulin put less importance on administration than insulin-naive T2D patients (3.1% vs. 47.5%; $p < 0.0001$). T2D patients who received diabetes education gave a priority to administration compared with those who did not (28.2% vs. 33.7%, respectively; $p < 0.0001$).

Conclusions

The insulin barriers perceived by patients with diabetes evolved with their disease experience. While administration was the primary preference driver for insulin-naive patients, patients were increasingly concerned with more clinically relevant barriers as they gained experience with insulin. The results obtained with this survey suggest that patients using insulin understand the importance of achieving an optimal balance between safety and efficacy.

> **COMMENT**
>
> The not unexpected results of this study show that treatment naive patients with diabetes have high barriers towards insulin. An interesting introduction into the results of this study can be found on the internet (http://www.youtube.com/watch?v=vHS4s0Ohqw4).

Survey of insulin site rotation in youth with type 1 diabetes mellitus

Patton SR[1,2], Eder S[1,2], Schwab J[2,3], Sisson CM[2,3]

[1] *Division of Child Behavioral Health, C.S. Mott Children's Hospital, Ann Arbor, MI, USA,* [2] *University of Michigan Medical School, Department of Pediatrics, Ann*

Arbor, MI, USA, and [3]*Division of Endocrinology, C.S. Mott Children's Hospital, Ann Arbor, MI, USA*

J Pediatr Health Care 2010; **24**: *365–71*

Background

Injection site rotation is known to be helpful in preventing lipodystrophy in patients with T1D. However, the question is, what do patients do in reality? The number of injection/infusion sites used by kids with T1D and their perceived barriers to insulin site rotation were evaluated.

Methods

Kids with T1D ($n = 201$) completed a 24-item survey about injection site rotation practices during a routine diabetes appointment.

Results

Fifteen per cent of the kids reported using at least four distinct sites in their rotation plan, while 22% reported using only one site. A negative correlation was found between number of sites used and the number of perceived barriers endorsed by kids on multiple daily injections. Fear of pain was the most common barrier stated.

Conclusions

In daily life many kids with T1D appear not to adhere to an adequate site rotation plan. During diabetes appointments regular assessment of insulin sites is needed. Also counselling regarding adequate site rotation should be part of regular practice.

COMMENT

Patients with diabetes (or they parents) receive many recommendations when participating in diabetes teaching and training programmes. It is interesting to see how limited the adherence of patients to such recommendations is, at least when it comes to injection site rotation. It appears as if in daily life patients most often inject the insulin into sites that are easily accessible. Another key aspect for patients with diabetes is discretion when applying insulin. At the end this results in the fact that certain skin areas (more precisely the subcutaneous tissue beneath the skin) are more prone to exhibit changes in structure (lipohypertrophy in most cases). The impact of such changes in the structure of the subcutaneous tissue on insulin absorption is not well studied. Also our knowledge about the prevalence of lipohypertrophy is limited. Diabetologists and diabetes nurses should much more often touch the injection sites of their patients to make sure that they have no lipohypertrophy; quite often such changes in the subcutaneous tissue are not visible but they are palpable.

REFERENCES

1. Patton JS, Brain JD, Davies LA, Fiegel J, Gumbleton M, Kim KJ, Sakagami M, Vanbever R, Ehrhardt C. The particle has landed – characterizing the fate of inhaled pharmaceuticals. *J Aerosol Med Pulm Drug Deliv* 2010; **23**: S71–87

2. Zarogoulidis P, Papanas N, Kouliatsis G, Spyratos D, Zarogoulidis K, Maltezos E. Inhaled insulin: Too soon to be forgotten? *J Aerosol Med Pulm Drug Deliv* 2011; **24**: 213–23

3. Cassidy JP, Amin N, Marino M, Gotfried M, Meyer T, Sommerer K, Baughman RA. Insulin lung deposition and clearance following Technosphere® insulin inhalation powder administration. *Pharm Res* 2011; **28**: 2157–64

4. Neumiller JJ, Campbell RK, Wood LD. A review of inhaled Technosphere insulin. *Ann Pharmacother* 2010; **44**: 1231–9

5. Neumiller JJ, Campbell RK. Technosphere insulin: an inhaled prandial insulin product. *BioDrugs* 2010; **24**: 165–72

6. Rubin RR, Peyrot M. Factors associated with physician perceptions of and willingness to recommend inhaled insulin. *Curr Med Res Opin* 2011; **27**: 285–94

7. Peyrot M, Rubin RR. Perceived medication benefits and their association with interest in using inhaled insulin in type 2 diabetes: a model of patients' cognitive framework. *Patient Prefer Adherence* 2011; **5**: 255–65

8. Landersdorfer CB, Jusko WJ. Pharmacokinetic/pharmacodynamic modeling of glucose clamp effects of inhaled and subcutaneous insulin in healthy volunteers and diabetic patients. *Drug Metab Pharmacokinet* 2010; **25**: 418–29

9. Potocka E, Baughman RA, Derendorf H. Population pharmacokinetic model of human insulin following different routes of administration. *J Clin Pharmacol* 2011; **51**: 1015–24

10. Potocka E, Cassidy JP, Haworth P, Heuman D, van Marle S, Baughman RA Jr. Pharmacokinetic characterization of the novel pulmonary delivery excipient fumaryl diketopiperazine. *J Diabetes Sci Technol* 2010; **4**: 1164–73

11. Potocka E, Amin N, Cassidy J, Schwartz SL, Gray M, Richardson PC, Baughman RA. Insulin pharmacokinetics following dosing with Technosphere insulin in subjects with chronic obstructive pulmonary disease. *Curr Med Res Opin* 2010; **26**: 2347–53

12. van Alfen-van der Velden AA, Noordam C, de Galan BE, Hoorweg-Nijman JJ, Voorhoeve PG, Westerlaken C. Successful treatment of severe subcutaneous insulin resistance with inhaled insulin therapy. *Pediatr Diabetes* 2010; **11**: 380–2

13. Mastrandrea LD. A breath of life for inhaled insulin: severe subcutaneous insulin resistance as an indication? *Pediatr Diabetes* 2010; **11**: 377–9

14. Lasagna-Reeves CA, Clos AL, Midoro-Hiriuti T, Goldblum RM, Jackson GR, Kayed R. Inhaled insulin forms toxic pulmonary amyloid aggregates. *Endocrinology* 2010; **151**: 4717–24

15. Bailey T, Edelman SV. Insulin pen use for type 2 patients – a clinical perspective. *Diabetes Technol Ther* 2010; **12** (Suppl 1): S86–90

16. Uslan M, Blubaugh M. Analysis: including visually impaired participants in validation design studies of diabetes technology. *J Diabetes Sci Technol* 2010; **4**: 1236–7

CHAPTER 7

Using Health Information Technology to Prevent and Treat Diabetes

Neal Kaufman

UCLA Schools of Medicine and Public Health, Los Angeles, CA, USA

INTRODUCTION

Patients with diabetes often need a complex set of services and support ranging from glucose monitoring, insulin and other medication management, psychotherapy and social support, to physical activity promotion, nutrition counselling and more. To be successful, patients must not only understand their condition, but also obtain the skills and attitudes to set goals, solve problems, monitor outcomes and overcome barriers to action. Patients and clinicians need to work together so patients with diabetes can adopt and sustain the health-promoting behaviours so necessary to assure good outcomes. Information technology is transforming the way patients receive education and support and clinicians need to utilise these approaches to maximise their reach and effectiveness.

Providers are increasingly expected to coordinate care for a panel of patients who live with incurable chronic conditions such as diabetes. Clinicians will have to collaborate with their patients and focus on improving their behaviours, because treating diabetes and other chronic conditions requires more than medication. Providers will need to put emphasis on supporting patients in the ongoing process of adopting and sustaining health-promoting habits. Integrating these supports into a patient's therapeutic regimen presents challenges that need to be addressed through a variety of strategies. Regrettably, given the significant time constraints of a busy medical practice, healthcare providers often do not have the time to adequately support all aspects of an effective behaviour change intervention. That is where information technology can have some of its greatest impact.

Int J Clin Pract 2012; **66** (Suppl. 175): 36–44

This chapter will present papers in which information technology has been used to improve the quality of care for patients with diabetes, to enable clinicians to more effectively manage their patients and to help patients self-manage their diabetes.

Web-based depression treatment for type 1 and type 2 diabetic patients: a randomised, controlled trial

van Bastelaar KM[1,2], Pouwer F[3], Cuijpers P[2,4], Riper H[5], Snoek FJ[1,2]

[1] *Department of Medical Psychology, VU University Medical Center, Amsterdam, The Netherlands,* [2] *Institute for Health and Care Research (EMGO Institute), VU University Medical Center, Amsterdam, The Netherlands,* [3] *Department of Medical Psychology and Neuropsychology, and* [4] *Center of Research on Psychology in Somatic diseases (CoRPS), Tilburg University, Tilburg, The Netherlands, and* [5] *Department of Clinical Psychology, VU University, Amsterdam, The Netherlands, Netherlands Institute of Mental Health and Addiction (Trimbos), Utrecht, The Netherlands*

Diabetes Care 2011; 34: 320–5

Aims

This study was an attempt to determine whether an internet-based intervention could successfully use an approach proven effective in person [cognitive behaviour therapy (CBT), coping with depression, developed by Lewinsohn] to improve depression symptoms in depressed patients with type 1 (T1D) or type 2 (T2D) diabetes. Primary outcomes were depressive symptoms. Secondary outcomes were diabetes-specific emotional distress and glycaemic control.

Methods

A total of 255 adult patients with clinical depression were randomised into the web-based intervention or to a 12-week waiting list control group. Assessments in the intervention group were scheduled after the participant completed or stopped the intervention and 1 month later. The web-based programme contained eight consecutive lessons that provided written and spoken information and videos of depressed patients explaining how they learned from the course. Coaches (certified psychologists) provided standardised concise and constructive feedback on homework assignments in <3 days. The feedback was meant to help the patient understand and apply CBT skills in their daily lives. Patients on the waiting list completed assessments 8 and 12 weeks post randomisation and were provided access to the web-based intervention 12 weeks post randomisation.

Results

The web-based CBT intervention was effective in reducing depressive symptoms and reduced diabetes-specific emotional distress but had no beneficial effect on glycaemic control.

Conclusions

This study demonstrated that web-based CBT can effectively lessen depressive symptoms for patients with T1D and T2D. It also demonstrated that a theory and research based in-person intervention can be successfully transformed for delivery via the internet.

COMMENT

It is encouraging to see that clinicians, researchers and technologists are embracing the approach that takes lessons learned from the non-technology world (e.g. in-person interventions) and transforms these successful approaches into effective interventions. While somewhat discouraging, it is not surprising that no changes in diabetes control were found given the short length of the study. The next phase in the research agenda is to identify the characteristics of individuals who are most likely to benefit from this approach and to determine the cost-effectiveness of these types of interventions. This information will be key as clinicians try to bring technology-enabled interventions to the widest and most appropriate audience possible.

An online community improves adherence in an internet-mediated walking programme. Part 1: Results of a randomised controlled trial

Richardson CR[1,2], Buis LR[3], Janney AW[1], Goodrich DE[2], Sen A[1,4], Hess ML[1], Mehari KS[1], Fortlage LA[1], Resnick PJ[5], Zikmund-Fisher BJ[6,7], Strecher VJ[8], Piette JD[2,6,9]

[1] *Department of Family Medicine, University of Michigan, Ann Arbor, MI, USA,* [2] *Health Services Research and Development Center for Clinical Management Research, Veterans Affairs Ann Arbor Healthcare System, Ann Arbor, MI, USA,* [3] *College of Nursing – Adult Health, Wayne State University, Detroit, MI, USA,* [4] *Department of Statistics, University of Michigan, Ann Arbor, MI, USA,* [5] *School of Information, University of Michigan, Ann Arbor, MI, USA,* [6] *Department of Internal Medicine, University of Michigan, Ann Arbor, MI, USA,* [7] *Department of Health Behaviour and Health Education, University of Michigan, Ann Arbor, MI, USA,* [8] *Center for Health Communications Research, University of Michigan, Ann Arbor, MI, USA, and* [9] *Michigan Diabetes Research and Training Center, University of Michigan, Ann Arbor, MI, USA*

J Med Internet Res 2010; **12***: e71*

Aims

This randomised control trial attempted to determine if providing web-based access to other overweight adults attempting to increase their physical activity would enhance the effectiveness of a 16-week web-based physical activity promotion programme.

Methods

Sedentary adults with at least one of body mass index ≥ 25 kg/mm^2, T2D or coronary artery disease were enrolled in a 16-week web-enabled intervention that provided four intervention components: uploading pedometers, step-count feedback, individually assigned and gradually incrementing step-count goals, and individually tailored motivational messages. Participants were instructed to wear their pedometers every day while awake and to log in at least once a week to view tailored messages and updated goals. Study subjects were randomised to have no additional online elements or access to a web-based community that focused on providing social support, encouraging social modelling of successes, and facilitating use of non-community components of the intervention. To promote sociability, participants were encouraged to post self-introductions, and research staff posted their own self-introductions. In addition, research staff posted open-ended questions encouraging participants to post messages modelling self-regulation strategies such as overcoming barriers and describing successes. Posts about pedometers, goals and graphs encouraged participants to pay attention to the non-online community components of the intervention. To generate more activity, contests were run with small rewards such as water bottles or bumper stickers for posting content. Assessments were done on all study subjects on entry and at the end of the intervention.

Results

A total of 324 subjects participated in the study; 70 were randomised to the activity website alone and 254 to the activity website plus the online community site. Both arms significantly increased their average daily steps between baseline and the end of the intervention period, but there were no significant differences in increase in step-counts between the two arms. The percentage of completers was 13% higher in the online community arm than the no online community arm (online community arm 79%, no online community arm 66%, p = 0.02). In addition, online community arm participants remained engaged in the programme longer than no online community arm participants [hazard ratio 0.47, 95% confidence interval (CI) 0.25–0.90, p = 0.02]. Participants with lower baseline social support posted more messages to the online community (p < 0.001) and viewed more posts (p < 0.001) than participants with higher baseline social support.

Conclusion

Adding online community features to an internet-mediated walking programme did not increase average daily step-counts but did reduce participant attrition. Participants with low baseline social support used the online community features more than those with high baseline social support. Thus, online communities may be a promising approach to reducing attrition from online health behaviour change interventions, particularly in populations with low social support. The authors suggest three possible mechanisms by which participation in an online community might impact programme attrition and step-counts.

1 *Increased social support*: Social support (defined as the structure and quality of social relationships) can improve health outcomes by improving adherence to healthy behaviours and by impacting emotions and mood.
2 *Social modelling*: The experiences of others, including the barriers they have overcome and the successes they have achieved, can serve as inspirational models. Reading the posts of others enables vicarious learning.
3 *Increased intervention website exposure*: Online communities can provide engaging and dynamic content that increases return visits and encourages use of non-online community components including self-regulation components such as goal setting, feedback and tailored motivational messages.

COMMENT

I chose this study to demonstrate that there are ways to thoughtfully investigate the impact of 'new technologies' on patient behaviours and outcomes. It is all the rage to add technology-enabled social networking to any intervention that moves...or gets patients to move. The real challenge is how to quickly study these innovations to see if the additional approach brings real value. This is made all the more difficult since whatever technology one studies is probably obsolete by the time the rigorous research study is completed and published. That is why we need to continue to increase our understanding of the core principles through which technology can have a positive impact on patient behaviours and outcomes.

Web-based interventions for the management of type 2 diabetes mellitus: a systematic review of recent evidence

Ramadas A[1], Quek KF[1], Chan CK[1], Oldenburg B[2]

[1] *School of Medicine and Health Sciences, Monash University Sunway Campus, Petaling Jaya, Malaysia, and* [2] *Department of Epidemiology and Preventive*

Medicine, Monash University Clayton Campus, Wellington Road, Clayton, VA, Australia

Int J Med Inform 2011; **80**: 389–405

Aims

The authors state that prior to this review it was known that (1) behavioural and self-monitoring interventions could assist T2D prevention and management effort; and (2) websites are a feasible medium for the delivery of behaviour interventions. The authors' aim was to analyse the state-of-the-evidence that web-based interventions can improve outcomes for patients with T2D.

Methods

A systematic literature review of English language papers published between 2000 and June 2010 was performed looking for papers (1) that describe exchange of information via the website between a healthcare provider and an individual with T2D; (2) that intervene in physical activity, nutrition, self-monitoring or weight loss; (3) that use a randomised controlled trial or quasi-experimental designs; (4) in which outcome measures include behaviour changes or biomarkers related to T2D.

Results

Twenty articles describing 13 different studies were found to meet the criteria and were the subject of this review. Constant tracking progress of participants, goal-setting, personalised coaching, interactive feedback and online peer support groups were some of the successful approaches which were applied in e-interventions to manage T2D. A strong theoretical background, use of other technologies and longer duration of intervention were proved to be successful strategies. As well, the use of other technologies such as mobile phones has been proved to improve compliance with an intervention.

Conclusion

Web-based interventions have demonstrated some level of favourable outcomes, provided they are further enhanced with proper e-research strategies.

COMMENT

This review furthers the conclusion that well designed and thoughtfully implemented interventions have the potential to generate long-term behaviour change and improve outcomes for patients with T2D. Not surprisingly, certain key elements associated with a positive impact are very similar to what has been shown to work when patients participate in face-to-face interventions.

Go figure…people are people no matter how they get their support. Technology is not going to change human nature. At its best it will make education and support more scalable and affordable for large numbers of patients.

Social cognitive determinants of nutrition and physical activity among web-health users enrolling in an online intervention: the influence of social support, self-efficacy, outcome expectations and self-regulation

Anderson-Bill ES[1], Winett RA[1], Wojcik JR[2]

[1]*Center for Research in Health Behaviour, Department of Psychology, Virginia Tech, Blacksburg, VA, USA, and* [2]*Exercise Science Program, Department of Physical Education, Sports and Human Performance, Winthrop University, Rock Hill, SC, USA*

J Med Internet Res 2011; 13: e28

Aims

This study attempts to increase the understanding of the characteristics of web-based users of a weight loss intervention to provide guidance regarding the development of effective, theory-based online behaviour change interventions. It focused on the influence of social support, self-efficacy, outcome expectations and self-regulation.

Methods

The demographic, behavioural and psychosocial characteristics of web-health users recruited for an online social cognitive theory (SCT) based nutrition, physical activity and weight gain prevention intervention, the Web-based Guide to Health (WB-GTH), were examined. Study subjects were directed to the WB-GTH site by advertisements through online social and professional networks and through print and online media. Participants were screened, consented and assessed with demographic, physical activity, psychosocial and food frequency questionnaires online (taking a total of about 1.25 h); they also kept a 7-day log of daily steps and minutes walked.

Results

From 4700 visits to the site, 963 web users consented to enrol in the study: 83% were female, mean age 44.4 years, 91% white, 61% college graduates; median annual household income was US$85,000. Daily step-counts were in the low active range and overall dietary measures were poor. The web-health users had good self-efficacy and outcome expectations for health behaviour change; however, they perceived little social support for making these changes and engaged in few self-regulatory behaviours. Perceived social support and use of self-regulatory behaviours were strong predictors of physical activity and nutrition behaviour. Web users' self-efficacy was also a good predictor of healthier levels of physical activity and dietary fat but not of fibre, fruits and vegetables. Social support and self-efficacy indirectly predicted behaviour through self-regulation, and social support had indirect effects through self-efficacy.

Conclusions

Results suggest web-health users visiting and participating in online health interventions will probably be middle-aged, well educated, upper middle class women whose detrimental health behaviours put them at risk of obesity, heart disease, some cancers and diabetes. The success of internet physical activity and nutrition interventions may depend on the extent to which they lead users to develop self-efficacy for behaviour change, and the extent to which these interventions help them garner social support for making changes. Success of these interventions may also depend on the extent to which they provide a platform for setting goals, planning, tracking and providing feedback on targeted behaviours.

COMMENT

This study of a self-selected population of users of a particular web-based programme demonstrated that, for educated, affluent, middle income, sedentary US women with poor nutrition habits, particular components can make a difference in outcomes. While this finding is of interest and perhaps helpful if one is building an intervention for the same target population, I included this paper more to show how research findings can be based on the specifics of a particular intervention. Of course the users of this web-based programme were of a particular demographic with particular needs generating unique conclusions. I assume that is the target population used in the creation and marketing of the programme. Unfortunately, from a logistics and cost-to-produce and implement perspective, every intervention needs to be created for a particular target population and ideally should be able to modify what the user experiences based on the user's characteristics (age, gender, ethnicity, readiness to change, psychological state, preferred style of learning, degree of social support etc.) and performance over time (met goals, specific outcomes obtained etc.).

Virtual reality and interactive digital game technology: new tools to address obesity and diabetes

Skip Rizzo A, Lange B, Suma EA, Bolas M

Institute for Creative Technologies, University of Southern California, Playa Vista, CA, USA

J Diabetes Sci Technol 2011; **5**: 256–64

Aims

This paper was an introduction to the field of clinical virtual reality and its ability to increase calorie expenditure as a way to help overweight individuals lose weight to improve health.

Methods

The authors present their personal opinions with reference to the virtual reality literature about the type, effectiveness and potential use of clinical virtual reality.

Results

The convergence of advances in virtual reality enabling technologies with a growing body of clinical research and experience has fuelled the evolution of the discipline of clinical virtual reality. This paper provides a brief overview of methods for producing and delivering virtual reality environments that can be accessed by users for a range of clinical health conditions. This includes interactive digital games and new forms of natural-movement-based interface devices (exergaming). Children using currently available exergames expend significantly more energy than sedentary activities (equivalent to a brisk walk). These activities currently do not reach the level of intensity that would match playing the actual sport, nor do they deliver the recommended daily amount of exercise for children.

Conclusions

These results provide some support for the use of digital exergames using the current state of technology as a complement to, rather than a replacement for, regular exercise. This may change in the future as new advances in novel full-body interaction systems for providing vigorous interaction with digital games are expected to drive the creation of engaging low-cost interactive game based applications designed to increase exercise participation in persons at risk for obesity.

COMMENT

See the end of the next paper for combined comments.

Integrative gaming: a framework for sustainable game-based diabetes management

Kahol K

Human Machine Symbiosis Laboratory, School of Biological and Health Systems Engineering, Center for Sustainable Health, BioDesign Institute, Arizona State University, Tempe, AZ, USA

*J Diabetes Sci Technol 2011; **5**: 293–300*

Aims

To highlight the opportunities for game-based diabetes management to help individuals adopt and sustain health programme behaviours and to describe an integrative gaming paradigm designed to combine multiple activities involving physical exercises and cognitive skills through a game-based storyline.

Methods

The authors review how games can address several unmet health and behavioural needs. Games can (1) address issues with compliance; (2) help address educational needs; (4) allow clinicians to keep track of patients through online monitoring of game play, scores etc.; (4) provide engaging environments to encourage exercise; and (5) be employed to encourage proper nutritional practices. The authors discuss previous work in each of these domains to identify the opportunities and challenges of employing games.

Results

Games can provide environments that seek a patient's attention, participation, motivation and retention, and offer dynamic adaptation. They provide a natural, easy and fun-to-use interface, seamlessly integrating recreation and disease management. A game's persuasive story acts as a motivational binder that enables a user to perform multiple activities such as running, cycling and problem solving. While performing the activities in the games, users wear sensors that can measure movement (accelerometers, gyrometers, magnetometers) and sense physiological measures (heart rate, oxygen saturation). These measures drive the game and are stored and analysed on a cloud computing platform.

A prototype integrative gaming system is described and design considerations are discussed.

Conclusions

Game-based diabetes management approaches are emerging as an effective method to help patients with diabetes adopt and sustain healthy behaviours. The reviewed system is highly configurable and allows researchers to build games for the system with ease and drive the games with different types of activities. The capabilities of the system allow for engaging and motivating the user for the long term. Clinicians can use the system to collect clinically relevant data in a seamless mode.

COMMENT

These two overview papers address similar issues and are included to give the reader a sense of what is about to become mainstream. All interventions – in person or technology-enabled – struggle with engaging users over time. People of all ages like to play games and to have exercise that is fun. Integrating gaming activities within a behaviour change intervention has the potential to transform the intervention. To be able to have these activities embedded within a theory-based and research-proven approach would presumably improve delivery of effective patient motivation and behaviour change and improve long-term outcomes. Stay tuned.

Review of Veterans Health Administration telemedicine interventions

Hill RD, Luptak MK, Rupper RW, Bair B, Peterson C, Dailey N, Hicken BL

Rural Health Resource Center, Veterans Administration Medical Center, Salt Lake City, UT, USA

*Am J Manag Care 2010; **16** (12 Suppl HIT): e302–10*

Aims

To describe the US Veterans Health Administration's (VHA) considerable experience with telemedicine to summarise their experience, identify outcomes and provide suggestions for other systems interested in providing telemedicine services.

Methods

The authors performed a comprehensive literature search and identified 19 exemplary peer-reviewed papers published between 2000 and 2009 of controlled, VHA-supported telemedicine intervention trials that focused on health outcomes.

Results

The VHA is the largest and most comprehensive managed healthcare system in the USA and includes approximately 150 medical centres and more than 900 outpatient clinics serving 5.1 million veterans nationwide. Among the many challenges facing the VHA is providing healthcare services to an increasingly diverse veteran population, many of whom are of advanced age, diagnosed with multiple disease conditions, and living in remote regions where transportation to VHA-facility-based clinics is difficult. Given the pressures on an infrastructure with finite – albeit still considerable – resources, for more than a decade the VHA has explored cost-effective healthcare delivery alternatives. These trials underscore the role of telemedicine in large managed healthcare organisations in support of (1) chronic disease management, (2) mental health service delivery through in-home monitoring and treatment and (3) interdisciplinary team functioning through electronic medical record information interchange. Telemedicine was found to be advantageous when ongoing monitoring of patient symptoms is needed, as in chronic disease care (e.g. for diabetes) or mental health treatment. Telemedicine appears to enhance patient access to healthcare professionals and provides quick access to patient medical information.

Conclusions

Since 2000, telemedicine has been a focus for VHA health service delivery funding. Telemedicine has been used to facilitate diagnosis, referral, monitoring, medical information interchange and intervention to offset higher costs associated with hard-to-access patients. The sustainability of telemedicine interventions for the broad spectrum of veteran patient issues and the ongoing technology training of patients and providers are challenges to telemedicine-delivered care.

COMMENT

Once again, the US Veterans Health Administration has demonstrated that it is one of the world's leaders in the effective use of technology to improve patient care and patient outcomes. Of course, the VHA is a massive organisation with extraordinary resources. Of course large bureaucracies are hard to change ... aren't we all? But what the VHA has been able to accomplish should give each of us encouragement – encouragement that, with the right political will, skilled and dedicated individuals can make a real difference especially when incentives are aligned and resources are made available.

Improved glycaemic control without hypoglycaemia in elderly diabetic patients using the ubiquitous healthcare service, a new medical information system

Lim S[1,2,3], Kang SM[1,2,3], Shin H[4], Lee HJ[1,5], Won Yoon J[1,2,3], Yu SH[6], Kim SY[1], Yoo SY[1], Jung HS[3], Park KS[3], Ryu JO[7], Jang HC[1,2,3]

[1]*Department of Medical Informatics, Seoul National University Bundang Hospital, Seongnam, Korea,* [2]*Department of Internal Medicine, Seoul National University Bundang Hospital, Seongnam, Korea,* [3]*Department of Internal Medicine, Seoul National University College of Medicine, Seoul, Korea,* [4]*Johns Hopkins Bloomberg School of Public Health, Baltimore, MD, USA,* [5]*Department of Radiology, Seoul National University Bundang Hospital, Seongnam, Korea,* [6]*Department of Internal Medicine, Hangang Sacred Heart Hospital, Seoul, Korea, and* [7]*Allmedicus Research Institute, Allmedicus Co. Ltd, Seoul, Korea*

*Diabetes Care 2011; **34**: 308–13*

Aims

To determine if elderly patients (>60 years old) with T2D will have improved outcomes while using a mobile phone based intervention.

Methods

The authors conducted a 6-month randomised, controlled clinical trial involving patients aged >60 years ($n = 144$). Participants were randomly assigned to receive routine care (control, $n = 48$), to the self-monitored blood glucose (SMBG, $n = 47$) group, or to the ubiquitous healthcare (u-healthcare) service group ($n = 49$). The u-healthcare system refers to an elderly-friendly, individualised medical service in which medical instructions are given through the patient's mobile phone. Patients receive a glucometer with a telephone-network-connected cradle that automatically transfers test results to a hospital-based server. Once the data are transferred to the server, an automated system, the Clinical Decision Support System (CDSS) rule engine, generates and sends patient-specific messages by mobile phone. The primary endpoint was the proportion of patients achieving A1c < 7% without hypoglycaemia at 6 months.

Results

After 6 months of follow-up, the mean A1c level was significantly decreased from 7.8% to 7.4% ($p < 0.001$) in the u-healthcare group and from 7.9% to 7.7% ($p = 0.020$) in the SMBG group, compared with 7.9% to 7.8% ($p = 0.274$) in the control group. The proportion of patients with A1c < 7% without hypoglycaemia was 30.6% in the u-healthcare

group, 23.4% in the SMBG group and 14.0% in the control group
(p < 0.05).

Conclusions

The CDSS-based u-healthcare service achieved better glycaemic control
with less hypoglycaemia than SMBG and routine care and may provide
effective and safe diabetes management in elderly patients with T2D.

COMMENT

See the combined comments at the end of the next paper.

Effect of mobile phone intervention for diabetes on glycaemic control: a meta-analysis

Liang X, Wang Q, Yang X, Cao J, Chen J, Mo X, Huang J, Wang L, Gu D

*Department of Evidence Based Medicine and Division of Population Genetics,
Cardiovascular Institute and Fu Wai Hospital, Chinese Academy of Medical
Sciences and Peking Union Medical College, Beijing, China*

*Diabet Med 2011; **28**: 455–63*

Aims

To assess the effect of mobile phone interventions on glycaemic control
in patients with diabetes.

Methods

The authors identified relevant papers from January 1990 through February 2010 in which the study (1) evaluated use of mobile phones for diabetes self-management; (2) reported mean values of pre-intervention
and post-intervention glycosylated haemoglobin (HbA1c) for each intervention group or the mean difference in HbA1c between intervention
groups; and (3) had one of the following study designs: randomised controlled trial, quasi-randomised trial (e.g. even- or odd-numbered medical records), controlled before–after trial or controlled crossover trial. The
authors conducted a systematic review and meta-analysis of the selected
papers to evaluate the effect of mobile phone use on glycaemic control in
diabetes self-management.

Results

A total of 22 trials were selected for the review. The mode of mobile phone intervention varied among the included trials with varying

degrees of use of the internet and in-person support in addition to texting (smart-phone use was not addressed). Contents of the mobile phone intervention were diverse with varying degrees of support provided for self-monitoring and transmitting blood glucose values, continuous education, reinforcement of diet, exercise and medication adjustment. Data of patients' self-monitoring of blood glucose, diet and medicine problems were transmitted daily or more often in 14 trials, weekly or more often in three trials, and with unspecified timing in four trials. Meta-analysis among 1657 participants showed that mobile phone interventions for diabetes self-management reduced HbA1c values by a mean of 0.5% over a median of 6 months follow-up duration. In subgroup analysis, 11 studies among T2D patients reported significantly greater reduction in HbA1c than studies among T1D patients (0.8% vs. 0.3%; p = 0.02). The effect of mobile phone intervention did not significantly differ by other participant characteristics or intervention strategies.

Conclusions

Results from the included trials provided strong evidence that mobile phone intervention led to statistically significant improvement in glycaemic control and self-management in diabetes care, especially for T2D patients.

COMMENT ON BOTH PAPERS

The first study showed that elderly individuals (since when is >60 elderly? I thought 60 is the new 50) show promising results. When a technology-enabled programme is designed for a specific target population – in this case patients older than 60 with T2D – it is much more likely to be effective. This is another study with the increasingly common conclusion that older people are quite capable of using technology for their own good.

While I am a fan of meta-analysis when the studies are actually comparable the only thing the studies had in common was the use of mobile phones as a delivery channel. This paper suffers from the challenge of mixing too many variables and too many completely different approaches to actually make a useful conclusion – even if it is one that we might want to find. I included this paper to demonstrate the current state-of-the art regarding the evidence surrounding mobile phone interventions and diabetes outcomes – not very good. This is completely understandable given the incredibly long time it takes to fund, plan, implement, analyse and publish a high quality research study. This is made all the more challenging by the rapid evolution of mobile technology – think smart web-enabled phones and thousands of smart-phone apps. While clinicians need good enough interventions for their patients, we also need to know that the approach used the guiding principles which have been shown to be effective – over time experiences tailored to the individual's characteristics and performance; support for goal setting, monitoring and tracking; getting and providing social support; being linked to, and receiving support from, a trusted therapeutic relationship. When those guiding principles are respected I believe the intervention is most likely to be effective.

The Diabeo software enabling individualised insulin dose adjustments combined with telemedicine support improves HbA1c in poorly controlled type 1 diabetic patients: a 6-month, randomised, open-label, parallel-group, multicentre trial (TeleDiab 1 Study)

Charpentier G[1], Benhamou PY[2], Dardari D[1], Clergeot A[3], Franc S[1], Schaepelynck-Belicar P[4], Catargi B[5], Melki V[6], Chaillous L[7], Farret A[8], Bosson JL[9], Penfornis A[3]; TeleDiab Study Group

[1] *Department of Diabetes and the Centre d'Etudes et de Recherche pour l'Intensification du Traitement du Diabète, Sud-Francilien Hospital, Corbeil-Essonnes, France,* [2] *Department of Endocrinology, University Hospital, Grenoble, France,* [3] *Department of Endocrinology, University Hospital, Besançon, France,* [4] *University Hospital Sainte Marguerite, Marseille, France,* [5] *Department of Endocrinology, CHU Bordeaux, Pessac, France,* [6] *Department of Diabetology, Toulouse Rangueil University Hospital, Toulouse, France,* [7] *Clinique d'Endocrinologie, Maladies Métaboliques et Nutrition, Institut du Thorax, Hôpital Laennec, Nantes, France,* [8] *Endocrinology Department, Centre Hospitalier Universitaire de Montpellier, Université de Montpellier, Montpellier, France, and* [9] *CIC-INSERM, Grenoble University Hospital, Grenoble, France*

Diabetes Care 2011; 34: 533–9

Aims

To demonstrate that the Diabeo software (a smart-phone that provides insulin adjustment advice via the internet) effectively enables individualised insulin dose adjustments and, with or without telemedicine support, significantly improves HbA1c in poorly controlled T1D patients.

Methods

Diabeo is a software uploaded onto smart-phones that works via an internet connection and provides the patient with (1) bolus calculators using validated algorithms, taking into account carbohydrate intake, pre-meal blood glucose and anticipated physical activity, (2) specific plasma glucose targets, (3) automatic algorithms for adjusting basal/bolus rates depending on glucose levels, and (4) data transmission to medical staff computers for analysis. In a 6-month open-label parallel-group, multicentre study, adult patients ($n = 180$) with T1D (>1 year), on a basal-bolus insulin regimen (>6 months), with HbA1c $\geq$ 8%, were randomised to usual quarterly follow-up, home use of a smart-phone recommending insulin doses with quarterly visits, or use of the smart-phone with short tele-consultations every 2 weeks but no clinic visit until the end of the study. The every 2-week tele-consultations consisted of web-based review of the participant's glucose values, diet and insulin treatment via automatically uploaded data from the smart-phone.

Results

Six-month mean HbA1c in the smart-phone plus telemedicine group (8.41%) was lower than in usual care group (9.10%; $p = 0.0019$). The smart-phone alone group displayed intermediate results (8.63%). The Diabeo system gave a 0.91% improvement in HbA1c over controls and a 0.67% reduction when used without tele-consultation. There was no difference in the frequency of hypoglycaemic episodes or in medical time spent for hospital or telephone consultations. However, patients in the usual care and the smart-phone alone group spent nearly 5 h more attending hospital visits than the smart-phone and tele-consultation group patients.

Conclusions

The Diabeo system, especially with additional tele-consultation, gives a substantial improvement to metabolic control in chronic, poorly controlled T1D patients without requiring more medical time and at a lower overall cost for the patient than usual care.

COMMENT

This study furthers the evidence base that patients are better able to self-manage their T1D when they are provided with real-time information and periodic access to a knowledgeable clinician. In this case using smart-phone technology was instrumental in providing patients with the just-in-time data and information needed to more effectively manage their blood sugars. This study also shows that helping patients change their behaviour is enhanced in the context of a therapeutic relationship. If that relationship can be facilitated by technology – in this case a website with relevant clinical information – clinicians can be not only more effective but at a lower overall cost.

Glycaemic control and health disparities in older ethnically diverse under-served adults with diabetes: five-year results from the Informatics for Diabetes Education and Telemedicine (IDEATel) study

Weinstock RS[1,2], Teresi JA[3,4,5], Goland R[4], Izquierdo R[1], Palmas W[4], Eimicke JP[3], Ebner S[4], Shea S[4]; IDEATel Consortium

[1] *SUNY Upstate Medical University, Syracuse, NY, USA,* [2] *Department of Veterans Affairs Medical Center, Syracuse, NY, USA,* [3] *Research Division, Hebrew Home at Riverdale, Riverdale, NY, USA,* [4] *Columbia University, New York, NY, USA, and* [5] *New York State Psychiatric Institute, New York, NY, USA*

*Diabetes Care 2011; **34**: 274–9*

Aims

To determine if ethnically diverse older adults with diabetes obtain different levels of benefit from a telemedicine intervention.

Methods

Informatics for Diabetes Education and Telemedicine (IDEATel) randomised between 2000 and 2007 Medicare beneficiaries with diabetes ($n = 1665$) to receive (1) home video visits with a diabetes educator and upload glucose levels every 4–6 weeks or (2) usual care. The home video visits consisted of self-management education, review of transmitted home blood glucose and blood pressure measurements, individualised goal setting, and access to educational web pages created by the American Diabetes Association. Annual measurements included body mass index, HbA1c (primary outcome) and completion of questionnaires (depression, social network, general health).

Results

Overall there was a reduction in HbA1c in the treatment compared to the usual care group. At baseline, HbA1c levels (mean ± SD) were 7.02 ± 1.25% in non-Hispanic whites ($n = 821$), 7.58 ± 1.78% in non-Hispanic blacks ($n = 248$) and 7.79 ± 1.68% in Hispanics ($n = 585$). Hispanics had the highest baseline HbA1c levels and showed the greatest improvement in the intervention but, unlike non-Hispanic whites, Hispanics did not achieve HbA1c levels <7.0% at 5 years. Over time, lower HbA1c levels were associated with more glucose uploads ($p = 0.02$) and female gender ($p = 0.002$). Blacks, Hispanics and insulin-users had higher HbA1c levels than non-Hispanic whites ($p < 0.0001$). Body mass index was not associated with HbA1c levels. Blacks and Hispanics had significantly fewer uploads than non-Hispanic whites over time.

Conclusions

Racial/ethnic differences were observed in this cohort of under-served older adults with diabetes. The IDEATel telemedicine intervention was associated with improvement in glycaemic control, particularly in Hispanics, who had the highest baseline HbA1c levels, suggesting that telemedicine has the potential to help reduce differences in diabetes management and improve outcomes.

COMMENT

It is always encouraging to see long-held but inaccurate biases proven most likely to be wrong. This study was able help dispel two myths in one: that older adults (1) will not do well with any intervention other than in-person encounter and (2) cannot, or will not, successfully use technology to improve their health. This particular study, completed in 2007, used what is now nearly obsolete technology. One can only imagine what we might find if the study were repeated with new and emerging approaches such as web-enabled mobile devices, automatic ways to monitor and collect biological information (think glucose sensors, accelerometers etc.) and methods to assess a patient's well-being and status frequently and easily (so-called ecological momentary assessment). The future is now – let's go after it.

Impact of electronic health record clinical decision support on diabetes care: a randomised trial

O'Connor PJ[1], Sperl-Hillen JM[1], Rush WA[1], Johnson PE[2], Amundson GH[1], Asche SE[1], Ekstrom HL[1], Gilmer TP[3]

[1] *HealthPartners Research Foundation and HealthPartners Medical Group, Minneapolis, MN, USA,* [2] *Carlson School of Management, University of Minnesota, Minneapolis, MN, USA, and* [3] *University of California at San Diego, San Diego, CA, USA*

*Ann Fam Med 2011; **9**: 12–21*

Aims

To assess the impact of an electronic health record based, clinician facing, diabetes clinical decision support system on the outcomes of patients with T2D.

Methods

The authors conducted a clinic-randomised trial from October 2006 to May 2007 in Minnesota. Patients were randomised either to receive or not to receive an electronic health record (EHR) based clinical decision support system (Diabetes Wizard) designed to improve care for those patients whose HbA1c, blood pressure or low-density lipoprotein cholesterol levels were higher than goal at any office visit. Diabetes Wizard provides recommendations in the following categories and suggests (1) specific changes in medications for patients not at treatment goals; (2) changes in treatment for patients with contraindications to existing treatments, or being treated with potentially risky drug combinations; (3) obtaining overdue laboratory tests; and (4) short follow-up intervals for patients not at goal.

Results

Included in the study were 11 clinics (six intervention, five control) with 41 consenting primary care physicians and the physicians' 2556 patients with diabetes. The intervention group physicians used the HER based decision support system at 62.6% of all office visits made by adults with diabetes. The intervention group diabetes patients had significantly better HbA1c (intervention effect −0.26%; 95% CI −0.06% to −0.47%; p = 0.01), better maintenance of systolic blood pressure control (80.2% vs. 75.1%, p = 0.03) and borderline better maintenance of diastolic blood pressure control (85.6% vs. 81.7%, p = 0.07), but not improved low-density lipoprotein cholesterol levels (p = 0.62) than patients of physicians randomised to the control arm of the study. Among intervention group physicians, 94% were satisfied or very satisfied with the intervention, and moderate use of the support system persisted for more than 1 year after feedback and incentives to encourage its use were discontinued.

Conclusions

EHR based diabetes clinical decision support significantly improved glucose control and some aspects of blood pressure control in adults with T2D.

COMMENT

This paper addresses a very critical area – how to improve the quality of care provided to patients with diabetes. Use of EHRs shows great promise but they will not reach nearly their potential if they are not coupled with (1) decision support as described in this paper for a range of clinicians; (2) ways to increase the efficiency and effectiveness of the team approach (including coordinating the variety of specialists); (3) ways for the patient to more actively participate in his or her own medical care; and (4) technology-enabled support that helps a patient self-manage his or her diabetes. Then we shall really see some tremendous improvements in outcomes.

TeleHealth improves diabetes self-management in an under-served community: diabetes TeleCare

Davis RM[1], Hitch AD[2], Salaam MM[2], Herman WH[3], Zimmer-Galler IE[4], Mayer-Davis EJ[5]

[1] *Department of Ophthalmology, University of North Carolina, Chapel Hill, NC, USA,* [2] *Department of Epidemiology and Biostatistics, Norman J. Arnold School of Public Health, University of South Carolina, Columbia, SC, USA,* [3] *Department of Internal Medicine, University of Michigan, Ann Arbor, MI, USA,* [4] *Wilmer Eye Institute, Johns Hopkins University Hospital, Baltimore, MD, and* [5] *Department of Nutrition, Gillings School of Global Public Health, University of North Carolina, Chapel Hill, NC, USA*

Diabetes Care 2010; **33***: 1712–7*

Aims

To evaluate a comprehensive diabetes self-management education (DSME) intervention delivered via telehealth (Diabetes TeleCare) on outcomes for adult patients with diabetes from an under-served community.

Methods

The authors conducted a 1-year randomised clinical trial of Diabetes TeleCare, administered by a dietitian and nurse/certified diabetes educator (CDE) in the setting of a federally qualified health centre in rural South Carolina. Diabetes TeleCare is a 12-month DSME intervention delivered via telehealth with 13 sessions, three individualised and 10 groups. The session sequentially addressed the following issues: welcome and healthy eating, goal setting, start stepping, be a food detective, know your medicines, shop smart, stick with it: positive thinking, foot care basic and know your numbers, healthy eating out, stress management, keeping well and healthy, community resources and social support, putting it all together.

Results

Individuals were randomised to the intervention ($n = 85$) or to usual care ($n = 80$). Results showed a significant reduction in HbA1c in the Diabetes TeleCare group from baseline to 6 and 12 months (9.4, 8.3 and 8.2, respectively) compared with usual care (8.8, 8.6 and 8.6, respectively). Low-density lipoprotein cholesterol was reduced at 12 months in the Diabetes TeleCare group compared with usual care. Although not part of the original study design, HbA1c was reduced from baseline to 12 and 24 months in the Diabetes TeleCare group (9.2, 7.4 and 7.6, respectively) compared with usual care (8.7, 8.1 and 8.1, respectively) in a *post hoc* analysis of a subset of the randomised sample who completed a 24-month follow-up visit.

Conclusions

Telehealth effectively created access to successfully conduct a 1-year re- mote DSME by a nurse CDE and dietitian that improved metabolic con- trol and reduced cardiovascular risk in an ethnically diverse and rural population. Factors which may have been related to the success of the intervention include high participant retention, modification of materials to be culturally sensitive, coordinating administrative functions with the primary care centres, and successful personalised interactions during the group sessions enabled by video conferencing.

COMMENTS

This well done and thoughtful programme successfully overcame some of the often insurmountable barriers to effectively support patients self-managing their diabetes. This is all the more impressive when the population is under- served and in this case rural. As in nearly all interventions, it is impossi- ble to know which components of the approach were the most impactful. My assumption is that adding technology-enabled social networking's abil- ity to provide social support would add much to these types of interven- tions, especially during the maintenance phase and after the programme is completed.

The Karlsburg Diabetes Management System: translation from research to e-health application

Salzsieder E, Augstein P

Institute of Diabetes Gerhardt Katsch Karlsburg, Karlsburg, Germany

J Diabetes Sci Technol 2011; 5: 13–22

Aims

To evaluate the acceptance, efficiency and cost-effectiveness of telemedicine-assisted personalised decision support (PDS) for physicians in routine outpatient diabetes care.

Methods

The authors did a retrospective analysis of data from adult patients with T2D who used or did not use the Diabetiva® programme of the German health insurance company BKK Taunus. KADIS® is part of the Diabetiva programme and was developed to improve the quality and cost-effectiveness of diabetes care and management for patients with T1D or T2D. KADIS is derived from the Karlsburg model of glucose–insulin interactions. It generates an *in silico* copy of the individual metabolic profile of a given patient (a personalised 'metabolic fingerprint') on the computer and allows testing of different therapeutic measures by interactive *in silico* simulation procedures aimed at quickly and safely identifying a regimen that may provide individually optimal glucose control. The results of the simulation procedure are summarised as patient-focused PDS for the responsible physicians. For implementation of KADIS-based PDS into routine diabetes care, the program is combined with continuous glucose monitoring (CGM) and a telemedicine-based communication and information platform (Diabetiva). Diabetiva offers telemedicine-based outpatient healthcare in combination with PDS generated by the Karlsburg Diabetes Management System, KADIS®. The analysis was based on data from the first year of running KADIS-based PDS in routine diabetes care. Participants were insured persons diagnosed with diabetes and cardiovascular diseases. For final analysis, patients were grouped retrospectively as users or non-users according to physician acceptance or not (based on questionnaires) of the KADIS-based PDS.

Results

A total of 538 patients participated for more than 1 year in the Diabetiva programme. Of these patients, 289 had complete data sets (two continuous glucose monitoring measurements, two or more haemoglobin HbA1c values, and a signed questionnaire) and were included in the final data analysis. According to the questionnaires completed by the participating physicians, there was an overall acceptance rate of approximately 74% (214/289). The acceptance of PDS was clearly related to HbA1c values at baseline. The highest acceptance rates were found for patients with baseline HbA1c values above 7.5% and the lowest for patients with baseline HbA1c values between 6.5% and 7.0%. If KADIS-based PDS was accepted, HbA1c decreased by 0.4% (7.1% to 6.7%). In contrast, rejection of KADIS-based PDS resulted in an HbA1c increase of 0.5% (6.8% to 7.3%). The insurance company revealed an annual cost reduction of about 900 € per participant in the Diabetiva programme.

Conclusions

KADIS-based PDS in combination with telemedicine has high potential to improve the outcome of routine outpatient diabetes care.

COMMENT

This study addressed the important issue of providing sophisticated computer modelling of patient diabetes control coupled with evidence-based support to clinicians so they can help patients better manage their diabetes. This is an example of an important step forward in that it can help clinicians do their jobs better. However, to make real and lasting changes in outcomes clinicians must support patients so they can make the day-to-day (and moment-to-moment) decisions patients with diabetes need to make all the time. Patients need the ability to get help with the 'micro decisions' they make. These decisions are about little things a patient needs to do, not one of which is really critical but the sum of which determine a patient's outcome. The capacity for new technologies to give such information and support will revolutionise the ways patients get the education and help they need to succeed on their own.

Effect of web-based lifestyle modification on weight control: a meta-analysis

Kodama S[1], Saito K[1], Tanaka S[2], Horikawa C[1], Fujiwara K[1], Hirasawa R[1], Yachi Y[1], Iida KT[3], Shimano H[1], Ohashi Y[4], Yamada N[1], Sone H[1]

[1] *Department of Internal Medicine, University of Tsukuba Institute of Clinical Medicine, Ibaraki, Japan,* [2] *Department of Clinical Trial, Design and Management, Translational Research Center, Kyoto University Hospital, Kyoto, Japan,* [3] *Department of Lifestyle Medicine, Ochanomizu University, Tokyo, Japan, and* [4] *Department of Biostatistic, Epidemiology and Preventive Health Sciences, University of Tokyo, Tokyo, Japan*

Int J Obes (Lond) 2011 Jun 21; doi: 10.1038/ijo.2011.121 [Epub ahead of print]

Aims

To systematically review the weight loss or maintenance effect of the internet component in obesity treatment.

Methods

The authors did a systematic literature search to identify studies published from 1980 through April 2011 which investigated the effect of web-based individualised advice on lifestyle modification on weight loss. Studies were included if (1) they were randomised controlled trials using a parallel design; (2) all participants were adults who were designated as overweight or obese by the study-specific definition; (3) they consisted of a web-user experimental group and non-web-user control group; (4) the intervention included controlling dietary intake and increasing physical activity; (5) the aim of using the internet was initial weight loss or weight maintenance; and (6) the effect was assessed by absolute body-weight change. The authors completed a meta-analysis of the selected papers. Weight changes in the experimental group in comparison with the control group were pooled with a random-effects model.

Results

A total of 23 studies comprising 8697 participants were included. Over-all, using the internet had a modest but significant additional weight loss effect compared with non-web-user control groups (-0.68 kg, $p = 0.03$). In comparison with the control group, stratified analysis indicated that using the internet as an adjunct to obesity care was effective (-1.00 kg, $p < 0.001$), but that using it as a substitute for face-to-face support was unfavourable ($+1.27$ kg, $p = 0.01$). An additional effect on weight control was observed when the aim of using the internet was initial weight loss (-1.01 kg, $p = 0.03$), but was not observed when the aim was weight maintenance ($+0.68$ kg, $p = 0.26$). The relative effect was diminished with longer educational periods (p trend $= 0.04$) and was insignificant (-0.20 kg, $p = 0.75$) in studies with educational periods of 12 months or more.

Conclusions

The meta-analysis indicated that the internet component in obesity treatment programmes has a modest effect on weight control. However, the effect was inconsistent, largely depending on the type of usage of the internet or the period of its use. The analyses indicated that those using the internet as a substitute for face-to-face support experienced a smaller weight loss than the control group. Another finding was that the web-based programmes did not have a significant additional weight loss effect unless their use was combined with face-to-face support. These results suggest that an in-person approach is superior to a technology-based approach from the viewpoint of the amount of weight loss; if used, an internet programme needs to include the component of a face-to-face programme for participants to achieve weight loss. It is known that social support is one of the important aspects of behavioural obesity treatment and is associated with better weight loss outcomes. One supposition for the superiority of face-to-face treatment is derived from the perception that the participants are supported by many staff members, as has been suggested by a previous study. It was reported that some participants felt uncomfortable using the internet even when compliance in using the internet for weight loss was maintained. Another supposition is that this feeling of discomfort could cause participants to lose enthusiasm for weight loss and negatively influence the effectiveness of the internet for this purpose.

> **COMMENT**
>
> It is encouraging that those who used the internet had some increased weight loss. Of more interest is the authors' conclusion that those who also received in-person support lost more weight than those who did not receive in-person support. This conclusion, if confirmed in prospective studies, would be important since it would modify how interventions are built and increase the cost to use technology-enabled interventions. I suspect that the answer will not be so clear. Most probably we will find that some interventions, when properly designed and implemented, can have significant impacts even without the addition of in-person components.

SUMMARY AND COMMENTS

Patients with diabetes need a complex set of services and supports. This chapter presented a cross-section of the year's publications regarding how information technology can help patients can get the services and supports they need to prevent or manage their diabetes. One of the key themes that emerges from these papers (and from my own experience) is that the challenge of integrating the array of services and supports into the diabetes regimen can be successfully overcome through *self-management support interventions that are clinically linked and technology-enabled*.

Why self-management support? A large proportion of the prevention and treatment of diabetes is dependent on the knowledge, attitudes, skills and behaviours of the individual, and providing education and needed support is so important in getting good outcomes.

Why interventions? Theory-based, evidence-proven, long-term, longitudinal programmes that are designed for each patient based on his or her unique characteristics, changing needs and performance over time are most likely to get the desired results.

Why clinically linked? Patients respond best and are more likely to adopt new behaviours when the approach is in the context of a trusted therapeutic relationship and within an effective medical care system.

Why technology-enabled? Capitalising on the amazing power of the ever-improving information technology landscape leads to the delivery of cost-effective, scalable, engaging and holistic solutions to complex clinical challenges such as the management of diabetes.

The future for these types of interventions is uncertain. What is known is that self-management education and support can change behaviours and when technology is used appropriately it can improve outcomes. Regardless of the structure of these interventions there are a core set of elements that need to be included in any intervention to maximise the effect. They include approaches to identify patients, encourage programme participation, assess baseline status, provide teaching and learning, set goals, motivate toward goal attainment, measure results towards goals, receive and provide social support, find needed help, provide coaching support.

Since the complexity of healthcare settings makes implementation challenging, there need to be efforts to understand how to implement these approaches in diverse clinical settings. One key issue is that clinicians need to be prepared for changes in their education and support roles. The cost to develop, implement and test these types of interventions is considerable, but once they are ready to go to scale the cost to bring them to large numbers of people is relatively low per patient. What is needed is the capital to build them and that will be available if there are ways to pay for an intervention once it is proven effective. Time will tell if the healthcare systems of the world will catch up to these innovative approaches and provide the financial coverage needed to be able to serve those who need education and support to improve diabetes outcomes.

CHAPTER 8

Technology and Pregnancy

Lois Jovanovic[1], Nicole A. Sitkin[1], Jennifer K. Beckerman[1] and Moshe Hod[2]

[1] Sansum Diabetes Research Institute, Santa Barbara, CA, USA
[2] Helen Schneider Hospital for Women, Rabin Medical Center, Petah Tikva, Israel

INTRODUCTION

Diabetes mellitus is a global epidemic that poses a host of health complications and life-long challenges. Some diabetes-associated complications include heart disease, stroke, blindness, kidney disease, neuropathy, amputation and premature death. Patients with diabetes also face the economic burdens associated with additional healthcare costs.

Women who become diabetic predispose their offspring to a range of health related complications associated with the disease. Current statistics reveal that 2%–10% of pregnant women develop gestational diabetes; however, scientists see a rapidly increasing trend and the newest diagnostic criteria project that 18% of pregnant women will develop gestational diabetes (1). The increased prevalence of diabetes indicates a bleak outlook for the health of future generations. However, first trimester diagnosis and treatment can minimise the effects of diabetes for both mother and child.

Over 65 papers – published from July 2010 to June 2011 – were reviewed during the compilation of this chapter. Ten papers were selected based on their contribution and relevance to the growing field of diabetes research. These papers illuminate the potential for utilising innovative technology and devices in order to treat gestational diabetes and to minimise the potential for diabetes onset during and after pregnancy.

Int J Clin Pract 2012; **66** (Suppl. 175): 45–51

Prediction of macrosomia at birth in type 1 and 2 diabetic pregnancies with biomarkers of early placentation

Kuc S[1,2], Wortelboer EJ[2], Koster MPH[1,2], de Valk HW[2,3], Schielen PCJI[1], Visser GHA[2]

[1] *Laboratory for Infectious Diseases and Screening, National Institute for Public Health and the Environment, Bilthoven, The Netherlands,* [2] *Department of Obstetrics, Wilhelmina Children's Hospital, University Medical Centre Utrecht, Utrecht, The Netherlands, and* [3] *Department of Internal Medicine, University Medical Centre Utrecht, Utrecht, The Netherlands*

BJOG 2011; **118***: 748–54*

Objective

The authors intended to explore the contribution of early placentation to the later development of macrosomia in the pregnancies of women with pre-gestational diabetes mellitus (PGDM). To this end, they measured the values of placental biomarkers previously associated with macrosomia (PAPP-A, fβ-hCG, ADAM12, PP13, P1GF and nuchal translucency) to determine their ability to predict the subsequent occurrence of neonatal macrosomia.

Methods

Through a national Trisomy 21 screening campaign conducted by the Dutch National Institute for Public Health and the Environment, serum samples were collected from women at 8–14 weeks' gestation. The samples were tested at the time of collection for PAPP-A and fβ-hCG, and trained sonographers using standardised techniques recorded fetal nuchal translucency and crown to rump length. Pregnancy outcomes, such as pregnancy complications, and neonate gender and weight were later recorded. Preserved serum samples identified as having originated from a woman with pre-gestational diabetes (for this study, a woman registered as receiving insulin in the first trimester) were retrieved from storage and tested for concentrations of PP13, P1GF and ADAM12 using automated time-resolved fluorescence (autoDELFIA or DELFIA Xpress; Perkin Elmer, Turku, Finland). Each PGDM serum sample was matched by gestational age at sampling, maternal weight, maternal age and sample date with a control serum sample that was subjected to the same testing. Serum marker levels were then expressed in terms of multiples of the gestation-specific normal medians (MoMs). Macrosomia was indicated by a birthweight greater than the 90th percentile. Percentiles were established by using the mean of the birthweight z-scores calculated using the Dutch Perinatal registry as weight for gestational age at the 50th centile.

Results

In comparison with the control group, the PGDM group had both a higher median birthweight centile (89 vs. 72, p $<$ 0.001) and a higher incidence of macrosomia (42.6% vs.18.3%, p $<$ 0.0001), concomitant with a younger gestational age at delivery. The median ADAM12 MoM was the only placental marker significantly lowered in the PGDM group in comparison with the control group (p $=$ 0.007). The median MoMs of PAPP-A and ADAM12 in the PGDM non-macrosomic subgroup were significantly lower than in all the other subgroups; the median P1GF in this subgroup was significantly lower than in the macrosomic PGDM subgroup.

Conclusions

As PAPP-A, ADAM12, PP13 and P1GF were found to be on average lower in the PGDM non-macrosomic subgroup than in the PGDM macrosomic subgroup, these placental markers may offer a means of predicting macrosomia as early as the first trimester in pregnancies complicated by PGDM. The authors also suggest that, as reduced levels of these placental markers may indicate impaired placentation, macrosomic birthweight in pregnancies with PGDM may relate to normal placentation and normal birthweight to impaired placentation. The authors further postulate that better glycaemic control, reflected in the normal concentration of insulin-like growth factor axis components such as PAPP-A and ADAM12, may translate to normal placentation and resulting macrosomia.

COMMENT

Macrosomia is associated with a greater rate of shoulder dystocia, brachial plexus injury and intrapartum asphyxia during labour, neonate hypoglycaemia and cardiomyopathy, and later childhood complications such as obesity, increased insulin resistance, hypertension and diabetes. The prevention of macrosomia is thus an important goal during a pregnancy complicated by diabetes. Current clinical care stresses the importance of strict glycaemic control in decreasing the prevalence of macrosomia. The potential early detection of macrosomic tendencies provided by these serum markers could play an important role in the future provision of care. However, the authors' postulation – that good glycaemic control, as reflected by the normal concentrations of certain placental markers, may actually increase the prevalence of macrosomia – demands further investigation, as it contradicts a key component of obstetrical care for diabetics. Also raised are the questions of what aspects of a PGDM woman's pregnancy other than hyperglycaemia may predispose the fetus to macrosomia, and what can be done to counteract the action of these factors.

Gestational diabetes mellitus screening based on the gene chip technique

Liang Z[1], Dong M[2], Cheng Q[2], Chen D[1]

[1]*Obstetrical Department, Women's Hospital, School of Medicine, Zhejiang University, Hangzhou, China, and* [2]*Central Laboratory, Women's Hospital, School of Medicine, Zhejiang University, Hangzhou, China*

*Diabetes Res Clin Pract 2010; **89**: 167–73*

Objective

The early detection of a genetic predisposition to gestational diabetes mellitus (GDM) would allow medical professionals to provide proper lifestyle guidance throughout the entire pregnancy, thus limiting the ability of behavioural factors to contribute to the later occurrence of GDM. Gene chips allow for quick, high throughput genetic analysis. This study aimed to identify single nucleotide polymorphisms (SNPs) associated with the occurrence of GDM and to design gene chips that could detect these SNPs and screen for GDM.

Methods

SNPs previously associated with diabetes were selected and then genotyped using 130 blood samples collected at the Women's Hospital School of Medicine at Zhejiang University – 50 from women with GDM, 80 from women without GDM. Relevant SNP patterns were identified, and gene chips were developed. Peripheral blood samples were then collected from 24 women with GDM and 24 women without. The samples were analysed using both gene chip technology and traditional polymerase chain reaction DNA sequencing.

Results

Following the initial genotyping and the application of Fisher's exact test, four SNPs – rs13266634, rs26679, rs3802177, rs9300039 – were identified as candidates for early detection. Of these four, the genotypes rs13266634, rs26679 and rs3802177 were significantly different ($p < 0.05$) between the 24 GDM and 24 non-GDM patients. These results are comparable with those obtained by polymerase chain reaction DNA sequencing.

Conclusions

Gene chips have thus demonstrated their diagnostic ability, and three loci with which to study GDM have been identified. The traditional method of diagnosis – an oral glucose tolerance test – can be unpleasant or inconvenient to administer, and may cause emesis in pregnant women. Gene chip identification of at-risk women is well tolerated, easy to administer, and may contribute to early identification and treatment of GDM.

COMMENT

Further studies must be conducted before gene chips can be put to clinical use. First, as there was a very small sample size (24), studies with a larger sample population must be conducted to verify that there is a significant difference in SNP patterns in GDM and non-GDM women. These trials also need to include a more heterogeneous patient population in order to determine if the findings are applicable to women with different ethnic backgrounds. Additionally, the predictive value of the SNPs in question must be established: does the presence of particular genotypes significantly predict the later occurrence of the disease?

Even once gene chip screening has been refined, it cannot replace an oral glucose tolerance test to determine if a woman has GDM. As GDM is a disease generated by the interaction of both genetic and lifestyle factors, a genetic predisposition to GDM may not translate to the onset of GDM. Gene chip screening can, however, identify at-risk women who may benefit from an oral glucose tolerance test and early intensive lifestyle counselling, even if they are currently asymptomatic.

Closed-loop insulin delivery during pregnancy complicated by type 1 diabetes

Murphy HR[1], Elleri D[1,2], Allen JM[1], Harris J[1], Simmons D[3], Rayman G[4], Temple R[5], Dunger DB[2], Haidar A[1], Nodale M[1], Wilinska ME[1,2], Hovorka R[1,2]

[1] *Institute of Metabolic Science, Metabolic Research Laboratories, University of Cambridge, Cambridge, UK,* [2] *Department of Paediatrics, University of Cambridge, Cambridge, UK,* [3] *Institute of Metabolic Science, Cambridge University Hospitals NHS Foundation Trust, Cambridge, UK,* [4] *Diabetes Centre, Ipswich Hospital NHS Trust, Ipswich, UK, and* [5] *Elsie Bertram Diabetes Centre, Norfolk and Norwich University Hospital NHS Trust, Norwich, UK*

Diabetes Care 2011; 34: 406–11

Objective

The hormonal changes associated with pregnancy can lead to fluctuating blood glucose levels and increasing insulin resistance. Even with educational and technological interventions, type 1 women spend an average of 10 h per day outside the optimal glycaemic range. Closed-loop insulin delivery systems may be beneficial in maintaining stricter glycaemic control. This study aims to assess the functionality of the FreeStyle Navigator continuous glucose monitor (CGM) and the model predictive control (MPC) algorithm in early and late pregnancy.

Methods

Ten pregnant type 1 women were observed during two 24-hour periods, one during early gestation (12–16 weeks) and the other during late gestation (28–32 weeks). A FreeStyle Navigator CGM was inserted the day before observation, and women were connected to an insulin pump delivering insulin aspart. An intravenous sampling cannula was inserted an hour before the start of observation, and venous samples were collected every 15 min. Patients were provided with two standardised meals during the observation period. The MPC algorithm calculated basal insulin infusion, and CGM readings were used to correct for model-based errors and carbohydrate availability. Insulin infusions were calibrated to obtain a sensor reading of 104.4 mg/dl. The mean time in glucose target range, above range, below range, and the insulin infusion rate were calculated with both plasma and sensor readings for each visit. The absolute difference between sensor and plasma readings was used to determine sensor accuracy.

Results

There were no significant differences in early and late gestation plasma glucose levels. Overnight glucose control, as measured by time spent in the optimal glucose range, was good: 84% in early pregnancy, 100% in late pregnancy. There were no significant differences in the prevalence of overnight hyperglycaemia (early gestation 7%, late gestation 0%, p = 0.25) and overnight hypoglycaemia, and no significant difference in pre- and post-meal glucose levels between early and late gestation. During both early and late gestation, there was a longer period of hyperglycaemia after breakfast than after dinner or during the overnight periods. In terms of sensor accuracy, the 93.6% and 95.6% values obtained, respectively, in early and late gestation were clinically acceptable according to Clarke error grid analysis.

Conclusions

The study has shown that the MPC algorithm can adapt insulin delivery to the physiological changes associated with pregnancy. The difficulties in controlling post-breakfast glucose levels highlight the complications associated with controlling postprandial hyperglycaemia. As the accuracy of the FreeStyle Navigator and MPC algorithm in type 1 pregnancies has been established, the authors plan to perform randomised controlled studies of closed-loop insulin delivery with tighter glycaemic goals, and to eventually perform a large, multicentre trial to compare closed-loop and sensor-augmented pump systems.

COMMENT

Closed-loop insulin delivery systems must be able to maintain strict glycaemic goals in order to protect the fetus from the harmful effects of maternal hyperglycaemia (macrosomia, neonatal hypoglycaemia etc.) While this study demonstrated the ability of the devices and algorithms used to keep blood glucose levels within the specified range for most of the time, that range is not representative of the optimal glucose goals for pregnant diabetic patients. Ideally, patients report a fasting glucose of 84 mg/dl, with a 2 h postprandial glucose < 120. This study defined a range of 63–140 mg/dl as normal. Furthermore, the target sensor glucose was set at 104.4 mg/dl. These glucose targets still place the fetus at risk for the complications associated with maternal hyperglycaemia.

Additionally, the excursions in blood glucose were not well controlled. These spikes are clearly evident both in the graph of plasma glucose concentrations and in the percentage of time spent in hyperglycemia following breakfast: 28% in early pregnancy, 44% in late pregnancy. As this closed-loop delivery system is intended to maintain near-normal glucose levels during pregnancy, such excursions indicate an ineffectiveness of the algorithm in use.

The definitions of early and late gestation could also be considered inaccurate. The early gestation observation was conducted between 12 and 16 weeks; however, the first trimester ends at 12 weeks. Glycaemic disturbances in the first trimester can lead to congenital abnormalities and spontaneous abortion. Any studies assessing a closed-loop system in early gestation must therefore assess glycaemic control in these first 12 weeks. Late gestation observations were obtained between 28 and 32 weeks, excluding analysis of the efficacy of the system in the latest stages of pregnancy (36 weeks or more). In effect, this study indicates only that the delivery system functions in the middle of pregnancy. Further study must be conducted to determine that it is also functional in the truly early and late stages of gestation.

Furthermore, the quantity of carbohydrates in the provided meals – 60 g for breakfast, 80 g for dinner – is on the higher side of what is recommended for diabetic patients. The argument can be made that a closed-loop delivery should be able to adjust for blood sugar spikes due to non-optimal carbohydrate intake. However, such high carbohydrate consumption should not be seen as the standard promoted by diabetes researchers, nor should it be the basis for all future research projects. As many diabetics are encouraged to adhere to a low carbohydrate diet, studies on a closed-loop system should assess its feasibility in conjunction with such a diet. It is also important to note that nowhere in this study is information provided on the amount of insulin administered. These data would be helpful in further understanding the research and its implications.

Maternal overweight and pregnancy outcome in women with type 1 diabetes mellitus and different degrees of nephropathy

Yogev Y[1], Chen R[1], ben-Haroush A[1], Hod M[1], Bar J[2]

[1] *Perinatal Division, Helen Schneider Hospital for Women, Rabin Medical Center, Sackler Faculty of Medicine, Tel Aviv, Israel, and* [2] *Department of Obstetrics and Gynecology, Wolfson Medical Center, Holon, Israel*

J Matern Fetal Neonatal Med 2010; **23**: *999–1003*

Objective

Despite advances in pre-pregnancy counselling, diabetic patients with associated nephropathy are still at greater risk for pre-eclampsia, intrauterine growth restriction, congenital abnormalities, pre-term labour, perinatal mortality and permanent deterioration of kidney function. This study aims to identify the risk factors for pregnancy complications in type 1 women with diabetic nephropathy.

Methods

This retrospective cohort study reviewed the medical records of 46 type 1 patients with nephropathy diagnosed before conception or in the first trimester of pregnancy. All patients were followed from preconception through delivery and received standardised care in accordance with the institute's guidelines. Pregnancy outcomes comprised at least one of the following: superimposed pre-eclampsia, pre-term delivery, small-for-gestational-age neonate (birthweight <10th centile), large-for-gestational-age neonate (birthweight > 90th centile), macrosomia (birthweight >4000 g), neonatal intensive care unit admission, first trimester abortion and stillbirth. Student's t-test, two-sided × 2 or Fischer's exact test, and multivariate logistic regression were used to analyse the data.

Results

Thirty-one patients (67% of the sample) experienced at least one pregnancy complication. There were no differences between the groups who did or did not have complications in terms of maternal age, duration of diabetes, pre-gestation creatinine levels, rate of pre-gestation care, pre-gestation and labour HbA1c, rate of retinopathy, or severity of proteinuria. The only statistically significant predictive factor for pregnancy complications was pre-pregnancy body mass index; maternal age, pre-existing hypertension, severity levels of proteinuria, retinopathy, duration of diabetes, treatment with angiotensin converting enzyme inhibitors, pre-pregnancy counselling, and HbA1c levels in the first trimester and at delivery were not statistically significant risk factors.

Conclusions

As body mass index was a significant predictor of future pregnancy complications, overweight and obese type 1 patients with nephropathy should receive information and advice on their increased risk for such conditions, and a focus on weight loss should be included in pre-pregnancy counselling.

COMMENT

An increasing percentage of type 1 patients are now diagnosed as overweight or obese. This study illustrates the impact of that interaction on pregnancy outcomes; further studies should investigate the impact of this comorbidity on other health outcomes. Additionally, the women included in this study primarily suffered from mild nephropathy. Future areas of study may be the determination of predictive factors for complications in patients with more severe forms of nephropathy, and what treatments are most useful for these women.

Association between 5 min Apgar scores and planned mode of delivery in diabetic pregnancies

Stuart AE[1,2], Mattheesen LS[1], Källén KB[2,3]

[1] Department of Obstetrics and Gynecology, Central Hospital, Helsingborg, Sweden, [2] Department of Obstetrics and Gynecology, Clinical Sciences Lund, Lund University, and [3] Reproductive Epidemiology Center, Lund University, Lund, Sweden

Objective

Increased rates of macrosomia, shoulder dystocia and other neonate morbidities are associated with pregnancies complicated by diabetes; such increased risk may indicate a benefit to elective caesareans. This study aimed to determine if an elective caesarean could prevent adverse neonate outcomes, as measured by the rate of infant 5 min Apgar scores <7 and the occurrence of long lasting neurological damage, as indicated by cerebral paresis and epilepsy.

Methods

The data of 13,491 singleton pregnancies complicated by type 1 diabetes or GDM were extracted from the Swedish Medical Birth Registry. The elective caesarean section group was defined as infants born at 38 weeks, before the commencement of labour. The planned vaginal delivery group was composed of all infants born at 39 weeks or more (regardless of final mode of delivery). The analysis of Apgar scores was completed for type 1 + GDM pregnancies, type 1 pregnancies, GDM pregnancies, and large-for-gestational-age pregnancies (regardless of type of diabetes). Infants weighing more than 2 SD above the mean centile were categorised as large for gestational age. Multivariate regression was used to rule out the effects of confounding variables.

Results

A significant difference in the risk of Apgar scores <7 between elective caesarean section and planned vaginal delivery was observed in the type 1 + GDM group (p = 0.021). No significant difference was observed in the type 1 or GDM group. There was also no significant difference in the odds ratio for the large-for-gestational-age group. The hazards ratio for a later neurological complaint – epilepsy or cerebral paresis – was 1.58 between the planned vaginal delivery group and the elective caesarean group. According to the necessary to treat calculation, 132 elective caesareans needed to be performed to prevent one infant from Apgar scores <7.

Conclusions

There were too few instances of cerebral paresis and epilepsy to make a significant assessment of the relative risks of later neurological damage. There was a significant decrease, however, in the risk of Apgar scores <7 with an elective caesarean. Despite the seemingly high need to treat number, it is important to keep in mind that many planned vaginal deliveries ultimately become emergency caesareans or instrument assisted deliveries. The study indicates that pre-term caesarean delivery may be the preferred option for diabetic mothers.

COMMENT

The study did not weigh the potential benefit for the infant vs. the risk for the mother. Caesarean deliveries can lead to blood transfusions, postoperative infection, postoperative pain, damage to pelvic organs, and an increased risk of miscarriage, ectopic gestation, placenta previa and placenta accreta in future pregnancies (2). Second, the study only included data on type 1 and GDM patients. Many GDM patients may have had undiagnosed type 2 or may go on to develop type 2; however, research must address type 2 patients with a pre-pregnancy diagnosis, as there are an increasing number of reproductive-age women entering this category. Last, as noted by the authors, diabetic patients may be good candidates for an elective caesarean because of their increased risk of macrosomia and the associated delivery complications. Yet if there is good glycaemic control throughout the pregnancy, macrosomia may be avoided and a caesarean indicated to a lesser degree. Sonographic methods must be improved to make the identification of macrosomic and large-for-gestational-age infants more precise, so that physicians can more accurately weigh the benefits and costs of an elective caesarean.

Lactation and maternal risk of type 2 diabetes: a population-based study

Schwarz EB[1,2], Brown JS[3], Creasman JM[4], Stuebe A[5], McClure CK[2], Van Den Eeden SK[6], Thom D[7]

[1] *Department of Medicine and Department of Obstetrics, Gynecology and Reproductive Sciences, University of Pittsburgh, PA, USA,* [2] *Department of Epidemiology, University of Pittsburgh, PA, USA,* [3] *Department of Obstetrics, Gynecology and Reproductive Sciences, Department of Urology and Department of Epidemiology, University of California, San Francisco, CA, USA,* [4] *Women's Health Clinical Research Center, University of California, San Francisco, CA, USA,* [5] *Department of Obstetrics and Gynecology, Division of Maternal-Fetal Medicine, University of North Carolina, Chapel Hill, NC, USA,* [6] *Division of Research, Kaiser Permanente, Oakland, CA, USA, and* [7] *Department of Family and Community Medicine, University of California, San Francisco, CA, USA*

Am J Med 2010; **123**: *863.e1–863.e6*

Background

A woman's decision to breastfeed her infant following birth poses great long-term consequences on the health of both the mother and child. A woman's vulnerability to developing type 2 diabetes mellitus after pregnancy is one such consequence. This study explored the relationship between lactation and the risk of developing type 2 diabetes mellitus for new mothers. Specifically, researchers looked at the association between the duration, exclusivity and consistency of breastfeeding to determine how these factors interact and affect the likelihood of a woman developing type 2 diabetes mellitus.

Methods

The Reproductive Risk Factors for Incontinence Study at Kaiser (RRISK) analysed the data for 2233 participants. The diverse sample group included women of various ages, races and diabetic backgrounds (and diabetic women were oversampled with 400 participants). The researchers collected data using self-reported questionnaires and in-person interviews, where they received detailed information on lactation from women who reported one or more live births. They inquired about the duration of lactation, duration of exclusive lactation and consistency of lactation, where consistency was broken up into three groups: women who consistently breastfed their children for more than 1 month, those who breastfed some (not all) of their children for more than 1 month, and those who never breastfed.

Results

Of the 2233 women studied, 1828 were mothers, and 56% of the mothers had breastfed an infant for at least 1 month. Duration of exclusive lactation was highly correlated with duration of total lactation (p < 0.001). On average, women breastfed each child for a total of 6.0 ± 5.7 months and breastfed exclusively for 3.0 ± 2.2 months. Women who had never breastfed an infant were more likely to be obese and have type 2 diabetes mellitus than women who had ever breastfed an infant. Women who had not exclusively breastfed were also more likely to have developed diabetes than mothers who had exclusively breastfed each of their children for an average of 1 or more months. Interestingly, the risk of type 2 diabetes mellitus among women who had consistently breastfed all of their children for at least 1 month remained similar to that of women who had never been pregnant (odds ratio 1.01; 95% confidence interval 0.56–1.81).

Conclusions

Women who do not breastfeed their children are more likely to develop type 2 diabetes mellitus. This is a consequence of maternal lactation patterns: lactation improves glucose and lipid metabolism levels which increases sensitivity to insulin. Furthermore, lactation may also decrease visceral adiposity built up during pregnancy, but mothers who breastfeed for shorter periods may not lose all their visceral fat acquired during pregnancy, greatly increasing their chances for developing type 2 diabetes mellitus.

COMMENT

The data collected for this study depended on the truthful responses of participants, who may have either over-reported or under-reported the duration and consistency of their lactation history due to error in subject recall. Although the study included racially diverse participants across a wide range of age groups, the study was limited by the fact that all women were recruited from the Kaiser Permanente Medical Care Program of Northern California. All participants came from the same geographic area and received comparable medical care through Kaiser's facilities, narrowing the applicability of the study.

First trimester pregnancy-associated plasma protein-A (PAPP-A) in pregnancies complicated by subsequent gestational diabetes

Beneventi F[1], Simonetta M[1], Lovati E[2], Albonico G[3], Tinelli C[4], Locatelli E[1], Spinillo A[1]

[1] *Department of Obstetrics and Gynecology, IRCCS Fondazione Policlinico San Matteo, University of Pavia, Pavia, Italy,* [2] *First Department of Medicine, IRCCS Fondazione Policlinico San Matteo, University of Pavia, Pavia, Italy,* [3] *Clinical Epidemiology and Biometric Unit, IRCCS Fondazione Policlinico San Matteo, University of Pavia, Pavia, Italy, and* [4] *Clinical Chemistry Laboratory, IRCCS Fondazione Policlinico San Matteo, University of Pavia, Pavia, Italy*

Prenat Diagn 2011; 31 : 523–8

Background

Metabolic markers of type 2 diabetes often change during the first trimester of pregnancy, signalling subsequent GDM. This study aimed to compare routine first trimester biomechanical and ultrasound markers between women who later developed GDM with women who experienced healthy pregnancies. Researchers measured pregnancy-associated plasma protein-A (PAPP-A) levels and the fetal crown to rump length to draw associations with other obstetric outcomes.

Methods

In all, 228 pregnant women were diagnosed with gestational diabetes during their second trimester of pregnancy, while 228 healthy pregnant women served in the control group. Subjects were selected from among a group of women seen for prenatal care and delivered at the Department of Obstetrics and Gynecology of the University Hospital of Pavia, Italy. These women underwent a routine second trimester screening for GDM at 24–28 weeks. A 50-g glucose challenge test with blood sugar >140 mg/dl was considered abnormal and was followed by a 100-g, 3-h glucose tolerance test. Normal values for the 100-g load were 95, 180, 155 and 140 mg/dl for the fasting, 1, 2 and 3 h postprandial respectively. Data was collected during the first trimester as well as at the time of delivery. Through statistical analysis, researchers utilised quantile regression models to analyse the relationship between maternal plasma PAPP-A multiple of the mean (MoM) and glucose intolerance. They derived models that indicated a correlation between PAPP-A levels and number of adverse birth effects in women who contracted GDM compared with those who experienced healthy pregnancies. Analyses also recorded factors such as pre-gestational body mass index, birthweight, fetal crown to rump length, maternal age, free β-hCG and nuchal translucency.

Results

The difference between actual and expected crown to rump length was less in women affected by gestational diabetes than the control group (0.2 mm vs. 1.4 mm; p = 0.003). Those who developed gestational diabetes experienced significantly lower first trimester median and adjusted multiple of median PAPP-A concentrations compared with the control group. Pregnancy complications were recorded in 9.6% of the healthy pregnant women and in 14.5% of the glucose-intolerant women (p = 0.114). In normal pregnancies, a weak linear negative correlation (r = −0.2; p < 0.001) was found between PAPP-A and maternal pre-gestational body mass index, and a weak negative correlation was found between PAPP-A and the birthweight (r = 0.2; p = 0.007), but this was not the case in women who developed gestational diabetes (r = 0.02; p = 0.791).

Conclusions

First trimester maternal PAPP-A concentrations were lower among pregnant women who developed second trimester gestational diabetes than in the control group. This study indicates that PAPP-A levels could be an early marker of glucose intolerance in pregnant women, thus predicting the onset of gestational diabetes. Lower PAPP-A levels correlate with a decreased difference in the actual and expected crown to rump length. Such outcomes suggest that first trimester fetal growth is more efficient among women with normal glucose tolerance, and low PAPP-A levels lead to less of a growth factor (insulin-like growth factor) – a key determinant in fetal growth.

COMMENT

The study fails to define a different set of normal PAPP-A levels for pregnant diabetic vs. pregnant non-diabetic women. Also, the study does not provide a minimum normal glucose value following the initial 50-g glucose challenge test. This study raises additional concerns related to the population sampled as well as the shifting criteria used to diagnose gestational diabetes. Because the subjects were chosen from the same hospital, they probably received comparable medical care minimising error due to treatment disparity. Yet, the homogeneity of the sampled population limits the applicability of the study's results to a defined group.

Also, the researchers recognise that the criteria used for diagnosing gestational diabetes have shifted, so the results must be verified through additional studies that employ the latest diagnostic criteria.

Relation of salivary antioxidant status and cytokine levels to clinical parameters of oral health in pregnant women with diabetes

Surdacka A[1], Ciężka E[1], Pioruńska-Stolzmann M[2], Wender-Ożegowska E[3], Korybalska K[4], Kawka E[4], Kaczmarek E[5], Witowski J[4]

[1]*Department of Conservative Dentistry and Periodontology, Poznan University of Medical Sciences, Poznan, Poland,* [2]*Department of General Chemistry, Poznan University of Medical Sciences, Poznan, Poland,* [3]*Department of Obstetrics and Gynecology, Poznan University of Medical Sciences, Poznan, Poland,* [4]*Department of Pathophysiology, Poznan University of Medical Sciences, Poznan, Poland, and* [5]*Department of Bioinformatics and Computational Biology, Poznan University of Medical Sciences, Poznan, Poland*

Arch Oral Biol 2011; **56***: 428–36*

Background

Both pregnancy and diabetes mellitus correlate with an increased incidence of oral health complications, putting diabetic pregnant women at greater risk for accelerated deterioration of oral health. Pregnancy may decrease the antioxidant capacity of saliva and gingival crevicular fluid, increasing susceptibility to dental caries and other periodontal diseases. Certain components of saliva may serve as biomarkers of both periodontal and systemic disease. This study analyses the antioxidant status and cytokine levels in saliva from pregnant women with and without diabetes in order to verify that the differences in the properties of saliva correspond with the patient's oral health.

Methods

Sixty-three women in their first trimester of pregnancy participated in the study; 30 women had diabetes and 33 women were healthy. The study classified the diabetic women into one of two subgroups according to duration as well as severity of diabetes. Group ABC included those who experienced recent onset, while group DFR characterised those who had suffered from the disease for a longer duration. These classifications are derived from White's criteria: class A refers to diabetes that began during pregnancy, and classes B, C and D correspond to diabetes that existed before pregnancy and lasted for less than 10 years, 10–19 years and more than 20 years, respectively. Class R refers to retinopathy and F to nephropathy. All participants completed an oral examination, which assessed clinical parameters related to dental and gingival status including the gingival index, sulcus bleeding index, probing depth, loss of clinical attachment level and the plaque index. Then, saliva samples were collected at regular intervals throughout the day and immediately analysed for particular antioxidants, cytokines and growth factors. The pH levels were also determined before the samples were stored.

Results

Both groups of pregnant and diabetic women revealed markedly increased indices of caries activity, plaque formation, gingival status and periodontal status compared with the control group. Also, saliva collected from the pregnant diabetic women contained significantly greater concentrations of proteins and an increased antioxidant capacity as well as elevated concentrations of several pro-inflammatory cytokines, growth factors (vascular endothelial growth factor, VEGF) and adhesion molecules. The results for the DFR group were more severe than the results for the ABC group when considering the variety of dental complications. These parameters were measured in relation to the patients' HbA1c levels, revealing a significant correlation between caries prevalence, plaque formation and salivary protein concentration. Results also revealed a significant negative correlation between the HbA1c level and both the saliva pH and flow rate. A positive correlation between the caries activity index and the salivary VEGF appeared in the pregnant diabetic patients, while a negative correlation surfaced between the contraction of caries disease and the presence of hepatocyte growth factor (HGF) (HGF and VEGF are two of the saliva cytokines). However, no such correlations surfaced in the healthy pregnant women.

Conclusions

Pregnant diabetic women are more prone to contracting caries disease than non-diabetic pregnant women due to salivary composition changes. These changes result from shifts in antioxidant capacity and cytokine concentrations, where total antioxidant capacity of the DFR group was more than double that of healthy subjects. Some of the differences are correlated with the intensity and duration of the subject's diabetes. Women who struggled longer with diabetes exhibited stronger results than the more recently diagnosed group.

COMMENT

This study failed to consider the varying degrees of the subjects' personal and professional dental care. The study also did not account for other factors that trigger oral health complications such as diet and oral hygiene.

Hypoglycaemia in type 1 diabetic pregnancy: role of preconception insulin aspart treatment in a randomised study

Heller S[1], Damm P[2], Mersebach H[3], Skjøth TV[3], Kaaja R[4], Hod M[5], Durán-García S[6], McCance D[7], Mathiesen ER[2]

[1] *Northern General Hospital, Sheffield, UK,* [2] *Rigshospitalet, University of Copenhagen, Copenhagen, Denmark,* [3] *Novo Nordisk, Soeborg, Denmark,* [4] *Helsinki University Central Hospital, Helsinki, Finland,* [5] *Rabin Medical Center, Tel-Aviv University, Petah-Tiqva, Israel,* [6] *University of Seville, Seville, Spain, and* [7] *Royal Victoria Hospital, Belfast, UK*

Diabetes Care 2010; 33: 473–7

Background

This randomised trial aimed to compare prandial insulin aspart (IAsp) with human insulin in type 1 diabetic pregnant women. It compared the rates of severe hypoglycaemia during pregnancy between women enrolled into the trial during pre-conception versus those enrolled during the first trimester of their pregnancy. The study observed how these two insulins affected the rate of severe hypoglycaemia in patients according to time of enrolment in the study, whether pre- or post-conception.

Methods

Study participants included women who had insulin treated type 1 diabetes for at least a year and were either planning to become pregnant or already were pregnant. Ninety-nine subjects (44 who received IAsp and 55 who received human insulin) were randomly assigned to the pre-conception group, while 223 subjects (113 given IAsp and 110 given human insulin) began treatment before 10 weeks of gestation. The IAsp groups injected their insulin immediately before each meal, and the human insulin groups injected 30 min before mealtime in combination with NPH insulin. Hypoglycaemic episodes were recorded throughout the pregnancy term. Participants were followed regularly each trimester and at 6 weeks postpartum. Severe hypoglycaemia was considered any event that demanded third party assistance or resulted in a plasma glucose level less than 3.1 mmol/l (or 56.4 mg/dl). Then, incidents of severe hypoglycaemia were compared between the pre-conception and early pregnancy groups as well as between those assigned to IAsp vs. those assigned human insulin treatment. The relative risk of severe hypoglycaemia was assessed with a gamma frailty model.

Results

Overall, 73 patients (or 23%) experienced severe episodes of hypoglycaemia at least once during the course of the study (rates peaked during early pregnancy). Rates of severe hypoglycaemia in subjects randomly assigned pre-conception vs. early pregnancy were 1.7 and 3.4 events per patient per year respectively during the first half of pregnancy (with a risk ratio of 1.70; p = 0.097), but the rates dropped to 0.8 vs. 0.9 events per patient per year in the second half of pregnancy (risk ratio was 1.35; p = 0.640). For subjects assigned pre-conception, the estimated risk for severe hypoglycaemia during the first and second halves of pregnancy was lower with IAsp than with human insulin (risk ratio 0.37 and p = 0.13 vs. risk ratio 0.20 and p = 0.16 respectively). The rates for hypoglycaemia among patients assigned to the pre-conception group who received IAsp vs. those who received human insulin before pregnancy, during the first half of pregnancy, during the second half of pregnancy, and postpartum were 0.9 vs. 2.4; 0.9 vs. 2.4; 0.3 vs. 1.2; and 0.2 vs. 2.2 respectively. Estimated risk for patients receiving IAsp insulin was 66% lower for those assigned to the pre-conception period. During pregnancy, average HbA1c levels among groups were comparable.

Conclusions

The data reveal that those who started injections pre-conception, rather than during early pregnancy, experienced a decreased incidence rate of hypoglycaemia. In fact, the estimated risk of severe hypoglycaemia was 70% higher in subjects randomly assigned early pregnancy as opposed to those assigned pre-conception and 66% lower for those assigned pre-conception while receiving IAsp insulin as opposed to human insulin. Results clearly show that rapid-acting insulin analogue (IAsp) and treatment before pregnancy minimise rates of hypoglycaemia.

COMMENT

Interestingly, although some groups experienced higher rates of hypoglycaemia, HbA1c levels remained comparable among the subjects assigned to different groups. In this case, HbA1c did not necessarily serve as a marker for predicting hypoglycaemia.

Early onset and high prevalence of gestational diabetes in PCOS and insulin resistant women before and after assisted reproduction

Bals-Pratsch M[1], Großer B[2], Seifert B[1], Ortmann O[3], Seifarth C[2]

[1] *Center for Reproductive Medicine, Regensburg, Germany,* [2] *Practice for Endocrinology, Regensburg, Germany,* [3] *Department of Gynecology and Obstetrics, University Hospital Regensburg, Regensburg, Germany*

*Exp Clin Endocrinol Diabetes 2011; **119**: 338–42*

Background

Pre-gestational metformin treatment is supported by the observation that rates of miscarriage and gestational diabetes are lower among women affected by polycystic ovary syndrome (PCOS) or insulin resistant diseases who conceive while taking metformin. However, these women often turn to assisted reproduction techniques (ART) in order to facilitate conception. The aim of this study is to analyse the frequency of impaired glucose tolerance or gestational diabetes in the first weeks of gestation after ART in women receiving metformin.

Methods

In all, 107 patients receiving metformin in order to treat PCOS, insulin resistance and a host of other fertility interfering disorders turned to ART. Those who scored less than 6 on the oral glucose tolerance test (OGTT) were categorised as insulin resistant. Within 4 weeks following conception, subjects received an oral 75-g 2-h OGTT in order to detect impaired glucose tolerance (IGT) or GDM. Those diagnosed as insulin resistant received dietary instruction and proper insulin treatment.

Results

Out of the 107 women receiving metformin and committed to ART treatment, 43 women developed GDM (40%) and 15 developed IGT (14%), while 49 (45.8%) maintained normal glucose levels within the first 7 weeks of pregnancy. Of the women who were insulin resistant before conception, 54% developed IGT or GDM, while 46% did not. Therefore, not all women with pre-conception insulin resistance developed GDM or IGT (the primary risk factor for both IGT and GDM was PCOS where p = 0.014). The frequency of GDM was 55% in the subgroup with pre-pregnancy confirmed insulin resistance not fulfilling the criteria for PCOS, 40.6% for PCOS women and 26.1% for women experiencing neither insulin resistance nor PCOS.

Conclusions

This study found that women undergoing ART showed a high rate of IGT and GDM in the first weeks of pregnancy. And, PCOS (rather than insulin resistance) is the main risk factor for IGT or GDM. Thus, metformin treatment through the seventh week of pregnancy is recommended for PCOS patients with pre-gestational insulin resistance to improve fertility. This study supports the recommendation that women should conduct OGTTs during the onset of pregnancy in order to maximise chances of a successful pregnancy. In addition to early detection, metformin coupled with proper treatment can stabilise glucose metabolism and reduce risk for miscarriage and gestational diabetes.

> **COMMENT**
>
> Results from this study reflect an older working definition of gestational diabetes. As the definition evolves over time, the study may lose its validity. Eventually, it may be necessary to revise and repeat a similar trial in the future to confirm the results.

CONCLUSION

Diabetes mellitus is a growing epidemic that seriously impacts the emotional, physical and financial well-being of those who have it. The current obesogenic environment – an environment that promotes low nutrient, calorie-dense foods, and low levels of exercise – will only increase the prevalence of people diagnosed with obesity and its common comorbid conditions, including type 2 diabetes. Recent research has even identified a potential link between early onset of type 1 diabetes and a greater childhood body mass index (3).

Prenatal programming puts children at an even greater risk of developing diabetes at a young age: poorly controlled diabetes during pregnancy primes the fetus for macrosomia and its resultant birth complications, childhood obesity and development of diabetes in childhood, adolescence or early adulthood. Those who develop diabetes early in life are at a greater risk for severe complications, as the duration of the disease is clearly linked with peripheral neuropathy, diabetic retinopathy, diabetic nephropathy and macrocardiovascular conditions. It is thus important to avoid such antenatal imprinting by controlling pregnancies complicated by diabetes as tightly as possible.

The research reviewed in this chapter covers new early-detection screening processes, developments in methods of glycaemic control during gestation, causes of comorbidities common to pregnancies complicated by diabetes, and optimal obstetrical care for diabetic pregnant women. All of these papers are part of a worldwide effort to reduce the impact of diabetes on both current and future generations. This goal will only be achieved by the dedicated research and collaborative efforts of researchers across the globe, from the UK and the USA to Israel and the People's Republic of China.

REFERENCES

1. Centers for Disease Control and Prevention. *National Diabetes Fact Sheet: National Estimates and General Information on Diabetes and Prediabetes in the United States*. Atlanta, GA: US

Department of Health and Human Services, 2011. Retrieved from http://www.cdc.gov/diabetes/pubs/factsheet11.htm?utm_source=WWW&utm_medium=ContentPage&utm_content=CDCFactsheet&utm_campaign=CON

2. Ecker J, Frigoletto F. Cesarean delivery and the risk–benefit calculus. *N Engl J Med* 2007; **356**: 885–8

3. Boyles S. Obesity linked to type 1 diabetes insulin resistance may explain disease increase in younger children. *WebMD Health News,* 2003. Retrieved from http://diabetes.webmd.com/news/20030926/obesity-linked-to-type-1-diabetes

CHAPTER 9

Type 1 Diabetes Mellitus: Immune Intervention

Jay S. Skyler

Division of Endocrinology, Diabetes, and Metabolism, and Diabetes Research Institute, University of Miami Miller School of Medicine, Miami, FL, USA

INTRODUCTION

This year saw the report of several major studies of immune intervention for type 1 diabetes (T1D). Immune intervention studies have been conducted both in patients with recently diagnosed T1D and earlier during the stage of evolution of the disease in individuals found to be at increased risk. This chapter of the *Yearbook of Advanced Technology and Treatments in Diabetes* reviews the key papers that have appeared in this field between July 2010 and June 2011. It includes only studies conducted in human beings.

Long-term outcome of individuals treated with oral insulin: Diabetes Prevention Trial Type 1 (DPT-1) oral insulin trial

Vehik K[1], Cuthbertson D[1], Ruhlig H[1], Schatz DA[2], Peakman M[3,4], Krischer JP[1]; DPT-1 and TrialNet Study Groups

[1] University of South Florida, Pediatrics Epidemiology Center, Tampa, FL, USA, [2] University of Florida, College of Medicine, Gainesville, FL, USA, [3] Department of Immunobiology, King's College London, London, UK, [4] National Institutes of Health Research Biomedical Research Centre at Guy's and St Thomas' NHS Foundation Trust and King's College London, London, UK

*Diabetes Care 2011; **34**: 1585–90*

Background

Insulin is an important antigen in T1D. Mucosal administration of antigens is thought to stimulate regulatory T-cells in preference to effector

---

T-cells. Thus, a number of studies have used mucosal administration of insulin in attempts to modulate the T1D disease process. These have included both oral and nasal administration of insulin. The DPT-1 Study Group had conducted a large study of oral insulin in individuals at risk of developing T1D (1). Although oral insulin did not delay the development of T1D in the group as a whole, it did show beneficial effects in a subgroup with higher levels of insulin autoantibodies ($\geq$80 nU/ml) at the time of enrolment. The current report is a follow-up of those subjects to evaluate the long-term intervention effects of oral insulin on the development of T1D and to assess the rate of progression to T1D before and after oral insulin treatment was stopped.

Methods

The follow-up included subjects who had participated in the DPT-1 oral insulin study (1994–2003) to prevent or delay T1D. In 2009, a telephone survey was conducted to determine whether T1D had been diagnosed and, if not, an oral glucose tolerance test (OGTT), HbA1c and autoantibody levels were obtained on subjects who agreed to participate. Originally, 372 subjects had been randomised, and 97 had developed T1D during the original trial. Subsequently, 75% of the remaining 272 subjects were contacted – 77 had been diagnosed with T1D and 54 others were evaluated with an OGTT.

Results

In subjects in the subgroup with benefit in the original study (those with insulin autoantibodies $\geq$ 80 nU/ml at enrolment), the overall benefit of oral insulin remained significant (p = 0.05). However, the hazard rate in this group increased (from 6.4% to 10.0%) after cessation of therapy, which approximated the rate of individuals treated with placebo.

Conclusion

The oral insulin treatment effect appeared to be maintained with additional follow-up in the subgroup with benefit in the original study. However, after therapy was stopped, the rate of developing diabetes in the oral insulin group increased to a rate similar to that of the placebo group.

Evidence that nasal insulin induces immune tolerance to insulin in adults with autoimmune diabetes

Fourlanos S[1,2,3], Perry C[2], Gellert SA[3], Martinuzzi E[4,5], Mallone R[4,5], Butler J[1], Colman PG[3], Harrison LC[1,2]

[1] *Autoimmunity and Transplantation Division, Walter and Eliza Hall Institute of Medical Research, Parkville, VA, Australia,* [2] *Burnet Clinical Research Unit, Royal Melbourne Hospital, Parkville, Australia,* [3] *Department of Diabetes and Endocrinology, Royal Melbourne Hospital, Parkville, Australia,* [4] *INSERM, U986, DeAR Laboratory Avenir, Saint Vincent de Paul Hospital, Paris, France, and* [5] *Université Paris Descartes, Faculté de Médecine René Descartes, Paris, France*

Diabetes 2011; **60***: 1237–45*

Background

A previous study (DIPP) followed genetically at-risk children from birth until the appearance of antibodies, at which point nasal insulin was administered, although without success (2). The authors of the current study had previously conducted a crossover study that suggested that nasal insulin might have beneficial effects on both the immune system and β-cell function in individuals at high risk of T1D (3). Therefore, the authors conducted this study to determine whether nasal insulin could induce immune tolerance.

Methods

The study recruited subjects diagnosed with diabetes in the previous 12 months, with glutamic acid decarboxylase (GAD) antibodies and fasting C-peptide >0.20 nmol/l, who had stable blood glucose control with diet and/or oral hypoglycaemic drug therapy but no previous insulin therapy. They randomised 52 subjects, aged 40–55 years, to nasal insulin ($n = 26$) or to placebo ($n = 26$). Intervention consisted of a metered dose nasal spray (two sprays per nostril, equivalent to 40 units of insulin) daily for 10 days and then on 2 consecutive days weekly for 12 months. Participants were assessed every 3 months for 24 months.

Results

Metabolic endpoints, β-cell function, both fasting and glucagon-stimulated C-peptide, HbA1c and fasting glucose, remained similar between nasal insulin and placebo groups. At 24 months, β-cell function had declined by 35%, and 23 of 52 participants (44%) progressed to insulin treatment. Insulin antibody response to injected insulin was significantly blunted in those who had received nasal insulin. In a small cohort, the interferon-γ response of blood T-cells to proinsulin was suppressed after nasal insulin.

Conclusion

The authors concluded that they had seen some evidence that nasal insulin induced immune tolerance to insulin. They assert that this provides a rationale for the use of nasal insulin to be studied to prevent diabetes in at-risk individuals.

COMMENT

Antigen-specific therapy is thought to be a highly desirable strategy to interrupt the immune processes that result in T1D. Such therapies are generally quite safe, are specific for T1D, and are not expected to alter generalised immune responses. Mucosal administration of antigen is thought to favour protective immunity over destructive immunity. Mucosal administration of insulin has been used by both the oral and the nasal route. However, to date, in recently diagnosed T1D, three studies of oral insulin and the Fourlanos *et al.* study of nasal insulin discussed above have all failed to alter metabolic function. In addition, studies of both oral and nasal insulin have failed in prevention studies, although the DPT-1 oral insulin prevention study did identify a subgroup that had a beneficial effect. Follow-up of those subjects in the report by Vehik *et al.* discussed above showed continued effect but, after cessation of oral insulin, regression to a rate of diabetes similar to the placebo group. The TrialNet Study Group is conducting an additional study with oral insulin on subjects with similar criteria to the subgroup that showed beneficial effect. Likewise, the Australian group is performing a prevention study with nasal insulin, and a dose-ranging study of both oral and nasal insulin is being conducted in newborns at risk of T1D. Dose determination is a vexing question that has hampered many studies with antigen-specific interventions, since translation of dose from rodents to human beings is fraught with much difficulty. Despite the lack of major success with mucosally based insulin administration, there remains hope that some form of antigen-specific therapy with insulin will ultimately prove beneficial.

Antigen-based therapy with glutamic acid decarboxylase (GAD) vaccine in patients with recent-onset type 1 diabetes: a randomised double-blind trial

Wherrett DK[1], Bundy B[2], Becker DJ[3], DiMeglio LA[4], Gitelman SE[5], Goland R[6], Gottlieb PA[7], Greenbaum CJ[8], Herold KC[9], Marks JB[10], Monzavi R[11], Moran A[12], Orban T[13], Palmer JP[14], Raskin P[15], Rodriguez H[4], Schatz D[16], Wilson DM[17], Krischer JP[2], Skyler JS[10]; Type 1 Diabetes TrialNet GAD Study Group

[1]*Hospital for Sick Children, University of Toronto, Toronto, ON, Canada,* [2]*University of South Florida, Tampa, FL, USA,* [3]*University of Pittsburgh, Pittsburgh, PA, USA,* [4]*Indiana University School of Medicine, Indianapolis, IN, USA,* [5]*University of California San Francisco, San Francisco, CA, USA,* [6]*Columbia University, New York, NY, USA,* [7]*University of Colorado Barbara Davis Center for Childhood Diabetes, Aurora, CO, USA,* [8]*Benaroya Research*

Institute, Seattle, WA, USA, [9] Yale University School of Medicine, New Haven, CT, USA, [10] Diabetes Research Institute, University of Miami Miller School of Medicine, Miami, FL, USA, [11] Children's Hospital Los Angeles, Los Angeles, CA, USA, [12] University of Minnesota, Minneapolis, MN, USA, [13] Joslin Diabetes Center, Boston, MA, USA, [14] University of Washington School of Medicine, Seattle, WA, USA, [15] University of Texas Southwestern Medical School, Dallas, TX, USA, [16] University of Florida, Gainesville, FL, USA, and [17] Stanford University, Stanford, CA, USA

*Lancet 2011; **378**: 319–27*

Background

GAD is another important antigen in T1D. In animal models, GAD has been an effective agent to modulate the T1D disease process. A previous pilot study of an aluminium-hydroxide-formulated GAD (GAD-alum) vaccine had modest effect (4). The current study was designed to determine whether GAD vaccine could preserve β-cell function in recent-onset T1D.

Methods

The study randomised 145 subjects (48 assigned to three injections of vaccine, 49 assigned to two injections of vaccine and one injection of placebo, and 48 assigned to three injections of placebo), aged 3–45, and randomised within 3 months of diagnosis of T1D. The primary endpoint was β-cell function – as measured by C-peptide – at 1 year, with 140 subjects included in the analysis.

Results

At 1 year, the mean level of C-peptide was similar in all three groups, with no evidence of a treatment effect. HbA1c levels, insulin use, and the occurrence and severity of adverse events did not differ between groups.

Conclusion

Antigen-based immunotherapy with two or three doses of subcutaneous GAD-alum did not alter the course of loss of insulin secretion during 1 year in patients with recently diagnosed T1D.

COMMENT

This paper tested another antigen-specific immunomodulatory approach in T1D, using GAD. As noted above in discussing insulin, antigen-specific therapy is thought to be a highly desirable strategy to interrupt the immune processes that result in T1D, and generally is both safe and specific for T1D.

Unfortunately, antigen-specific therapies have had more failures than successes. Indeed, in addition to this study, there have been press releases announcing the failure of two phase 3 studies using the same GAD-alum vaccine (5,6). However, in the case of GAD, it is important to note that the benefits seen in animals used a number of routes of administration, but not as a subcutaneous vaccine. Moreover, they used GAD for prevention, not to slow the loss of β-cell function in recent-onset T1D. This raises the question of whether GAD should be considered in prevention studies in human beings. It may also be appropriate to consider GAD as one component of a combination therapeutic approach in T1D.

Teplizumab for treatment of type 1 diabetes (Protégé Study): 1-year results from a randomised, placebo-controlled trial

Sherry N[1], Hagopian W[2], Ludvigsson J[3], Jain SM[4], Wahlen J[5], Ferry RJ Jr[6], Bode B[7], Aronoff S[8], Holland C[9], Carlin D[9], King KL[9], Wilder RL[1,10], Pillemer S[1,11], Bonvini E[9], Johnson S[9], Stein KE[9], Koenig S[9], Herold KC[1,12], Daifotis AG[9]; Protégé Trial Investigator

[1]Massachusetts General Hospital, Boston, MA, USA, [2]Pacific Northwest Diabetes Research Institute, Seattle, WA, USA, [3]Division of Pediatrics, Department of Clinical and Experimental Medicine, Faculty of Health Sciences, Linköping University, Linköping, Sweden, [4]TOTALL Diabetes Hormone Research Institute, Indore, Madhya Pradesh, India, [5]Endocrine Research Specialists, Ogden, UT, USA, [6]Division of Pediatric Endocrinology and Metabolism, Le Bonheur Children's Hospital and University of Tennessee Health Science Center, Memphis, TN, USA, [7]Atlanta Diabetes Associates, Atlanta, GA, USA, [8]Research Institute of Dallas, Dallas, TX, USA, [9]MacroGenics, Rockville, MD, USA, [10]PAREXEL International, Durham, NC, USA, [11]American Biopharma Corporation, Gaithersburg, MD, USA, and [12]Yale University, New Haven, CT, USA

*Lancet 2011; **378**: 487–97*

Background

Previous reports have shown that, with a short course of humanised anti-CD3 monoclonal antibody (either teplizumab or otelixizumab), there was preservation of β-cell function – as measured by C-peptide – and lower insulin doses with either better or equivalent glycaemic control (7,8). The short course of treatment, initiated soon after diagnosis, resulted in beneficial effects that extended for 2–4 years (9,10). The current report describes a phase 3 study using teplizumab.

Methods

The study randomised 516 subjects (209 assigned a 14-day course of full-dose teplizumab, 102 assigned a 14-day course of low-dose teplizumab, 106 assigned a 6-day course of full-dose teplizumab, and 99 assigned placebo). Treatment was given at baseline and at 26 weeks. Subjects were aged 8–35 and randomised within 3 months of diagnosis of T1D. The study is designed to last 2 years, with the current report giving outcome at 1 year. The primary outcome measure was a composite of the percentage of patients with insulin use of <0.5 U/kg per day and HbA1c of <6.5% at 1 year.

Results

The primary outcome did not differ between groups at 1 year. However, 5% (19/415) of patients in the teplizumab groups were not taking insulin at 1 year, compared with no patients in the placebo group at 1 year (p = 0.03). Moreover, exploratory analyses suggested that teplizumab could help preserve β-cell function – as measured by C-peptide – at 1 year, and might decrease the amount of insulin needed for glycaemic control, particularly in subgroups such as children. Similar proportions of patients had adverse events and serious adverse events. The most common clinical adverse event in the teplizumab groups was rash.

Conclusion

Anti-CD3 therapy did not impact the primary outcome measure but exploratory analyses suggested that anti-CD3 therapy could help preserve β-cell function. The authors concluded that this should influence the design of future studies.

COMMENT

Earlier studies had shown that relatively short courses of treatment (6 or 14 days) with an anti-CD3 monoclonal antibody can have sustained effects on β-cell function – as measured by C-peptide. Therefore, both of the anti-CD3 antibodies used (teplizumab and otelixizumab) were studied in full-scale phase 3 trials for potential commercialization for use in recent-onset T1D. The Protégé Study, discussed here, unfortunately selected a primary outcome measure that had not been used either in earlier trials of anti-CD3 or in other major immunotherapy trials discussed in this chapter or its predecessors in the previous two editions of this *Yearbook*. The Protégé Study also enrolled subjects in South Asia. Although these subjects met the clinical criteria used for enrolment, it is important to note that typical immune-mediated T1D (also called type 1A diabetes) is a disease principally of European Caucasians. Enrolment of Asian subjects may have confounded the results. It also turns out that the phase 3 DEFEND-1 Study using otelixizumab in T1D also did not meet its primary endpoint, as was announced by a press release on 11 March 2011 (11). The DEFEND-1 Study unfortunately selected a dose (3.1 mg total dose) dramatically lower than that used in the original teplizumab study (48 mg). Thus, there are lessons to be learned about clinical trial design, in terms of dose selection, population studied and outcome measure chosen. Nonetheless, the fact that beneficial effects were observed in the earlier studies, and suggested by the exploratory analyses in the Protégé Study, should be taken as encouraging for this therapeutic approach. Nonetheless, in the original trials with both of these antibodies, there is progressive decline in β-cell function, suggesting that there may be a need for repeated courses of administration. This was being tested in the Protégé Study and probably needs further examination. Moreover, these antibodies remain candidates to be used in combination therapy with another agent (or agents).

Co-stimulation modulation with abatacept in patients with recent-onset type 1 diabetes: a randomised, double-blind, placebo-controlled trial

Orban T[1], Bundy B[2], Becker DJ[3], DiMeglio LA[4], Gitelman SE[5], Goland R[6], Gottlieb PA[7], Greenbaum CJ[8], Marks JB[9], Monzavi R[10], Moran A[11], Raskin P[12], Rodriguez H[4], Russell WE[13], Schatz D[14], Wherrett D[15], Wilson DM[16], Krischer JP[2], Skyler JS[9]; Type 1 Diabetes TrialNet Abatacept Study Group

[1] Joslin Diabetes Center, Boston, MA, USA, [2] University of South Florida, Tampa, FL, USA, [3] University of Pittsburgh, Pittsburgh, PA, USA, [4] Indiana University School of Medicine, Indianapolis, IN, USA, [5] University of California San Francisco, San Francisco, CA, USA, [6] Columbia University, New York, NY, USA, [7] University of Colorado Barbara Davis Center for Childhood Diabetes, Aurora, CO, USA, [8] Benaroya Research Institute, Seattle, WA, USA, [9] University of Miami Diabetes Research Institute, Miami, FL, USA, [10] Children's Hospital Los Angeles, Los Angeles, CA, USA, [11] University of Minnesota, Minneapolis, MN, USA, [12] University of Texas Southwestern Medical School, Dallas, TX, USA, [13] Vanderbilt University, Nashville, TN, USA, [14] University of Florida, Gainesville, FL, USA, [15] Hospital for Sick Children, University of Toronto, Toronto, ON, Canada, and [16] Stanford University, Stanford, CA, USA

*Lancet 2011; **378**: 412–19*

Background

To be fully active, immune T-cells need a co-stimulatory signal in addition to the main antigen-driven signal. Abatacept modulates co-stimulation and prevents full T-cell activation. Studies in both animals and human beings have shown that interruption of the co-stimulatory second signal beneficially affects autoimmunity. Co-stimulation blockade has been effective in psoriasis, rheumatoid arthritis, juvenile rheumatoid arthritis and control of allograft rejection. This study used abatacept to modulate co-stimulation in recent-onset T1D.

Methods

The study randomised 112 subjects (77 assigned to abatacept, 35 assigned to placebo), aged 6–45, and randomised within 3 months of diagnosis of T1D. The primary endpoint was β-cell function – as measured by C-peptide – at 2 years, with 103 subjects included in the analysis. Intervention consisted of infusions of abatacept (or placebo) on days 1, 14 and 28, and then monthly for a total of 27 infusions.

Results

At 2 years, the mean level of C-peptide was significantly higher in the abatacept group than in the placebo group, and declined at a slower rate. The difference between groups was present throughout the trial, with an estimated 9.6 months' delay in C-peptide reduction with abatacept, even though abatacept treatment was continued for the entire 2 years. The abatacept group also had significantly lower A1c levels and required less insulin in the aggregate during the total course of the study. Adverse effects were minimal and there was no increase in infections or in neutropenia.

Conclusion

The co-stimulation modulator abatacept showed beneficial effects on β-cell function in recent-onset T1D. Further observation will determine whether the beneficial effect continues after cessation of abatacept infusions.

COMMENT

This study demonstrates that treatment with the co-stimulation modulator abatacept can have beneficial effects on β-cell function – as measured by C-peptide – at 2 years. Nonetheless, there is progressive decline in β-cell function, despite continued monthly infusions of abatacept. Since abatacept works to block T-cell activation and does not impact memory T-cells, this suggests that T-cell activation lessens with time. It will be important to see what happens in the follow-up of the participants in this trial, after abatacept was discontinued. A future study might be desirable to see whether a shorter course of abatacept (e.g. 6 or 9 months) would offer similar effects. In addition, the development of a subcutaneous version of abatacept would make administration far easier, and would be mandatory if abatacept was to be explored for use in high risk subjects for delay or prevention of T1D. Abatacept might also be useful in combination therapy with another agent.

No protective effect of calcitriol on beta-cell function in recent-onset type 1 diabetes: the IMDIAB XIII trial

Bizzarri C[1], Pitocco D[2], Napoli N[3], Di Stasio E[2], Maggi D[3], Manfrini S[3], Suraci C[4], Cavallo MG[5], Cappa M[1], Ghirlanda G[2], Pozzilli P[3]; IMDIAB Group

[1] *Department of Endocrinology and Diabetes, Bambino Gesù Children's Hospital, Rome, Italy,* [2] *Department of Diabetology, Catholic University, Rome, Italy,* [3] *Department of Endocrinology and Diabetes, University Campus Bio-Medico, Rome, Italy,* [4] *Department of Diabetology, Sandro Pertini Hospital, Rome, Italy, and* [5] *Department of Medical Therapy, University Sapienza, Rome, Italy*

Diabetes Care 2010; 33: 1962–3

Background

Vitamin D deficiency has been associated with T1D, and epidemiological studies suggest that vitamin D supplementation in early childhood may decrease risk of developing T1D. A previous study (discussed in last year's *Yearbook*) evaluated whether $1,25(OH)_2D_3$ (calcitriol) improves β-cell function in adults with recent-onset T1D. The current study included younger individuals.

Methods

The study randomised 34 subjects, aged 11–35, and randomised within 3 months of diagnosis of T1D. Intervention consisted of calcitriol or placebo daily for 2 years. The primary endpoint was β-cell function – as measured by C-peptide – at 2 years, with 27 subjects included in the analysis (15 in the calcitriol group, 12 in the placebo group).

Results

Outcome measures were assessed at 6, 12 and 24 months. HbA1c and insulin use were similar in both groups. Fasting C-peptide declined similarly in both groups. Stimulated C-peptide was measured at baseline and 12 months, and was similar in both groups.

Conclusion

Calcitriol did not have a beneficial effect in recent-onset T1D.

COMMENT

As noted in last year's *Yearbook*, the potential role of vitamin D as a preventative intervention for T1D has been suggested for some time. Unfortunately, in the studies conducted to date in recent-onset T1D, $1,25(OH)_2D_3$ has failed to show a beneficial effect. The real question of whether vitamin D might have an effect in prevention of T1D has not been explored. Given the tendency towards nearly routine supplementation with vitamin D, it is uncertain whether a controlled study of its use in prevention can actually be conducted.

Dietary intervention in infancy and later signs of beta-cell autoimmunity

Knip M[1,7], Virtanen SM[3,8], Seppä K[1,6], Ilonen J[9,10], Savilahti E[1], Vaarala O[4], Reunanen A[5], Teramo K[2], Hämäläinen AM[1,11], Paronen J[1], Dosch HM[1,12], Hakulinen T[1,6], Akerblom HK[1]; Finnish TRIGR Study Group

[1]*Hospital for Children and Adolescents and* [2]*Department of Obstetrics and Gynecology, University of Helsinki and Helsinki University Central Hospital, Helsinki, Finland,* [3]*Nutrition Unit,* [4]*Immune Response Unit and* [5]*Department of Health and Functional Capacity, National Institute for Health and Welfare, Helsinki, Finland,* [6]*Finnish Cancer Registry, Helsinki, Finland,* [7]*Department of Pediatrics and* [8]*Research Unit, Tampere University Hospital, and Tampere School of Public Health, University of Tampere, Tampere, Finland,* [9]*Immunogenetics Laboratory, University of Turku, Turku, Finland,* [10]*Department of Clinical Microbiology, University of Kuopio, Kuopio, Finland,* [11]*Department of Pediatrics, Jorvi Hospital, Espoo, and Department of Pediatrics, University of Oulu, Oulu, Finland, and* [12]*Hospital for Sick Children, Research Institute, University of Toronto, Toronto, Canada*

N Engl J Med 2010; **363**: *1900–8*

Background
Short duration of breastfeeding and/or early exposure to complex dietary proteins have been implicated as potential risk factors for β-cell autoimmunity and T1D.

Methods
The study randomised 230 infants to receive either a casein hydrolysate formula or a conventional, cow's-milk based formula (control) whenever breast milk was not available during the first 6–8 months of life. Eligible infants had human leucocyte antigen (HLA) conferred susceptibility to T1D and at least one family member with T1D. Children were followed for 10 years for the development of diabetes related autoantibodies and for development of T1D.

Results
The group assigned to casein hydrolysate formula had a reduced risk of development of β-cell autoimmunity (appearance of one or more antibodies).

Conclusion

Dietary intervention during infancy appears to have a long-lasting effect on markers of β-cell autoimmunity.

COMMENT

Epidemiological studies have suggested that either short duration of breast-feeding and/or early exposure to cow's milk increases the risk of T1D. It would be unethical to randomise subjects to breastfeeding vs. no breastfeeding. Thus, focus has been on avoidance of cow's milk at the time of weaning from breast milk. The Finnish TRIGR Study Group reports on the appearance of diabetes autoantibodies and has found that these are reduced by half. Under way is the full Trial to Reduce Insulin-dependent Diabetes Mellitus in the Genetically at Risk (TRIGR), a true primary prevention study (12). TRIGR has recruited 5606 newborn infants with a family member affected by T1D and enrolled 2159 eligible subjects who carried a risk-conferring HLA genotype. Eighty per cent of the participants were exposed to the study formula. The overall retention rate over the first 5 years was 87%, and protocol compliance was 94%. The full TRIGR has the development of T1D as its primary outcome. The study will conclude in 2017 when the last subject reaches age 10. To this writer, it seems appropriate to always encourage breastfeeding for as long as reasonable. TRIGR will determine whether cow's milk formulas should be avoided. If the Finnish TRIGR study results are replicated – and extended to result in reduced incidence of T1D – it will change feeding habits, probably not just for those with a family history of T1D but perhaps also for the population at large.

Residual beta cell function in newly diagnosed type 1 diabetes after treatment with atorvastatin: the randomised DIATOR trial

Martin S[1], Herder C[1], Schloot NC[1,2], Koenig W[3], Heise T[4], Heinemann L[4], Kolb H[1], on behalf of the DIATOR Study Group

[1] *Institute for Clinical Diabetology, German Diabetes Center, Leibniz Center for Diabetes Research at Heinrich Heine University, Düsseldorf, Germany,*
[2] *Departments of Medicine and Metabolic Diseases, University Hospital, Düsseldorf, Germany,* [3] *Department of Internal Medicine II – Cardiology, University of Ulm Medical Center, Ulm, Germany,* [4] *Profil Institute for Metabolic Research, Neuss, Germany*

PLoS One 2011; 6: e17554

Background

There is some evidence suggesting that the lipid-lowering agent atorvastatin also has immunomodulatory effects. Thus, the current study was undertaken to determine whether atorvastatin might alter the course of T1D.

Methods

The study randomised 89 subjects (46 to atorvastatin, 43 to placebo), aged 18–39, and randomised within 3 months of diagnosis of T1D. Intervention consisted of atorvastatin or placebo daily for 18 months. The primary endpoint was β-cell function – as measured by C-peptide – at 18 months, with 63 subjects included in the analysis.

Results

Outcome measures were assessed at 12 and 18 months. Fasting and stimulated C-peptide levels were not significantly different between groups at 18 months. However, in secondary analyses, both fasting and median stimulated C-peptide declined over time more slowly in the atorvastatin group than in the placebo group when the groups were considered independently.

Conclusion

Atorvastatin did not have a beneficial effect in recent-onset T1D. Some secondary analyses suggest that additional studies may be warranted.

COMMENT

This small provocative study did not meet its primary outcome (difference in C-peptide between groups at 18 months). However, when the authors examined the decline in C-peptide within the atorvastatin group, there was a non-significant decline, whereas the decline in C-peptide within the placebo group was significant. This may indicate that further evaluation of atorvastatin is warranted. Statins are widely used for the treatment of hypercholesterolaemia and reduction of cardiovascular risk. Atorvastatin will soon be generic. If an orally administered, commonly used, generic drug could slow the course of T1D that would be worthwhile. Thus, this writer would be enthusiastic to see a full-scale trial of atorvastatin in T1D.

Phase I (safety) study of autologous tolerogenic dendritic cells in type 1 diabetic patients

Giannoukakis N[1,2], Phillips B[1], Finegold D[3], Harnaha J[1], Trucco M[1]

[1] Division of Immunogenetics, Department of Pediatrics, University of Pittsburgh School of Medicine, Pittsburgh, PA, USA, [2] Department of Pathology, University of Pittsburgh School of Medicine, Pittsburgh, PA, USA, and [3] Department of Human Genetics, University of Pittsburgh School of Medicine, Pittsburgh, PA, USA

*Diabetes Care 2011; **34**: 2026–32*

Background

This phase 1 study investigated the safety of autologous dendritic cells, stabilised into an immunosuppressive state, in established T1D.

Methods

The study randomised 10 subjects (three to unmanipulated 'control' autologous dendritic cells and seven to autologous dendritic cells engineered *ex vivo* toward an immunosuppressive state). Subjects were aged 18–60 and were randomised after at least 5 years of T1D, all with undetectable C-peptide. All subjects received four rounds of autologous dendritic cells administered intradermally once every 2 weeks. The primary endpoint was the proportion of patients with adverse events over 12 months, based on physician global assessment, haematology, biochemistry and immune monitoring.

Results

There were no discernible adverse events in any patient during the study. The only measurable difference, compared with baseline, was a significant increase in peripheral B220+ CD11c B-lymphocytes, mainly seen in the recipients of engineered dendritic cells.

Conclusion

Treatment with autologous dendritic cells, in a native state or directed *ex vivo* toward a tolerogenic immunosuppressive state, is safe and well tolerated.

COMMENT

Autologous tolerogenic dendritic cells theoretically may be a major novel approach in arresting the course of T1D. The current study was initiated to determine whether administration of such cells might result in unexpected adverse effects that would limit their use. The answer is that no obvious adverse effects emerged. Hopefully this will pave the way for use of autologous dendritic cells engineered *ex vivo* toward an immunosuppressive state in recent-onset T1D, to see whether they have the potential to alter the course of the disease. We eagerly await the initiation of such studies.

Beta cell function during rapamycin monotherapy in long-term type 1 diabetes

Piemonti L[1], Maffi P[1], Monti L[2], Lampasona V[3], Perseghin G[4,5], Magistretti P[1], Secchi A[1,6], Bonifacio E[1,7]

[1] Diabetes Research Institute (HSR-DRI), San Raffaele Scientific Institute, Milan, Italy, [2] Cardiodiabetes and Core Lab, Division of Metabolic and Cardiovascular Sciences, San Raffaele Scientific Institute, Milan, Italy, [3] Unit of Genomics for the Diagnosis of Human Pathologies, Center for Genomics, Bioinformatics and Biostatistics, San Raffaele Scientific Institute, Milan, Italy, [4] Unit of Obesity and Metabolic Related Diseases, Division of Metabolic and Cardiovascular Sciences, San Raffaele Scientific Institute, Milan, Italy, [5] Department of Sport, Nutrition and Health Sciences, Università degli Studi di Milano, Milan, Italy, [6] Unit of Clinical Transplant, Division of Immunology, Transplantation and Infectious Diseases, Università Vita-Salute San Raffaele, Milan, Italy, and [7] Center for Regenerative Therapies Dresden, Dresden University of Technology, Dresden, Germany

Diabetologia 2011; **54**: 433–9

Background

The authors sought to determine whether immunosuppression therapy can reinstate β-cell function in patients with long-term T1D.

Methods

The study measured β-cell function in 22 subjects aged 30–48 with long-standing (17–35 years' duration) T1D, on a waiting list for islet transplantation, who received rapamycin monotherapy as pre-conditioning. As a comparison group, the study measured β-cell function in 14 subjects aged 20–68, with long-standing (11–22 years' duration) T1D, also on a waiting list for islet transplantation, but who did not receive rapamycin pre-conditioning.

Results

During rapamycin treatment, the proportion of patients with detectable fasting C-peptide increased from 4 of 22 prior to rapamycin therapy to 13 of 22 ($p = 0.01$). Exogenous insulin requirement decreased in those who were C-peptide responsive. These variables remained unchanged in the 14 control patients.

Conclusion

The authors concluded that therapies to reinstate β-cell function may be applicable to patients with long-term C-peptide negative T1D.

COMMENT

This is a provocative study that found that patients who were awaiting islet cell transplantation and were pre-treated with rapamycin had an increase in β-cell function. Since it is generally not thought possible to restore β-cell function in long-standing T1D, this study raises new questions about the potential reversibility of the disease. In last year's *Yearbook*, we commented on an autopsy study (13) that demonstrated that some patients with long-standing apparent T1D had normal-appearing islets, intact C-peptide, absence of high risk HLA, and lack of antibodies at the time of death. Other studies also suggest that there may be persistent β-cell function in long-standing T1D. The current study suggests that such persistent β-cell function may be enhanced by immune intervention. Although such intervention is unlikely to fully re-store β-cell function, studies of this type raise many new questions about our understanding of T1D.

OVERALL COMMENTARY

This year has raised concerns amongst many, due to the highly visible press releases concerning failure to achieve the primary outcome mea-sure in two phase 3 studies with anti-CD3 (Protégé and DEFEND-1) and two phase 3 studies with GAD-alum. As noted in the above commen-taries, all is not so bleak. As discussed, there were crucial design flaws in the anti-CD3 studies, and the GAD-alum studies perhaps used the wrong formulation (with adjuvant), by the wrong route (subcutaneous) and at the wrong time (after clinical diagnosis of T1D). To this writer, it would be premature to bury either anti-CD3 or GAD as potential interventions, particularly if they are used in prevention of T1D or as components of combination therapy. Indeed, all of the trials of immunotherapy that have achieved their primary outcome still have showed loss of effect over time, so that it is unlikely that any single therapy alone will dramatically alter the course of T1D. As discussed in a recent 'Perspective', stopping T1D will probably not only involve a combination of therapies but also re-quire either replacement of β-cells or use of agents that stimulate β-cell regeneration or at the least enhance β-cell function (14). Fortunately, there is much progress in conducting the pre-clinical studies needed to advance such concepts into clinical trials. Over the next few years, we should begin seeing such clinical trials being conducted.

REFERENCES

1. Effects of oral insulin in relatives of patients with type 1 diabetes. The Diabetes Preven-tion Trial – Type 1. The Diabetes Prevention Trial – Type 1 Study Group. *Diabetes Care* 2005; **28**: 1068–76
2. Näntö-Salonen K, Kupila A, Simell S, Siljander H, Salonsaari T, Hekkala A, Korhonen S, Erkkola R, Sipilä JI, Haavisto L, Siltala M, Tuominen J, Hakalax J, Hyöty H, Ilonen J, Veijola R, Simell T, Knip M, Simell O. Nasal insulin to prevent type 1 diabetes in chil-dren with HLA genotypes and autoantibodies conferring increased risk of disease: a double-blind, randomised controlled trial. *Lancet* 2008; **372**: 1746–55
3. Harrison LC, Honeyman MC, Steele CE, Stone NL, Sarugeri E, Bonifacio E, Couper JJ, Colman PG. Pancreatic β-cell function and immune responses to insulin after

administration of intranasal insulin to humans at risk for type 1 diabetes. *Diabetes Care* 2004; **27**: 2348–55

4. Ludvigsson J, Faresjö M, Hjorth M, Axelsson S, Chéramy M, Pihl M, Vaarala O, Forsander G, Ivarsson S, Johansson C, Lindh A, Nilsson NO, Aman J, Ortqvist E, Zerhouni P, Casas R. GAD treatment and insulin secretion in recent-onset type 1 diabetes. *N Engl J Med* 2008; **359**: 1909–20

5. http://www.diamyd.com/docs/pressClip.aspx?section=investor&ClipID=578780

6. http://www.diamyd.com/docs/pressClip.aspx?section=investor&ClipID=584435

7. Herold KC, Hagopian W, Auger JA, Poumian-Ruiz E, Taylor L, Donaldson D, Gitelman SE, Harlan DM, Xu D, Zivin RA, Bluestone JA. Anti-CD3 monoclonal antibody in new-onset type 1 diabetes mellitus. *N Engl J Med* 2002; **346**: 1692–8

8. Keymeulen B, Vandemeulebroucke E, Ziegler AG, Mathieu C, Kaufman L, Hale G, Gorus F, Goldman M, Walter M, Candon S, Schandene L, Crenier L, De Block C, Seigneurin JM, De Pauw P, Pierard D, Weets I, Rebello P, Bird P, Berrie E, Frewin M, Waldmann H, Bach JF, Pipeleers D, Chatenoud L. Insulin needs after CD3-antibody therapy in new-onset type 1 diabetes. *N Engl J Med* 2005; **352**: 2598–608

9. Herold KC, Gitelman SE, Masharani U, Hagopian W, Bisikirska B, Donaldson D, Rother K, Diamond B, Harlan DM, Bluestone JA. A single course of anti-CD3 monoclonal antibody hOKT3gamma1(Ala-Ala) results in improvement in C-peptide responses and clinical parameters for at least 2 years after onset of type 1 diabetes. *Diabetes* 2005; **54**: 1763–9

10. Keymeulen B, Walter M, Mathieu C, Kaufman L, Gorus F, Hilbrands R, Vandemeulebroucke E, Van de Velde U, Crenier L, De Block C, Candon S, Waldmann H, Ziegler AG, Chatenoud L, Pipeleers D. Four-year metabolic outcome of a randomised controlled CD3-antibody trial in recent-onset type 1 diabetic patients depends on their age and baseline residual beta cell mass. *Diabetologia* 2010; **53**: 614–23

11. http://www.gsk.com/media/pressreleases/2011/2011_pressrelease_10039.htm

12. Knip M, Virtanen SM, Becker D, Dupré J, Krischer JP, Åkerblom HK for the TRIGR Study Group. Early feeding and risk of type 1 diabetes: experiences from the Trial to Reduce Insulin-dependent diabetes mellitus in the Genetically at Risk (TRIGR). *Am J Clin Nutr* 2011 Jun 8; doi:10.3945/ajcn.110.000711

13. Gianani R, Campbell-Thompson M, Sarkar SA, Wasserfall C, Pugliese A, Solis JM, Kent SC, Hering BJ, West E, Steck A, Bonner-Weir S, Atkinson MA, Coppieters K, von Herrath M, Eisenbarth GS. Dimorphic histopathology of long-standing childhood-onset diabetes. *Diabetologia* 2010; **53**: 690–8

14. Skyler JS, Ricordi C. Stopping type 1 diabetes: attempts to prevent or cure type 1 diabetes in man. *Diabetes* 2011; **60**: 1–8

CHAPTER 10

Advances in Exercise, Physical Activity and Diabetes Mellitus

Howard Zisser[1,2], Mark Sueyoshi[1], Kelsey Krigstein[1], Andrei Szigiato[3] and Michael C. Riddell[3]

[1] Sansum Diabetes Research Institute, Santa Barbara, CA, USA,
[2] University of California at Santa Barbara, Santa Barbara, CA, USA
[3] School of Kinesiology and Health Science, York University, Toronto, ON, Canada

INTRODUCTION

Diet and exercise form a solid foundation for the prevention and treatment of diabetes mellitus. Regular physical activity increases insulin sensitivity, improves pharmacotherapy, lowers blood sugar concentrations, reduces body fat content, builds muscle and improves cardiovascular fitness and function. A number of recent studies have demonstrated the effectiveness of regular exercise in improving metabolic control and overall health in persons with diabetes, although the clinical management of physically active patients with type 1 diabetes (T1D) remains a challenge. This year, we highlight a number of papers, published between 1 July and 30 June 2011, that are valuable contributions to the field of exercise and diabetes management.

Acute hypoxia and exercise improve insulin sensitivity (S_I^{2*}) in individuals with type 2 diabetes

Mackenzie R[1], Maxwell N[2], Castle P[3], Birckley G[2], Watt P[2]

[1] School of Life Sciences, Department of Human and Health Sciences, University of Westminster, London, UK, [2] Chelsea School Research Centre, University of Brighton, Eastbourne, UK, and [3] Department of Sport and Exercise Science, University of Bedfordshire, Bedford, UK

Diabetes Metab Res Rev 2011; 27: 94–101

Int J Clin Pract 2012; 66 (Suppl. 175): 58–60

Aims

Similar to muscular contractions, hypoxia has been suggested to stimulate glucose uptake into skeletal muscle independent of insulin signalling. However, hypoxia has also been shown to cause insulin resistance in rodents, due to a sympathoadrenal-induced epinephrine release, thereby reducing glucose disposal. The aim of the study was to examine the effects of acute hypoxia, with and without exercise, on insulin sensitivity (S_I^{2*}), glucose effectiveness (S_G^{2*}) and β-cell function in individuals with type 2 diabetes mellitus (T2D).

Methods

Eight sedentary males with T2D, who were not on exogenous insulin and who were diagnosed within the last 5 years, were recruited for this study. Following an overnight fast and baseline blood sampling, subjects completed the following in a randomised order (each visit separated by 7–14 days): (1) normoxic rest; (2) hypoxic rest (inspired $O_2 =$ 14.6%); (3) normoxic exercise; and (4) hypoxic exercise (inspired $O_2 =$ 14.6%). The exercise performed was at a work load equivalent to 90% of normoxic lactate threshold. Arterialised venous blood samples were taken every 10 min during the tests. A 4-h intravenous glucose tolerance test was administered immediately following each test under normoxic conditions.

Results

The tests demonstrated increased insulin sensitivity following hypoxic rest compared with normoxic rest [$S_I^{2*}=$ 2.25 ± 0.50 vs. 1.39 ± 0.08 × 10^{-4} μU/ml (mean ± SEM), respectively] ($p < 0.05$), greater insulin sensitivity following hypoxic exercise compared with normoxic exercise ($p < 0.05$), and a lower acute insulin response to glucose following hypoxic rest compared with normoxic rest ($p = 0.014$). Blood lactic acid tests showed no differences between groups. Arterialised blood glucose tests showed a significantly greater decrease in glycaemia during hypoxic exercise (−1.82 ± 0.64 mmol/l) compared with normoxic exercise (−0.91 ± 0.35 mmol/l) ($p < 0.05$). With respect to insulin levels, hypoxic rest showed no change, while hypoxic exercise caused insulin levels to decrease from baseline but with no difference compared with normoxic exercise. The ability of glucose to use the muscle-contraction-stimulated pathway, as measured by glucose effectiveness (S_G^{2*}), showed no differences between conditions.

Conclusion

Hypoxic conditions improve glucose tolerance, via insulin-mediated and non-insulin-mediated mechanisms, in the hours following exposure.

Hypoxic exercise enhances insulin sensitivity over normoxic exercise in patients with T2D.

COMMENT

Based on this study, acute hypoxia during rest and particularly during exercise provides improvements in short-term insulin sensitivity and glycaemic control for patients with T2D. While this study is an interesting and innovative approach to the treatment of diabetes, its applications and uses are limited with respect to economic and clinical practicality. Applying acute hypoxia to patients with T2D is expensive and cumbersome as a treatment. Research into long-standing hypoxia with respect to insulin sensitivity and glycaemic control may be useful in high elevation areas such as mountain climbing for those with diabetes. However, as a treatment for more sedentary diabetics on a wider scale, it is probably impractical at this stage of technological development (i.e. hypoxic environmental chambers). Moreover, a 2004 study that looked at 2658 participants in a sleep-disordered breathing state or sleep apnoea, which involves periods of hypoxia, found that sleep-related hypoxia was associated with glucose intolerance rather than improved insulin sensitivity, independent of age, gender, body mass index and waist circumference (1). Similarly, in a smaller study with 13 non-diabetic volunteers who underwent 5 h of intermittent hypoxia over 2 days, insulin sensitivity deteriorated (2). Thus, it remains unclear if hypoxia is good or bad for insulin sensitivity for patients with T2D.

Effect of an intensive exercise intervention strategy on modifiable cardiovascular risk factors in subjects with type 2 diabetes mellitus: a randomised controlled trial. The Italian Diabetes and Exercise Study (IDES)

Balducci S, Zanuso S, Nicolucci A, De Feo P, Cavallo S, Cardelli P, Fallucca S, Alessa E, Fallucca F, Pugliese G; for the Italian Diabetes Exercise Study (IDES) Investigators

Diabetes Division, Sant'Andrea Hospital, Rome, Italy

*Arch Intern Med 2010; **170**: 1794–803*

Aims

Cardiorespiratory fitness is inversely related to rates of cardiovascular-related mortality in patients with T2D. The aim of this study was to assess the efficacy of an exercise intervention strategy combining supervised exercise with exercise counselling on increasing physical activity (PA) levels, lowering HbA1c levels and improving other cardiovascular risk factors in a large T2D cohort in Italy.

Methods

In all, 606 eligible sedentary patients with T2D were enrolled in 22 outpatient diabetes clinics across Italy and were randomised to the exercise plus counselling group (EXE, $n = 303$) or the counselling-only group (CON, $n = 303$). The study period was 12 months and counselling was given every 3 months for both groups. The EXE group underwent mixed aerobic and resistance training twice a week for a total of 150 min of supervised exercise per week. Efficacy was measured primarily by HbA1c levels, while secondary outcomes were measures of other modifiable cardiovascular risk factors. Baseline PA levels were established by the Minnesota Leisure-time Physical Activity Questionnaire and PA levels were estimated in metabolic equivalents [1 MET = 1 kcal/(kg h); sleeping is 0.9 MET, running a 5.5 min mile is 18 METs]. Unsupervised PA levels were prospectively evaluated through daily diaries.

Results

Compared with the CON group, the EXE group had double the total PA levels during the intervention (mean ± SD: 10.0 ± 8.7 vs. 20.0 ± 0.9 MET hours per week). The EXE group also had significant improvements in HbA1c levels [mean difference (95% confidence interval): −0.30% (−0.49% to −0.10%); $p < 0.001$], systolic [−4.2 mmHg (−6.9 to −1.6 mmHg); $p = 0.002$] and diastolic [−1.7 mmHg (−3.3 to −1.1 mmHg); $p = 0.03$) blood pressures; high-density lipoprotein levels [3.7 mg/dl (2.2–5.3 mg/dl); $p < 0.001$]; low-density lipoprotein levels [−9.6 mg/dl (−15.9 to −3.3 mg/dl); $p = 0.003$]; waist circumference [−3.6 cm (−4.4 to −2.9 cm); $p < 0.001$]; body mass index [−0.78 (−1.07 to −0.49); $p < 0.001$]; and C-reactive protein levels [−1.0 mg/l (−1.4 to −0.7 mg/l); $p < 0.001$]. Moreover, risk scores as measured by the 10-year Coronary Heart Disease UK Prospective Diabetes Study [−3.1 (−4.2 to −2.0); $p < 0.001$] and 10-year fatal algorithms [−2.4 (−3.3 to −1.5); $p = 0.01$] also improved in the EXE group.

Conclusion

This type of exercise intervention (supervised and unsupervised together) is effective in improving exercise adherence, cardiorespiratory fitness and cardiovascular risk factors, while lowering HbA1c levels in patients with T2D. In contrast, although PA counselling alone may promote some increases in PA patterns, this is probably insufficient to reduce the cardiovascular risk profile in these high risk individuals.

COMMENT

This large-scale study included several centres across Italy, thereby reducing the influence of local factors (e.g. urban vs. rural living) that are often thought to influence PA adherence. These results are promising for a 1-year intervention, with potentially better outcomes had the study continued. The study provides strong support for the combination of PA counselling with supervised training rather than counselling alone to lower HbA1c and other cardiovascular risk factors. The success in reinforcing PA through this mixed method may be applied to dietary counselling. What the study does not reveal are the social effects of interacting with other patients with diabetes on a regular basis in an exercise setting. In a large 2011 meta-analysis that compared PA counselling alone with structured exercise training with instruction, it was found that only the latter was associated with improvements in HbA1c while PA 'advice only' lowered HbA1c when combined with dietary advice (3). Another study that looked at 70 inactive T2D patients found that giving PA counselling at baseline, 6 and 9 months with follow-up calls at 1, 3, 6 and 9 months resulted in clinically significant decreases in HbA1c, blood pressure, fibrinogen and cholesterol levels (4). Thus, regular reinforcement of PA by a trained exercise counsellor, as opposed to intermittent advice during medical appointments, is probably of considerable benefit for patients with diabetes. When PA is not a familiar daily activity, we think it unreasonable to expect individuals to suddenly change sedentary behaviours after a 15-min medical appointment, once every 3 months.

Exercise treadmill test in detecting asymptomatic coronary artery disease in type 2 diabetes mellitus

Kim MK, Baek KH, Song KH, Kwon HS, Lee JM, Kang MI, Yoon KH, Cha BY, Son HY, Lee KW

Department of Internal Medicine, Catholic University of Korea School of Medicine, Seoul, Korea

*Diabetes Metab J 2011; **35**: 34–40*

Background

In T2D patients, asymptomatic coronary artery disease (CAD) has higher cardiac mortality risk because CAD often becomes symptomatic at an advanced stage. In a large autopsy study of diabetic patients with asymptomatic CAD, about 50% less than 65 years and 75% older than 65 years had high-grade coronary atherosclerosis with no evidence prior to death (5). Although it is debatable whether to screen all T2D patients for asymptomatic CAD, appropriate screening criteria using an evidence-based diagnostic approach for high risk patients may identify individuals who could benefit from early detection.

Aims

The aim of the study was to develop appropriate criteria for screening patients with T2D for asymptomatic CAD using a diagnostic approach of an exercise treadmill test (ETT) and then a coronary angiogram if the ETT was positive for myocardial ischaemia.

Methods

T2D outpatients ($n = 213$) with no previous history of cardiovascular disease or severe systemic disease with poor prognosis were enrolled. The ETT was performed using the Bruce graded exercise protocol. The study also tested, using the ETT, T2D patients ($n = 53$) who had reported chest discomfort. Patients ceased taking beta blockers and calcium channel blockers 72 h prior to the test. A 12-lead electrocardiogram (ECG) was used during the test and blood pressure was monitored every 2 min during exercise and recovery. The ETT was considered positive when a horizontal or down-sloping ST segment with a depression ≥ 1 mm occurred 0.08 s after the J point at 85% of the predicted maximal heart rate for the patient's age. Coronary angiography was performed only when the ETT was positive. Positive asymptomatic was defined as objective evidence of ischaemia during the ETT. Flow-limiting CAD was defined as a stenosis of 70%+ on coronary angiography.

Results

A total of 186 patients successfully completed the tests, with 31 (16.6%) patients with a positive ETT and 155 (83.3%) having a negative ETT. Of the 31, two had no defects on a thallium scan and six refused further evaluation. Within the remaining 23 patients, 11 patients were found to have coronary stenosis $\geq 70\%$ via coronary angiogram. Both age (63.1 $\pm$ 9.4 years vs. 53.7 $\pm$ 10.1 years, p = 0.008) and duration of diabetes (16.0 $\pm$ 7.5 years vs. 5.5 $\pm$ 5.7 years, p < 0.001) predicted the results of the ETT and coronary angiography. When the authors analysed the results for 60+ years of age and a 10-year duration of diabetes, they found that a positive predictive value using the ETT was 87.5%. With respect to patients who presented with chest discomfort or exertional dyspnoea, 13 of the 17 patients with a positive ETT underwent coronary angiography; 10 of 13 (76.9%) of those had coronary stenosis >70%.

Conclusion

The authors concluded that the ETT had a higher success rate and thus improved cost-effectiveness if used to screen for asymptomatic CAD, age $\geq$ 60 years with a duration of T2D $\geq$ 10 years.

COMMENT

Despite some acknowledged limitations (sample size, retrospective design etc.), this study shows that the ETT is a cost-effective means for determining if CAD is present in older patients with T2D who have prolonged disease duration (>10 years). Indeed, the ETT demonstrates the heart's actual work capacity and health status more accurately than a pharmacological stress test, at least for those who can complete the exercise, and it does not expose the patient to ionising radiation. The European Society of Cardiology and International Olympic Committee recently endorsed a standardised screening evaluation method which utilises a 12-lead ECG along with a detailed history and physical examination to detect underlying causes of sudden cardiac death. The USA lacks a standardised screening system and is in need of well designed studies to demonstrate the effectiveness of the ECG for identifying underlying cardiovascular abnormalities in young athletes (6). In an assessment of appropriateness for stress echocardiography in detecting CAD in asymptomatic patients with high coronary heart disease risk, which includes anyone with diabetes, the study scored the diagnostic approach 6 out of 9 for appropriateness, with a score of 7 being considered as a generally acceptable approach (7). In a 1990 study with 136 diabetic patients, it was found that ETT for diabetic persons yielded angiographically demonstrable asymptomatic coronary heart disease in 9% (8). Based on this study's results, the use of ETT to diagnose asymptomatic CAD may be justified with its 48% success rate for all patients. As the paper notes, the best approach seems to redefine the screening protocol to patients' age $\geq$ 60 and with at least a decade long history of diabetes.

Preventing exercise-induced hypoglycaemia in type 1 diabetes using real-time continuous glucose monitoring and a new carbohydrate intake algorithm: an observational field study

Riddell MC, Milliken J

School of Kinesiology and Health Science, Muscle Health Research Centre, Physical Activity and Diabetes Unit, York University, Toronto, ON, Canada

*Diabetes Technol Ther 2011; **13**: 819–25*

Background

Physical activity for individuals with T1D is coupled with a risk of hypoglycaemia that can be difficult to predict, much less prevent. Symptoms of hypoglycaemia are often masked by physical activity. In order to better prevent a hypoglycaemic event, individuals with T1D must know the duration and intensity of activity beforehand to adjust insulin administration and carbohydrate intake. There are currently no guidelines on carbohydrate intake to prevent hypoglycaemia when glucose levels are within the appropriate range, but still dropping. Real-time continuous glucose monitoring (RT-CGM) offers a solution to reduce the likelihood of hypoglycaemic events for individuals during and after exercise, but only if appropriate amounts of carbohydrate are ingested during exercise.

Aims

This study assessed the use of a novel carbohydrate intake algorithm to be used with RT-CGM, which takes into account both the interstitial glucose concentration and the rate at which glucose is dropping during exercise.

Methods

At a youth sports camp in Canada, 25 youth (12 girls and 13 boys, 8–18 years old) with T1D participated in this field study. A baseline capillary glucose was taken each morning and intermittently throughout the day and interstitial glucose was measured with RT-CGM for 2–6 days of physical activity. The sports performed (basketball, tennis, soccer and track and field) varied from moderate to vigorous activity throughout the day. Using the RT-CGM algorithm, the researchers provided a dose of fast-acting oral carbohydrate (8 g, 16 g or 20 g) based on the measured glycaemia and the RT-CGM downward trend arrows predicting ensuing biochemical hypoglycaemia (glucose < 3.9 mml/l). Participants stopped their sporting activity if interstitial levels dropped below 5 mml/l or if they felt symptoms of hypoglycaemia.

Results

Of the 25 participants, six were excluded because of sensor loss or insufficient data and one was excluded because of a hypoglycaemic event where he infused insulin on his own agency after a fast-acting oral carbohydrate intake. From the 18 volunteers included in the analyses, 35 algorithm events were captured with an average sensor use time of 2.9 days. When glucose levels were already below target (<5.0 mmol/l) and carbohydrates were consumed, five out of 13 possible cases of mild hypoglycaemia occurred. Mild hypoglycaemia occurred only twice of 22 times when the RT-CGM alerted participants of dropping glucose levels during exercise and when the new carbohydrate intake algorithm was used.

Conclusion

The use of RT-CGM with a novel carbohydrate intake algorithm that implements directional rate of change arrows appears to reduce the risk of hypoglycaemic events and helps maintain euglycaemia in physically active youth with T1D. This study also found fairly consistent glycaemic responses to fast-acting carbohydrates despite age and body size differences. Smaller doses of carbohydrates (8 g, 16 g) were sufficient to

prevent hypoglycaemia, while larger does (20 g) had a more variable glucose response when the glucose was rapidly dropping. The algorithm is
designed to help 'fine tune' glucose levels already in the targeted range.
In all cases when the algorithm was used, participants maintained a near
euglycaemic state for 30 min before carbohydrate intake and 60 min after. Because of a small test group and lack of a control group, however,
the recommendations are difficult to generalise.

COMMENT

Previous exercise trials have shown that patients with T1D exhibit a wide variability in interstitial glucose profiles before, during and after physical exercise
(9). In the same vein, this study also revealed more variable responses to higher
amounts of ingested glucose (20 g) and thus the need for person-specific
glucose intake protocols, or perhaps a higher CGM threshold for pending
hypoglycaemia in order to avoid needing large doses of glucose that would
yield different responses from person to person. A small June 2011 study on
low glucose alarms on CGMs found that increasing the alarm warning from
4.0 mmol/l to 5.5 mmol/l reduced the occurrence of hypoglycaemic events
by half with no cases of false alarms (10). That particular study did not use a
carbohydrate intake algorithm to prevent a future hypoglycaemic event, but
raising the threshold in which the RT-CGM alerts the individual may eliminate
occurrences of even mild hypoglycaemia and/or allow for slower acting food
carbohydrates to be used rather than the relatively costly fast-acting oral dex-
trose tabs. Based on this preliminary work, it may be that RT-CGM would be
most beneficial to younger individuals with T1D with less experience in managing exercise and glycaemia or those who begin or change their exercise
regimen because of lack of experience with their body's response to exercise
and glucose doses.

Metformin and exercise in type 2 diabetes: examining treatment modality interactions

Boule NG[1], Robert C[1], Bell GJ[1], Johnson ST[2], Bell RC[3], Lewanczuk RZ[4], Gabr RQ[5], Brocks DR[5]

[1] *Faculty of Physical Education and Recreation, University of Alberta, Edmonton, Canada,* [2] *Centre for Nursing and Health Studies, Athabasca University, Athabasca, Canada,* [3] *Department of Agricultural, Food and Nutritional Science, University of Alberta, Edmonton, Canada,* [4] *Faculty of Medicine, Division of Endocrinology, University of Alberta, Edmonton, Canada, and* [5] *Faculty of Pharmacy and Pharmaceutical Sciences, University of Alberta, Edmonton, Canada*

*Diabetes Care 2011; **34**: 1469–74*

Background

Metformin is regularly prescribed with regular physical activity for the management of T2D. However, the few studies conducted on therapy that combines metformin with lifestyle modification do not show an additive benefit. Both muscle contraction and metformin have been shown to activate AMP-activated protein kinase (AMPK) and thus the oral agent has been termed an 'exercise mimetic'. Metformin has also been shown to improve exercise tolerance in non-diabetic women with clinically defined angina.

Aims

This study had three objectives: (1) to examine the effect of metformin on acute metabolic and hormonal responses to exercise; (2) to examine the effect of exercise on plasma metformin concentrations; and (3) to examine the interaction between metformin and acute exercise on subsequent response to a standardised meal.

Methods

Ten T2D volunteers (eight men and two post-menopausal women) were included in this study. The participants were between the ages of 30 and 65; not taking glucose-lowering medication or insulin; HbA1c $\leq 8\%$, resting blood pressure $\leq 140/90$ mmHg, low-density lipoprotein ≤ 3.5 mmol/l, and total high-density lipoprotein ≤ 5.0; and consistent activity levels, medications and diet within the last 3 months with no intent to change over the course of the study. The study used a factorial design with each participant exposed to four conditions: (1) metformin and no exercise; (2) metformin and exercise; (3) placebo and no exercise; and (4) placebo and exercise. Metformin and placebo conditions were given in 28-day increments. On the last 2 days of each condition, participants were assessed for baseline glucose levels during a non-exercise day followed by an exercise day. During the non-exercise day, participants remained at rest for the test period. On exercise days, blood samples were taken before, during and after (up to 2 h) the exercise test. On both days, metabolic outcomes such as V_{O_2} and V_{CO_2} were measured and blood samples were taken.

Results

Plasma metformin concentrations were higher on the exercise day compared with the non-exercise day both before (1897 ± 352 vs. 1594 ± 363 ng/ml, p = 0.02) and after (2230 ± 335 vs. 1893 ± 323 ng/ml, p = 0.01) exercise. Metformin increased heart rate and plasma lactate levels during exercise (p ≤ 0.01) and lowered the respiratory exchange ratio (p = 0.03) but did not affect total energy expenditure. Glycaemic response to the standardised meal was reduced by metformin, but the effect was minimised when exercise was added (p = 0.05). In the metformin and exercise condition, glucagon levels were the highest. Throughout all sessions, lactate concentrations were higher in the metformin condition compared with the placebo (p ≤ 0.05).

Conclusion

Metformin and exercise increased heart rate, sustained higher plasma metformin concentrations and had no additive effects on the glycaemic response to meals. Under the study conditions, exercise appeared to interfere with the glucose-lowering effect of metformin. Other metformin interactions included increased lipid oxidation and increased lactate concentrations during exercise.

COMMENT

A similar study looking at the short-term treatment with metformin also found that the combination of metformin treatment with acute exercise did not enhance insulin sensitivity in insulin resistant individuals. Interestingly, the combination of the two may reduce the positive effects of exercise alone (11). While in this particular study it was found that metformin increased heart rate, a previous study with 17 participants found a statistically significant reduction in peak heart rate with metformin (–2.0%). The findings of that study are consistent that metformin reduces respiratory exchange ratio (–3.0%) (p < 0.05) (12). The authors state that the lack of improvement in post-meal (lunch) plasma glucose concentrations on the exercise days should not discourage the use of exercise as a treatment modality. While metformin has no additive glycaemic benefit when used with exercise, this study emphasises that it may be important to consider the timing of exercise and meals to obtain optimal glycaemic benefits.

Endurance athletes and type 1 diabetes

Devadoss M, Kennedy L, Herbold N

Milton Hospital, Milton, MA, USA

*Diabetes Educ 2011; **37**: 193–207*

Aims

The aim of this study was to gather information about the diabetes management practices of endurance athletes with T1D, and then to compare these findings with the current American Diabetic Association (ADA) recommendations regarding physical activity performed by individuals with T1D.

Methods

A total of 94 endurance athletes (long-distance runners, swimmers, cyclists, cross-country skiers and triathletes) aged 18 and older with T1D participated in this study. Participants were instructed to complete an anonymous online survey that consisted of 38 questions regarding their carbohydrate ingestion, insulin regimen, injection site, insulin range, exercise routine and eating habits. The questions were derived from ADA guidelines, literature on the topic of athletes with T1D and the researchers' own experiences working with athletes with diabetes. The majority of Likert scale questions inquired how closely participants believed they followed ADA guidelines on exercise and diabetes. A link to the questionnaire was posted on the Diabetes Exercise and Sports Association website from 20 February to 20 March 2010.

Results

Male participants made up 52.7% of respondents. Only 13% of participants claimed to adhere to ADA recommendations when planning their meals, while 46% reported not knowing the guidelines and 41% said they did not follow the guidelines. With regard to current clinical recommendations for athletes with T1D, participants reported following about 50% 'most of the time' or 'almost always'. Forty per cent of respondents claimed they followed the recommendations 'sometimes' or 'most of the time'. When duration of exercise was divided into 0–1 h, 1–1.5 h and more than 1.5 h, analysis showed that the occurrence of low blood glucose increased with longer duration of exercise ($p = 0.012$). Occurrence of low blood glucose corresponds to the following scale: 1, almost never; 2, rarely; 3, sometimes; 4, most of the time; 5, almost always. For 0–1 h of exercise, this value was 2.17 ± 0.761. For 1–1.5 h, the value was 2.57 ± 0.647. For more than 1.5 h of exercise, the value increased to 2.73 ± 0.691. Twenty-eight of the 94 participants (35.9%) reported that they did not decrease their basal insulin dosage on exercise days. Of the athletes who did reduce basal insulin, 20.5% ($n = 16$) reduced it by at least 50%. However, data analysis did not reveal a correlation between reduction of basal insulin and the occurrence of low blood glucose. Athletes who consumed carbohydrate 'almost always' prior to exercise when their blood glucose was less than 100 mg/dl reported fewer episodes of hypoglycaemia 0–4 h after exercise compared with those who responded 'sometimes' or 'almost never/rarely'. However, these results were not statistically significant ($p = 0.222$). While most of the participants followed ADA recommendations for monitoring blood glucose before (90%) and after (85.7%) exercise, only 46 participants (50%) reported monitoring glucose during exercise. Lastly, 72% of athletes who completed the survey claimed that they exercise when their blood glucose is 250 mg/dl or greater.

Discussion

Perhaps one of the most significant findings from this study was that longer duration of exercise increases the likelihood of low blood glucose in individuals with T1D. This result was expected, given that hepatic glycogen stores become depleted during exercise and/or hepatic glucose production fails to match peripheral glucose utilisation in patients with T1D who do not lower their circulating insulin levels. Importantly, data from this study suggest that reducing basal insulin levels on days of exercise helps to decrease the prevalence of hypoglycaemia during the post-exercise period. In addition to lowering pre-exercise insulin levels, the ADA also recommends consumption of carbohydrates before, during and after endurance exercise to help prevent the occurrence of exercise-induced hypoglycaemia (13). While the findings of this study are consistent with ADA recommendations, the results were not statistically different from those who do not lower basal insulin levels. Only half of these athletes indicated that they follow the ADA guideline to check blood glucose during exercise, and almost three-quarters of them admitted to exercising with high blood glucose values (>250 mg/dl). The ADA suggests that athletes should discontinue exercise with blood glucose values higher than 250 mg/dl if ketones are present in the urine, and if there are no ketones present they should exercise with caution. Such a high prevalence of exercising with high blood glucose may be explained by the idea that athletes intentionally compete with hyperglycaemia in order to prevent exercise-induced hypoglycaemia.

COMMENT

While physical activity promotes insulin sensitivity and improved metabolic control, it also promotes hypoglycaemia, which is a barrier for participation (14). Normally, the pancreas secretes less insulin in response to prolonged aerobic exercise. However, athletes who rely on exogenous insulin often experience hyperinsulinaemia and consequent hypoglycaemia as a result of not properly lowering their insulin dosage prior to exercise. The risk of hypoglycaemia may last for 24–36 h post-exercise due to increased insulin sensitivity that helps to replenish muscle and liver glycogen levels (15). However, proper glucose control is often challenging for athletes, as the fear of hypoglycaemia during physical activity can lead to intentional hyperglycaemia prior to exercise which may hinder training performance. Thus, the ADA provides detailed guidelines for endurance athletes in order to better maintain glycaemia during and after exercise (13). However, the results of this study show that many athletes are not aware of these guidelines or that they are aware but simply do not follow them. In addition, despite these guidelines, most athletes frequently experience hypoglycaemia. Thus, better evidence-based dissemination tools are needed to better educate athletes with T1D who are facing challenges in glucose control during sport.

Resistance exercise and glycaemic control in women with gestational diabetes mellitus

de Barros MC, Lopes MAB, Francisco RPV, Sapienza AD, Zugaib M

Department of Obstetrics and Gynecology, University of Sao Paulo School of Medicine, Sao Paulo, Brazil

*Am J Obstet Gynecol 2010; **203**: 556.e1–6*

Aims

Insulin resistance that is first diagnosed during pregnancy is known as gestational diabetes mellitus (GDM). The aim of this study was to evaluate the effect of a resistance exercise (RE) programme with an elastic band on insulin requirements and glycaemic control in patients diagnosed with GDM. The hypothesis that RE would reduce the number of women who require insulin during their gestation was tested.

Methods

A randomised control trial of 64 women with GDM was conducted. The women were placed into two groups: an exercise group (EG) that underwent an RE programme during pregnancy and a control group (CG) that was not enrolled in an exercise programme. After the initial GDM diagnosis, made by a 3-h oral glucose tolerance test, the patients were instructed to self-monitor their blood glucose concentration, with the objective of maintaining a fasting glucose of 95 mg/dl or less according to ADA guidelines. All women received dietary instructions from a nutritionist. EG patients were given written guidelines on how to perform each resistance exercise, which consisted of using an elastic band to exercise the main muscle groups. These patients were required to perform the exercises three times each week on non-consecutive days for approximately 30–40 min. EG women were contacted by telephone weekly and met with the main researcher each week to make sure that they adhered to the exercise programme. The CG followed the standard prenatal care routine, as they attended weekly return outpatient visits with their doctor. Each patient's glycaemic profile was reviewed weekly, and insulin was introduced when more than 30% of glucose readings were above the recommended value or when 20%–30% of the measurements were hyperglycaemic and fetal weight (as determined monthly) was above the 75th percentile.

Results

The EG patients participated in an average of 2.4 ± 0.4 (mean ± SD) RE sessions per week, each lasting 30–40 min. RE was associated with a decreased need for initiating insulin therapy as treatment for GDM, as seven out of 32 EG patients (21.9%) required insulin during gestation compared with 18 of 32 CG patients (56.3%) (p = 0.005). In the EG, the percentage of weeks spent in the target blood glucose range as suggested by the ADA was higher (p = 0.006) than for patients in the CG, the mean being 0.63 ± 0.30 in the EG compared with 0.41 ± 0.31 in the CG. No significant difference in mean glucose levels was observed between the two groups. There were no recorded cases of post-exercise hypoglycaemia, and RE did not seem to interfere with safety of the mother or the fetus, as there were no significant differences observed in body mass index, pregnancy weight gain, gestational age at delivery and the number of caesarean sections between the two groups. Newborn birthweight greater than 4000 g occurred in one EG patient and three CG patients. Pre-term delivery, in which the delivery took place at 35–36 weeks of gestation, occurred in three patients in each group

Discussion

The results of this study indicate that RE with an elastic band may be an effective therapy for women with GDM, as it significantly reduced the number of patients who required insulin and improved their glycaemic control compared with standard care. Further studies with a larger number of subjects should be conducted to provide more conclusive evidence of the effects of RE on women with GDM, and should compare the effectiveness of RE on metabolic control to the effects of aerobic exercise.

COMMENT

Adequate blood glucose control is necessary in order to minimise the risk of complications during pregnancy and delivery resulting from GDM. Studies have shown that even subtle degrees of hyperglycaemia during pregnancy result in a higher incidence of fetal complications including macrosomia, hypoglycaemia, hyperbilirubinaemia, hypocalcaemia, polycythaemia and major congenital anomalies (16). Skeletal muscles have been found to be one of the major sites of insulin resistance in women with GDM (17). Thus, it follows that exercise may be a safe and effective method for stimulating glucose uptake, resulting in good glycaemic control. While previous studies have shown the effectiveness of aerobic exercise in treating GDM, little is known about the effect of RE on this worrisome condition. The results of this study showed tighter glucose control in women who performed RE multiple times each week during gestation, as women in the RE group spent significantly more time within the proposed target glucose range. Furthermore, consistent RE reduced the need to begin insulin therapy, as 56.3% of women in the CG required insulin compared with only 21.9% of women in the EG (p = 0.006). Thus, further studies on this subject may reaffirm RE as a safe, cost-effective and beneficial alternative to insulin for improving metabolic control in women with GDM, and may result in a reduction in fetal complications resulting from the disease.

Comparison of different heat modalities for treating delayed-onset muscle soreness in people with diabetes

Petrofsky J[1,2], Batt J[2], Bollinger JN[2], Jensen MC[2], Maru EH[2], Al-Nakhli HH[1]

[1] *Loma Linda University, Loma Linda, CA, USA, and* [2] *Azusa Pacific University, Azusa, CA, USA*

Diabetes Technol Ther 2011; **13***: 645–55*

Aims

This study examined the severity of delayed-onset muscle soreness (DOMS) post-exercise in people with diabetes compared with age-matched controls. The authors further compare the effectiveness of three different heat modalities in treating DOMS.

Methods

A total of 120 subjects were used in this study. They were divided into three cohorts of 40 subjects each. The first cohort comprised younger subjects in the age range 20–45 years. The second cohort consisted of older adults, aged 45–70 years. The last cohort included subjects with T2D from 45 to 70 years old. Within each cohort, subjects were divided randomly into four groups of 10 subjects who underwent different heat treatments: 10 subjects tested dry heat wraps (ThermaCare); 10 tested chemical moist heat (ThermaCare 24-cell product); 10 tested hydrocollator heat wraps (silica pack placed in 49 °C); and the last 10 subjects in each cohort were controls to whom no heat was applied. Before exercise, the subjects first rested for 15 min during which time baseline data of skin temperature, skin blood flow and soreness [as indicated by the subjects using a visual analogue scale (VAS)] of the abdominal region were taken. The subjects then followed 60 min of p90X workout routines. The exercise consisted of a 44-min core workout and a 16-min abdominal workout. Subjects were instructed to complete the workout with the highest intensity variation of each exercise that they could. They were given four 3-min breaks to rest and hydrate during the hour-long video. Twenty-four hours after completing the exercise routine, thermal images of subjects' abdomen and skin blood flow were taken. Subjects were then asked to measure their level of muscle soreness using the VAS. The control group laid supine for 2 h, filling out VAS scores at 60 min and 120 min. The other three groups were instructed also to lie supine for 2 h, each having a different heat modality (hydrocollator wraps, dry heat or moist heat) applied to their abdomen. The soreness VAS was filled out by each subject immediately prior to heat treatment, and at 60 min and 120 min after treatment began. Subjects also filled out a comfort VAS along with the soreness VAS. Abdominal thermal photos and skin blood flow readings were taken post heat therapy. VASs, skin temperature and blood flow measures were repeated at 48 h post-exercise.

Results

While the younger and older groups had no soreness or discomfort prior to exercise, the T2D group showed soreness before the study began. The mean soreness on the VAS for the diabetes cohort after exercise (mean ± SEM 73.3 ± 16.2) was significantly higher ($p < 0.01$) than for the younger (41.5 ± 9.3) and older (56.1 ± 15.1) groups. Across all three cohorts, reduction of muscle soreness was greatest when moist heat was used for treatment, both immediately after heat was applied and up to 2 days after exercise. Moist heat reduced pain in older subjects by 52.3%, by 30.5% in the subjects with diabetes and by 33.3% in the younger subjects. ThermaCare dry heat wraps reduced pain by about 30% in older subjects, about 20% in the subjects with T2D and about 25% in the younger subjects. The hydrocollator heat wraps, which are often used in physical therapy, were almost as effective as moist heat at reducing pain, but the effect wore off within 2 h after the modality was applied. Average blood flow in the younger cohort before exercise was 81.3 ± 9.2 flux, significantly higher than the other two cohorts [$p < 0.01$, analysis of variance (ANOVA)]. In the younger control group, this value did not change significantly during the 2-day study. The younger group that used moist heat exhibited the greatest increase in blood flow, as it increased by 503.1 ± 83.2 when the modality was applied. Mean blood flow in the older group was 59.5 ± 15.2 flux, and this value did not change significantly during the 2-day period for the control group. The older group using moist heat similarly experienced the greatest increase in blood flow after the modality, as the mean increased by 423 ± 79.5 flux. For the diabetes group, the initial mean blood flow of 45.7 ± 11.8 flux was significantly lower ($p < 0.01$, ANOVA) than that of the younger and older cohorts. As with the other cohorts, skin blood flow in subjects with diabetes increased the most in the group using moist heat, as it resulted in a mean increase of 352 ± 38.7 flux. Across all cohorts, moist heat wraps caused the greatest increase in blood flow, followed by hydrocollator heat, and then dry heat. Blood flow remained elevated 2 h after moist heat was applied, but returned to near normal values by 48 h after the modality was used.

Discussion

In individuals with diabetes, exercise performance and training are often impaired due to a high prevalence of endothelial dysfunction. In this study, subjects with T2D had mild muscle soreness even before starting the exercise routine and experienced the greatest increase in soreness between 1 and 2 days post-exercise compared with the other two groups. Hydrocollator packs are most often used clinically to reduce muscle pain. Importantly, this study found that moist heat wraps resulted in the greatest increase in blood flow and reduction in muscle soreness compared with dry heat and hydrocollator modalities.

COMMENT

DOMS is a condition that results from physical activity in people who do not exercise frequently or in those who exceed their physical limits (18). Symptoms of DOMS can range from mild muscle tenderness to severe pain. Normally, the intensity of the pain peaks between 24 h and 72 h after exercise, and the pain does not disappear until 5–7 days following exercise. Often, patients with T2D have impaired endothelial function that consists of reduced tissue blood flow, resulting in impaired tissue healing. Thus, based on the physiology, it may be expected that DOMS would be more severe in people with diabetes. The results of this novel study indicate that those with T2D had significantly higher levels of muscle pain both before and after exercise compared with age-matched non-diabetic controls. These findings prove somewhat problematic because resistance exercise is often recommended for patients with diabetes to help maintain lower A1c levels and improve musculoskeletal fitness. This research also provides reasonably effective strategies to limit DOMS, which include moist heat wrap applications. Indeed, this simple technique enhanced local blood flow and reduced pain in approximately 30% of subjects with diabetes. Because exercise is an important component of treating T2D, it is imperative that individuals with diabetes participate in some form of physical activity. If solutions for the ensuing muscle pain are provided, as they were in this study, perhaps these patients will be more inclined to exercise and gain better glycaemic control as a result.

The impact of resistance exercise training on the mental health of older Puerto Rican adults with type 2 diabetes

Lincoln AK[1,2], Shepherd A[1,2], Johnson PL[2,3], Castaneda-Sceppa C[1]

[1] Health Sciences Department, Northeastern University, Boston, MA, USA,
[2] Sociology Department, Northeastern University, Boston, MA, USA, and
[3] Division of Psychiatry, Boston Medical Center, MA, USA

J Gerontol B Psychol Sci Soc Sci 2011 May 12 [Epub ahead of print]

Aims

The aim of this study was to investigate the impact of resistance exercise on depression among older Hispanic patients with T2D. The authors hypothesised that an exercise intervention designed to improve glycaemic control would additionally improve mental health.

Methods

Fifty-eight Puerto Rican men ($n = 21$) and women ($n = 37$) older than 60 years of age (mean 67.1 ± 7.8 years) with T2D were recruited to participate in the study. Subjects reported having lived in the USA for a mean of 23 (±13) years. All subject interviews took place in Spanish, as 94% of subjects reported Spanish as their primary language. Subjects were randomly assigned to either the intervention group ($n = 29$) that underwent progressive resistance exercise training (PRT) or the control group ($n = 29$). Patients in the PRT group exercised three times each week under supervision for a total of 16 weeks. Each exercise session lasted approximately 45 min. Subjects in the control group received phone calls every other week and performed one-repetition maximum testing during baseline and at weeks 9 and 16 to measure the heaviest load they could lift once in good form and through the full range of motion. The authors measured two primary outcomes. The first was the Geriatric Depression Scale (GDS), which consists of 30 items and is used to assess depression in older adult populations. Scores ranging from 0 to 9 are considered normal, 10 to 19 indicate mild depressive symptoms and 20 to 30 signify severe depression. The second test was the Short-Form 36 Health Survey Questionnaire (SF-36) which is commonly used to assess different domains of health: general and mental health, physical and social functioning, bodily pain, and vitality, each ranging from 0% to 100%, with higher scores indicating better quality of life. The mental component summary score (MCS) of the SF-36 was determined for each subject. Both the GDS and the SF-36 have been validated in Spanish and have been shown to be reliable indicators of mental health. MCS and SF-36 scores were taken before intervention and again at 16 weeks. Statistical analysis of mental health scores was performed.

Results

Among the subjects, 33% used insulin treatments and 60% used oral glycaemic medications. Patients were also taking medications prescribed for mood problems (17%) or other medications known to affect mood (91%). There were no significant correlations between the types of medications used and GDS and MCS scores. GDS and MCS values were not different between the two groups at baseline. At week 0, the PRT group had a mean GDS score of 11.5 ± 7.5 and the control group had a mean value of 11.1 ± 7.4. At week 16 after intervention, the mean GDS score for subjects in the PRT group decreased to 3.1 ± 3.5, indicating dramatically improved mental health, compared with a mean of 12.4 ± 8.0 for the control group (p < 0.0001). The mean MCS score at week 0 in the PRT group was 44.2 ± 10.6 and 47.9 ± 9.3 in the control group. At week 16, the mental health of the PRT subjects also improved, as the mean score increased to 54.4 ± 6.9. This MCS score was significantly higher than the mean score of 44.5 ± 10.1 in the control group at 16 weeks (p < 0.0001).

Discussion

The initial GDS and MCS scores indicate that older Puerto Ricans with T2D exhibit depressive symptoms and poor mental health. Before intervention, approximately 50% of subjects reported levels of depressive symptoms considered to be indicative of clinical depression. This study demonstrated that participation in PRT not only improves glycaemic control, as has previously been shown (19), but also improves mental health in older individuals with diabetes. The authors theorise that perhaps some of the improvement in mental health in the PRT group may be attributed to increased social interaction due to the exercise programme.

COMMENT

People with diabetes are twice as likely to have clinical depression as matched controls without the disease (20). This study used a subject pool of older Puerto Ricans, as Puerto Ricans have significantly higher rates of diabetes than non-Hispanic whites. Furthermore, depression and diabetes occur together more frequently in older Hispanic/Latinos than in other populations, even though they are less likely than non-Hispanic whites to be diagnosed and treated for depression. A randomised control trial performed in 2002 found that resistance exercise significantly improved glycaemic control and insulin sensitivity in patients with T2D (19). Other researchers have found that regular exercise can be as effective as antidepressants for treating depression (20,21). While earlier studies have documented the effect of exercise on depression and the effect of exercise on diabetes separately, this study examined the impact of resistance exercise training on people with T2D. The authors found that in addition to greatly improving glycaemic control, exercise was highly effective at reducing the prevalence of depression and poor mental health in older diabetic individuals. This study provides much insight into an especially at-risk group and reveals the high rate of depression among them. The results indicate that perhaps healthcare professionals should focus on improving the mental health of their diabetic patients in addition to glycaemic control. Exercise appears to be an effective means to accomplish both goals and consequently improve quality of life.

An innovative telemedical support system to measure physical activity in children and adolescents with type 1 diabetes mellitus

Shiel R, Thomas A, Kaps A, Bieber G

MEDIGREIF-Inselklinik Heringsdorf GmbH, Department of Diabetes and Metabolic Diseases, Seeheilbad Heringsdorf, Germany

Exp Clin Endocrinol Diabetes 2011 Apr 6 [Epub ahead of print]

Aims

The aim of this study was to observe the applicability and effectiveness of a new telemedical support system, which consisted of a continuous glucose monitor (CGM) and a sensor detecting physical activity (DiaTrace), in children with T1D. This feasibility trial sought to observe the use of this innovative technology in a clinical setting. The ultimate goal of the project was to investigate the acceptance of the technology by the patients, to analyse correlations between physical activity and blood glucose, and also to define algorithms to improve the adjustment of insulin dosage.

Background

DiaTrace, a new technology originally developed in 2008, consists of a sensor that measures physical activity that is integrated into a cell phone containing a digital camera. Using pre-programmed algorithms, DiaTrace analyses the type, intensity and duration of physical activity. This system has been proved reliable in previous studies, as the accuracy rates of identification were 99.38% for walking, 99.72% for running, 97.01% for cycling and 98.79% for driving (22).

Methods

A total of 16 adolescents (mean age 14.5 ± 2.2 years) with T1D participated in this study. Each subject received the DiaTrace system integrated into a mobile phone to assess physical activity. All subjects also received a CGM (Medtronic GmbH) to be used in conjunction with DiaTrace. The patients used the telemedical system for a total of 3 days, beginning at 6:00 am on the first day and ending at 10:30 pm on the last day. Statistical analysis of the relationship between physical activity and blood glucose values was performed.

Results

All patients used the technical devices for the duration of the trial without any complaints. During the study period, the mean duration of physical activity was 204.9 ± 66.5 min/day (mean $\pm$ SEM). Physical activity consisted of walking (102.5 ± 62.5 min/day), running (7.4 ± 5.8 min/day), cycling (39.2 ± 32.7 min/day), driving (36.0 ± 18.6 min/day) and non-specific physical activity (57.0 ± 29.7 min/day). Periods without physical activity lasted for 386.5 ± 187.2 min/day. Energy expenditures were 1964.1 ± 185.5 kcal/day. Physical activity (activity units, AU) measured by DiaTrace and blood glucose values obtained from the CGM were documented graphically for each patient. There was a direct correlation between physical activity and blood glucose levels in six out of 16 subjects, with Pearson's correlation coefficients ranging between 0.59 and 0.99 (median 0.91). In 10 of the 16 children there were no significant correlation coefficients. These results indicate the high variability in individual reactions to physical activity. There was no association between the kind of insulin therapy used (continuous subcutaneous insulin infusion or multiple daily injections) and the correlation between blood glucose values and physical activity.

Discussion

The results of this feasibility study indicate that there may be a direct correlation between physical activity and blood glucose values, as six of the 16 patients demonstrated near linear relationships between the two parameters. The fact that statistical analysis of exercise and blood glucose yielded a variety of correlation coefficients reflects the wide range of insulin sensitivity in diabetic individuals. While further studies should be conducted with larger subject pools and for longer duration, the DiaTrace/CGM system may prove to be useful to improve insulin dose adjustment during physical activity for children and adults. None of the subjects reported problems using the new technology during the 3-day trial, demonstrating that this telemedical system could be integrated into diabetes therapy easily.

COMMENT

Many researchers have previously sought to determine the relationship between physical activity and insulin sensitivity, with some trials reporting an inverse association between the two (23). Such studies observing the effect of physical activity on certain parameters largely rely on subjective patient self-reports. However, the new DiaTrace system seems accurately and objectively to assess duration, intensity and type of physical activity, allowing for greater precision and accuracy for experiments involving exercise. While the results of this study are inconclusive, the innovative combination of the Dia-Trace system and a CGM sets a precedent for future research. Because exercise increases the risk of hypoglycaemic episodes in individuals with T1D, insulin dose adjustment prior to physical activity may often be difficult to determine accurately. This new DiaTrace/CGM system may provide useful information about changes in insulin sensitivity during exercise and may allow adolescents and adults with T1D to better understand and more safely control their blood glucose levels during periods of physical activity.

Short-term aerobic exercise reduces nitroglycerin-induced orthostatic intolerance in older adults with type 2 diabetes

Madden KM, Lockhart CK, Potter TF, Cuff DJ, Meneilly GS

ITALITY Research Laboratory, Division of Geriatric Medicine, Department of Medicine, University of British Columbia, Vancouver, BC, Canada

*J Cardiovasc Pharmacol 2011; **57**: 666–71*

Aims

Syncope due to orthostatic intolerance is a common problem for older adults, leading to many hospitalisations in Canada and the USA. The presence of T2D further increases the risk of fainting, especially in patients with vasoactive medications. There have been mixed findings in the literature about the benefits of aerobic training on improving orthostatic intolerance. This study examined whether short-term aerobic exercise reduces orthostatic intolerance in older adults with T2D who were given nitroglycerin as a short-acting vasoactive medication.

Methods

Forty-six adults above the age of 65 (28 males and 18 females) who had been diagnosed with T2D for at least 5 years were recruited for this study, excluding those that had any history of angina, myocardial infarction, stroke, chronic pulmonary disease, were currently smoking, or had an exercise limiting orthopaedic impairment. Orthostatic intolerance was measured via the tilt table test, before and after exercise intervention. Subjects were randomly selected into either an aerobic training (AT) group or a non-aerobic (NA) group. The aerobic training sessions consisted of moderate to vigorous intensity exercise (heart rate set at 60%–75% of heart rate reserve, based on the Karvonen formula) on a treadmill and cycle ergometer for 60 min, three times a week for 3 months. Non-aerobic training consisted of non-strenuous exercise ball and dumb-bell exercises. At 24 h following the last training session subjects were given a tilt table test, where 400 μg of nitroglycerin was administered sublingually and then each subject was placed in a 70° head-up tilt for 30 min. The test was considered positive if the subject experienced presyncopal symptoms and more than a 30 mmHg drop in blood pressure. V_{O_2} max, body mass index and hip to waist ratio were also measured on all subjects pre- and post-intervention.

Results

At baseline, subjects in both groups were equally likely to develop syncope or presyncope during the tilt table test (AT vs. NA group, p = 0.366). After the exercise intervention, eight in the AT group and 15 in the NA group experienced syncope and presyncope, the difference in syncope/presyncope rates being significantly different between groups (p = 0.027). Tilt table duration between groups was not significantly different at baseline (AT vs. NA group, p = 0.719), but average tilt table tolerance was significantly longer in the AT group after the training programme (AT = 22.29 ± 2.32 min, NA = 13.22 ± 2.07 min, p = 0.006). No training effect on maximal haemodynamic changes was observed during upright tilting. The training intervention did not result in any significant changes in V_{O_2} max, body mass index, waist to hip ratio or fasting blood glucose.

Discussion

After only 3 months of aerobic training, upright nitroglycerin tolerance was improved in older adults with T2D. These improvements occurred without any significant changes in physical fitness, body mass index, fasting blood glucose or waist to hip ratio, suggesting that the effects of aerobic exercise on orthostatic tolerance are independent of those other well known benefits of exercise. Most studies showing negative or no improvements to orthostatic tolerance after exercise had used young athletes, exercising at a very intense level. The only study that supported these current findings used young adult military recruits (non-athletes), who also gained a large improvement in orthostatic tolerance after aerobic exercise. Orthostatic intolerance is thought to be more in common in elderly populations because of the increased vascular stiffness that accompanies old age, resulting in lower baroreflex sensitivity. Previous studies have shown that aerobic exercise reduces vascular stiffness in middle aged and older adults with T2D, as well as reducing sympathetic tone, both of which can explain a training-related improvement in baroreflex sensitivity.

COMMENT

Falls due to orthostatic intolerance are a concern for older adults, especially those with T2D; 233 per 100,000 people in this age group are hospitalised annually in the USA (24). The underlining neuropathies associated with T2D and the addition of commonly prescribed vasodilatory medications make this population especially vulnerable to this condition. It is encouraging to see that a simple aerobic exercise programme can have lasting, positive effects on orthostatic tolerance, indicating that exercise can be easily used as a first line of defence against orthostatic intolerance.

Effects of an exercise program on balance and trunk proprioception in older adults with diabetic neuropathies

Song CH[1], Petrofsky JS[2], Lee SW[1], Lee KJ[1], Yim JE[2]

[1] *Department of Physical Therapy, Sahmyook University, Seoul, Korea, and* [2] *Department of Physical Therapy, School of Allied Health Professions, Loma Linda University, Loma Linda, CA, USA*

Diabetes Technol Ther 2011; 13: 803–11

Aims

So far, little research has been done on the treatment of diabetes induced peripheral neuropathies using exercise. The aim of this study was to test the effect of a balance training exercise programme on improving balance and trunk proprioception in older adults with T2D.

Methods

In all, 38 older adults with diabetic peripheral neuropathies were randomly assigned into either an experimental exercise group (19 participants, 72.9 ± 5.6 years old) or a control group (19 participants, 73.2 ± 5.4 years old). The exercise programme consisted of 10 min of warm-up activity, 40 min of balance training and 10 min of cool-down activities, conducted twice a week for 8 weeks. Balance training exercises were done with eyes open and closed, plus an additional three activities were done in a group or with partners to challenge participants to improve their balance. Health education sessions were also given to participants once a week for the 8-week intervention, focusing on diabetes disease progression and the importance of diet and exercise in managing their diabetes. Dynamic force and pressure distribution during walking and standing were measured with a Zebris multifunction force measuring plate. Balance was assessed by the one leg standing (OLS) test and the Berg balance scale (BBS). Dynamic balance and functional mobility were measured by the functional reach test (FRT) and the timed up and go (TUG) test, respectively. Walking speed was measured using a 10 m walking test. The trunk repositioning errors test was used to assess trunk proprioception.

Results

There was no difference in any of the tests for balance and trunk proprioception between control and exercise groups at baseline. After intervention, the exercise group showed improvements in static balance (lower body sway distance with eyes opened or closed; longer time spent in OLS test in all conditions) and dynamic balance (higher BBS score, longer FRT distance, shorter TUG time and faster 10 m walk speed), and had fewer trunk repositioning errors (for all differences, $p < 0.05$). There were no significant improvements in any of the tests for patients in the control group.

Conclusion

Diabetes is the main cause of peripheral neuropathies, which can disrupt proprioceptive feedback from the lower limbs and make it harder for one to keep on balance, especially when the impairments in neurological control and muscle weakness that accompany old age are taken into account. This study has shown that 8 weeks of balance exercises are enough to improve static and dynamic balance as well as trunk proprioception in older adults with T2D, which could be enough to help prevent falls and help patients lead more active, independent lives.

COMMENT

This is yet another solid paper that demonstrates the power of an exercise programme to reduce the risk of falls, this time by working to improve balance and proprioception in older T2D adults. The exercises performed by the participants were something that could easily be incorporated at low cost into a daily routine, while providing a considerable benefit. This is the first study to show the effects of exercise on improving trunk proprioception and it has shown promising results. It will be valuable to see more studies performed on larger subject groups to support these data which could ultimately be used to improve the quality of life of elderly patients with this condition.

Exercise training improves physical fitness and vascular function in children with type 1 diabetes

Seeger JP[1,2], Thijssen DH[1,3], Noordam K[4], Cranen ME[1], Hopman MT[1], Nijhuis-van der Sanden MW[2,5]

[1]*Department of Physiology, Radboud University Nijmegen Medical Centre, Nijmegen, The Netherlands,* [2]*Paediatric Physical Therapy, Radboud University Nijmegen Medical Centre, Nijmegen, The Netherlands,* [3]*Research Institute for Sport and Exercise Science, Liverpool John Moores University, Liverpool, UK,*

[4]*Department of Paediatrics, Radboud University Nijmegen Medical Centre, Nijmegen, The Netherlands, and* [5]*Scientific Institute for Quality of Healthcare, Radboud University Nijmegen Medical Centre, Nijmegen, The Netherlands*

Diabetes, Obesity Metab 2011; 13: 382–4

Aims

Even at a young age, patients with T1D are known to have impaired endothelial function or even increases in carotid artery wall thickness, both of which are thought to be early signs of atherosclerosis and cardiovascular disease. This study examines the effect of an 18-week exercise programme on vascular function and structure in children with T1D.

Methods

Nine children with T1D (ages 8–12; four boys, five girls; mean duration of diabetes 2.7 ± 3.1 years) were placed in an exercise intervention for 18 weeks, with predominantly running exercises for 60 min twice a week. One training day was guided by a coach while the other was individually paced at home. Brachial artery endothelial function and carotid artery wall thickness, measured using a high-resolution ultrasound machine, were assessed on all children before and after the 18-week intervention. Aerobic fitness and heart rhythm were measured during a maximal exhaustive running test using a three-lead electrocardiogram.

Results

Aerobic capacity increased after the exercise programme, while maximal heart rate at peak oxygen consumption did not change. Flow mediated dilatation of the brachial artery was significantly higher after training, but no change in baseline diameter was observed. There was no difference in common carotid artery diameter, wall thickness or wall to lumen ratio pre- and post-exercise training.

Discussion

This study has shown that two exercise sessions per week for 18 weeks was sufficient in increasing physical fitness and improving endothelial function in young children with T1D. Endothelial dysfunction, which is a precursor to atherosclerosis and adverse cardiovascular events, is linked to physical inactivity in diabetic youth but these data have shown that even modest amounts of exercise can reverse it. The lack of change in carotid wall thickness, however, could be attributed to a short duration of T1D, not enough time to develop wall thickening, or to a brief exercise intervention, with not enough time spent exercising to cause structural remodelling of blood vessels.

COMMENT

This study further emphasises the benefits of exercise for a growing child with T1D, and the need for exercise programmes for these youth in order to prevent cardiovascular risk factors from developing early in life. Exercising with this condition is not without risks, most notably for hypoglycaemic events, but the benefits gained to the cardiovascular, muscular and endocrine systems far outweigh them.

REFERENCES

1. Punjabi, NM, Shahar E, Redline S, Gottlieb DJ, Givelber R, Resnick HE, and the Sleep Heart Health Study Investigators. Sleep-disordered breathing, glucose intolerance, and insulin resistance: the sleep heart health study. *Am J Epidemiol* 2004; **160**: 521–30

2. Louis, M, Punjabi NM. Effects of acute intermittent hypoxia on glucose metabolism in awake healthy volunteers. *J Appl Physiol* 2009; **106**: 1538–44

3. Umpierre D, Ribeiro PAB, Kramer CK, Leitão CB, Zucatti ATN, Azevedo MJ, Gross JL, Ribeiro JP, Schaan BD. Physical activity advice only or structured exercise training and association with HbA1c levels in type 2 diabetes: a systematic review and meta-analysis. *JAMA* 2011; **305**: 1790–9

4. Kirk A, Mutrie N, MacIntyre P, Fisher M. Effects of a 12-month physical activity counselling intervention on glycaemic control and on the status of cardiovascular risk factors in people with type 2 diabetes. *Diabetologia* 2004; **47**: 821–32

5. Alexander CM, Landsman PB, Teutsch SM. Diabetes mellitus, impaired fasting glucose, atherosclerotic risk factors, and prevalence of coronary heart disease. *Am J Cardiol* 2000; **86**: 897–902

6. Seto CK, Pendleton ME. Preparticipation cardiovascular screening in young athletes: current guidelines and dilemmas. *Curr Sports Med Rep* 2009; **8**(2); 59–64.

7. Douglas PS *et al.* ACCF/ASE/ACEP/AHA/ASNC/SCAI/SCCT/SCMR 2008 appropriateness criteria for stress echocardiography: a report of the American College of Cardiology Foundation Appropriateness Criteria Task Force, American Society of Echocardiography, American College of Emergency Physicians, American Heart Association, American Society of Nuclear Cardiology, Society for Cardiovascular Angiography and Interventions, Society of Cardiovascular Computed Tomography, and Society for Cardiovascular Magnetic Resonance endorsed by the Heart Rhythm Society and the Society of Critical Care Medicine. *J Am Coll Cardiol* 2008; **51**: 1127–47

8. Koistmen MJ. Prevalence of asymptomatic myocardial ischemic in diabetic subjects. *MBJ* 1990; **301**: 92–5

9. Kapitza C, Hövelmann U, Nosek L, Kurth H-J, Essenpreis M, Heinemann L. Continuous glucose monitoring during exercise in patients with type 1 diabetes on continuous subcutaneous insulin infusion. *J Diabetes Sci Technol* 2010; **4**: 123–31

10. Iscoe KE, Davey RJ, Fournier PA. Increasing the low-glucose alarm of a continuous glucose monitoring system prevents exercise-induced hypoglycemia without triggering any false alarms. *Diabetes Care* 2011; **34**: e109

11. Sharoff CG, Hagobian TA, Malin SK, Chipkin SR, Yu H, Hirshman MF, Goodyear LJ, Braun B. Combining short-term metformin treatment and one bout of exercise does not increase insulin action in insulin-resistant individuals. *AJP – Endo* 2010; **298**: E815–23

12. Braun B, Eze P, Stephens BR, Hagobian TA, Sharoff CG, Chipkin SR, Goldstein B. Impact of metformin on peak aerobic capacity. *Appl Physiol Nutr Metab* 2008; **33**: 61–7

13. Wasserman DH, Zinman B. Exercise in individual with type-1 IDDM. *Diabetes Care* 1994; **17**: 924–37

14. Brazeau AS, Rabasa-Lhoret R, Strychar I, Mircescu H. Barriers to physical activity among patients with type 1 diabetes. *Diabetes Care* 2008; **31**: 2108–9

15. Guelfi KJ, Jones TW. New insights into managing the risk of hypoglycaemia associated with intermittent high-intensity exercise in individuals with type 1 diabetes mellitus. *Sports Med* 2007; **37**: 937–46

16. Hod M, Merlob P, Friedman S, Schoenfeld A, Ovadia J. Gestational diabetes mellitus. A survey of perinatal complications in the 1980s. *Diabetes* 1991; **40**: 74–8

17. Barbour LA, McCurdy CE, Hernandez TL, Kirwan JP, Catalano PM, Friedman JE. Cellular mechanisms for insulin resistance in normal pregnancy and gestational diabetes. *Diabetes Care* 2007; **30**: S112–19

18. Cheung K, Hume PA, Maxwell L. Delayed onset muscle soreness: treatment strategies and performance factors. *Sports Medicine* 2003; **33**: 145–64

19. Castaneda C, Layne JE, Munoz-Orians L, Gordon PL, Walsmith J, Foldvari M, Roubenoff R, Tucker KL, Nelson ME. A randomized controlled trial of resistance exercise training to improve glycemic control in older adults with type 2 diabetes. *Diabetes Care* 2002; **25**: 2335–41

20. Lin EHB, Katon W, Von Korff M, Rutter C, Simon GE, Oliver M, Ciechanowski P, Ludman EJ, Bush T, Young B. Relationship of depression and diabetes self-care, medication adherence, and preventive care. *Diabetes Care* 2004; **27**: 2154–60

21. Singh NA, Clements KM, Fiatarone MA. A randomized controlled trial of progressive resistance training in depressed elders. *J Geront Ser A: Biol Sci Med Sci* 1997; **52**: 27–35

22. Schiel R, Kaps A, Bieber G. Identification of determinants for weight reduction in children and adolescents with overweight and obesity. *J Telemed Telecare* 2010; **16**: 368–73

23. Hawley JA, Gibala MJ. Exercise intensity and insulin sensitivity: how low can you go? *Diabetologia* 2009; **52**: 1709–13

24. Shibao C, Grijalva CG, Raj SR, Biaggioni I, Griffin MR. Orthostatic hypotension-related hospitalizations in the United States. *Am J Med* 2007; **120**: 975–80

CHAPTER 11

Diabetes Technology and Treatment in the Paediatric Age Group

Shlomit Shalitin[1] and H. Peter Chase[2]

[1] Jesse Z and Lea Shafer Institute of Endocrinology and Diabetes, National Center for Childhood Diabetes, Schneider Children's Medical Center of Israel, Petah Tikva, Israel

[2] Barbara Davis Center for Childhood Diabetes, University of Colorado, Denver, CO, USA

INTRODUCTION

Type 1 diabetes (T1D) predominantly occurs in young patients with an increasing rate in the last decades (1). Paediatric patients with T1D, their families and care providers face the challenge of maintaining blood glucose levels in the near to normal range over years, which was proved to be important for prevention of long-term microvascular and macrovascular complications (2) and to avoid the acute complications of severe hypoglycaemia (SH) and diabetic ketoacidosis. Exercise is important for all youth, but unfortunately has been identified as a major precursor of SH in youth. In one of the papers reviewed below, it was shown that modification of basal insulin rates in youth using insulin pumps could eliminate the 48% incidence of nocturnal hypoglycaemia (blood glucose <60 mg/dl; <3.2 mmol/l) after heavy exercise. In another report reviewed below, the Juvenile Diabetes Research Foundation study group was unable to find good predictors of SH other than the well known recent SH episode.

The never-ceasing challenge faced by diabetic patients and their caregivers has through the years inspired continuing efforts to find ways and means for achieving better control of blood glucose levels. The new modern advanced technologies may help to attain the aim of maintaining the metabolic control goals for youth with T1D.

The use of insulin pump therapy and different insulin analogues has become a common practice in the treatment of young patients with T1D.

Int J Clin Pract 2012; **66** (Suppl. 175): 61–67

Frequent blood glucose tests per day were shown to be an important factor related to metabolic control in patients with T1D (3). Standard use of glucose meters for self-monitoring of blood glucose (SMBG) provides only intermittent single blood glucose levels, without illustrating the glucose variability during the 24 h. Therefore, the use of a device such as real-time continuous glucose monitoring (RT-CGM) that provides continuous glucose measurements may have the potential to increase the proportion of patients who are able to maintain target HbA1c values, to decrease glucose excursions and to decrease the risk of SH.

In the last year many studies (including several reviewed below) that included paediatric patients evaluated the implications and advantages of using CGM. Insulin pumps and RT-CGM have recently been combined into the sensor-augmented pump (SAP) system, with evaluation of its clinical use.

T1D is characterised by immune-mediated pancreatic β-cell destruction. Screening for autoantibodies to insulin, glutamic acid decarboxylase (GAD) and protein tyrosine IA-2 is the mainstay of risk prediction for T1D. The attempt to identify the most significant predictors of progression to diabetes is presented below.

A major goal in T1D is in the area of prevention. Most studies countered the diabetes process by immunomodulation and/or enhancement of β-cell proliferation and regeneration. However, most attempts to use immune intervention to preserve residual β-cell function have achieved limited benefits or have been associated with adverse effects. In an important study reviewed below, the sensor augmented pump (SAP) was used from the onset of T1D and showed preservation of fasting C-peptide levels in youth 12–16 years of age. Further studies focusing on preservation of C-peptide will be important.

Accumulating evidence suggests that β-cell autoimmunity may be induced early in life (4). Food content in early life may modify the risk of T1D. Early exposure to complex dietary proteins is postulated to increase the risk of β-cell autoimmunity and T1D in children with genetic susceptibility (5). Thus, early nutritional intervention may help to prevent T1D.

The process we have used for choosing the papers to be included in our chapter included a Medline search for papers dealing with the following topics: diabetes technology, insulin pump therapy (CSII), CGM, open- and closed-loop systems, and new therapies (immunomodulation etc.) in T1D relating to the paediatric age group (0–18 years). Our review of the literature was centred on the recent key papers that offer some insight into these issues.

CONTINUOUS SUBCUTANEOUS INSULIN INFUSION THERAPY

The impact of baseline haemoglobin A1c levels prior to initiation of pump therapy on long-term metabolic control

Pinhas-Hamiel O, Tzadok M, Hirsh G, Boyko V, Graph-Barel C, Lerner-Geva L, Reichman B

Maccabi Juvenile Diabetes Center, Raanana, Israel

*Diabetes Technol Ther 2010; **12**: 567–73*

Background

Many studies have shown increased benefits of using an insulin pump over multiple daily injections (MDI) in patients with T1D. However, there is controversy over long-term effects on metabolic control while using pump therapy. This retrospective study sought to identify the various factors that influence long-term metabolic control in children and adolescents using insulin pumps.

Methods

The medical files of 113 patients with T1D, aged 9.7 ± 5.1 years, who had been treated with an insulin pump for up to 7 years (mean 3.8 ± 6.1 years) were reviewed. The linear trends for HbA1c levels were followed based on gender, metabolic control prior to pump initiation, time from diagnosis until pump therapy, age of initiation and duration of pump therapy.

Results

HbA1c values at baseline had a significant effect on follow-up values. Patients with HbA1c values at baseline below 7.5% had lower levels during follow-up than those who had moderate or poor metabolic control. The mean value at follow-up for patients initially below 7.5% was $7.2\% \pm 0.9\%$. Patients with moderate metabolic control at baseline (7.5% to <9%) had a mean value of $8.1\% \pm 0.9\%$ during follow-up. Patients with poor metabolic control at baseline (>9%) had a mean value of $8.2\% \pm 1.1\%$ (p = 0.0001) at follow-up. Although subjects with the poorest metabolic control did not achieve target HbA1c levels, they did benefit by a decline of more than 1%. In the multivariate analyses, a baseline HbA1c level $\leq 7.5\%$, duration of ≤ 1 year between diagnosis of diabetes and pump initiation, and younger age at pump initiation were independently associated with lower HbA1c levels during long-term follow-up.

Conclusions

The long-term response to pump treatment was impacted by baseline metabolic control. In addition, lower HbA1c values occurred when insulin pump treatment was started at a young age and within 1 year of diagnosis.

COMMENT

Not surprisingly, families doing better with glycaemic control prior to pump initiation also did better while receiving CSII. It was surprising to find the decline in HbA1c levels >1.0% in the most poorly controlled subjects. This suggests that they did better in receiving insulin boluses while on CSII compared with insulin injections. The authors suggest that initiation of pump therapy at a young age and within 1 year of diagnosis will result in later improved long-term metabolic control. This is in contrast to a previous report (6) in which subjects initiating pump therapy in the pre-teen years did not maintain better HbA1c levels in comparison to subjects initiating pump therapy in the teen-aged years. Further research is needed to determine the effects of initiating insulin pump therapy in the first year post-diagnosis. These studies will need to include C-peptide levels to determine whether insulin production can be maintained.

Preventing post-exercise nocturnal hypoglycaemia in children with type 1 diabetes

Taplin CE, Cobry E, Messer L, McFann K, Chase HP, Fiallo-Scharer R

University of Colorado, Barbara Davis Center for Childhood Diabetes, Aurora, CO, USA

J Pediatr 2010; **157***: 784–8*

Background

One important goal of diabetes is to maintain normal blood glucose levels with few or no episodes of hypoglycaemia. However, hypoglycaemia and nocturnal hypoglycaemia are common after exercise. The goal of this study was to determine the effects of alterations in insulin-pump basal insulin or of a bedtime dose of terbutaline on post-exercise nocturnal hypoglycaemia.

Methods

This crossover study enrolled youth (mean age 13.3 ± 1.8 years) who had T1D for 6.9 ± 3.5 years and who were on insulin pumps. The subjects underwent three overnight study visits. Each visit included a 60-min exercise session in which blood glucose levels were taken every 30 min.

For all visits, the basal insulin was discontinued during exercise, followed by a 50% decrease in basal rate for 45 min after the exercise. Patients were randomised to bedtime treatment with terbutaline, 2.5 mg, or to a 20% basal insulin reduction for 6 h (9 pm to 3 am), or to no bedtime treatment.

Results
While treatment with terbutaline eliminated blood glucose values <80 mg/dl, there were significantly more readings ≥250 mg/dl than in the control visit (p < 0.001) or the basal reduction visit (p < 0.001). The basal rate reduction from 9 pm to 3 am resulted in fewer blood glucose readings <80 and <70 mg/dl and no values <60 mg/dl. During the control visit (no night-time basal rate reduction) there were five separate episodes of hypoglycaemia.

Conclusions
These specific interventions had an impact on preventing both exercise and delayed (nocturnal) hypoglycaemia. While the terbutaline was effective in preventing nocturnal hypoglycaemia, the 2.5 mg dose often caused hyperglycaemia. The cessation of basal insulin during exercise combined with night-time basal insulin reduction was safe and effective in raising nocturnal blood glucose levels and in eliminating nocturnal hypoglycaemia (<60 mg/dl).

COMMENT

This report is one of the first studies in youth to show that delayed nocturnal hypoglycaemia after exercise can be prevented. The use of no basal insulin during exercise and a 20% reduced basal dose from 9 pm to 3 am resulted in no nocturnal blood glucose levels <60 mg/dl (<3.3 mmol/l). In contrast, a previous DirecNet investigation using the same exercise protocol (7) found 48% of children to have nocturnal glucose levels <60 mg/dl (3.3 mmol/l) when insulin dosages were not reduced. Many would now conclude that one of the major benefits of insulin pump therapy is modification of insulin delivery during and after exercise to prevent later hypoglycaemia.

CONTINUOUS GLUCOSE MONITORING

Patients' evaluation of nocturnal hypoglycaemia with GlucoDay continuous glucose monitoring in paediatric patients

Meschi F, Bonfanti R, Rigamonti A, Giulio F, Battaglino R, Viscardi M, Poscia A, Chiumello G

Paediatric Department, Scientific Institute H San Raffaele, Vita-Salute University, Milan, Italy

Acta Diabetol 2010; **47***; 295–300*

Background

The goal of this study was to evaluate the accuracy of the GlucoDay continuous glucose monitoring system (CGMS) to assess nocturnal hypoglycaemia in adolescents with T1D over 48 h, compared with a seven-time capillary blood glucose profile.

Methods

Twenty subjects (mean age 13.5 ± 2.3 years; six males) with T1D (duration 5.3 ± 3.3 years) and poor metabolic control (HbA1c 9.7 ± 1.68%) were hospitalised for 4 days. Equal doses of intermediate insulin (NPH) were administered at 19:00 and 22:00 on the first and second nights of the study, respectively. GlucoDay subcutaneous glucose measurements were compared with plasma glucose values.

Results

The accuracy of the GlucoDay was good, with a correlation coefficient of 0.94 ($R^2 = 0.817$) in comparison with capillary measurements. Classical Clark error grid analysis showed 98.3% of the values in the A and B areas. Nocturnal hypoglycaemia (<60 mg/dl) was detected in 12 of 18 patients (mean time 29 min). The administration of NPH insulin at 19:00 h (day 1) vs. 21:00 h (day 2) resulted in less nocturnal hypoglycaemia during the second night.

Conclusions

This was the first evaluation of the GlucoDay CGMS in children and adolescents. The authors concluded that the system was accurate compared with conventional glucose determinations as well as other CGM devices currently available. The high incidence of asymptomatic nocturnal hypoglycaemia was again confirmed.

COMMENT

The authors note that the actual dimensions of the GlucoDay machine limit its use in real life for children and adolescents. Perhaps home use during sleep will be possible, particularly when size is not as critical. Although the use of NPH insulin at dinner or at bedtime is now less frequent in developed countries, it was again noted to result in a reduced incidence of nocturnal hypoglycaemia when administered at bedtime compared to dinner.

Use of integrated real-time continuous glucose monitoring/insulin pump system in children and adolescents with type 1 diabetes: a 3-year follow-up study

Scaramuzza AE[1], Iafusco D[2], Rabbone I[3], Bonfanti R[4], Lombardo F[5], Schiaffini R[6], Buono P[7], Toni S[8], Cherubini V[9], Zuccotti GV, for the Diabetes Study Group of the Italian Society of Paediatric Endocrinology and Diabetology (ISPED)[1]

[1]*Department of Pediatrics, Azienda Ospedaliera, University of Milano, 'Ospedale Luigi Sacco', Milano, Italy,* [2]*Department of Pediatrics, Second University of Naples, Naples, Italy,* [3]*Department of Pediatrics, University of Turin, Turin, Italy,* [4]*Department of Pediatrics, Endocrine Unit, Scientific Institute Hospital San Raffaele, Vita-Salute University, Milan, Italy,* [5]*Department of Pediatric Sciences, University of Messina, Messina, Italy,* [6]*Endocrinology and Diabetes Unit, University Department of Pediatric Medicine, Bambino Gesù Children's Hospital, Rome, Italy,* [7]*Department of Pediatrics, University Federico II, Naples, Italy,* [8]*Juvenile Diabetes Centre, Anna Mayer Children's Hospital, Florence, Italy, and* [9]*Regional Center for Diabetes in Children and Adolescents, Department of Pediatrics, Polytechnic University of Marche, Salesi Hospital, Ancona, Italy*

Diabetes Technol Ther 2011; 13: 99–103

Background

The availability of CGM has allowed the patient to monitor real-time glucose values, review trend graphs for the latest hours and receive alarms/alerts for impending hypoglycaemia or hyperglycaemia. Insulin pumps and RT-CGM devices have been combined into the SAP system.

Aim

The aim of the study was to evaluate the clinical use and safety of SAP in a large population of paediatric patients with T1D.

Methods

This was a multicentre observational study. A questionnaire was administered in 65 paediatric diabetic centres in Italy. The study included patients with T1D aged ≤18 years using the SAP for ≥6 months. Each centre filled out a questionnaire, and the data were collected from the medical records. The primary endpoint was the change in HbA1c between baseline and the end of the observation period. Insulin requirement, body mass index, episodes of severe hypoglycemia and diabetic ketoacidosis, and days of sensor use were also evaluated.

Results

Among all patients using an insulin pump, 129 patients aged 13.5 ± 3.8 years with disease duration of 6.3 ± 3.4 years have been using SAP for 1.4 ± 0.7 years, representing 9% of the total population. The control group consisted of 493 patients aged 12.9 ± 4.3 years with disease duration of 6.2 ± 3.3 years using conventional insulin pump therapy for 1.7 ± 0.5 years. Primary reasons for SAP initiation were HbA1c $> 8\%$ in 45% of patients, recurrent hypoglycaemia in 25%, involvement in competitive sports in 10%, wide glycaemic variability in 10%, and patient and/or family request in 10%. Median glucose sensor usage was 13.4 days/month, without a difference in sensor use between children and adolescents and without a significant correlation with HbA1c. After 0.5–3 years of using SAP or conventional insulin pump therapy, HbA1c significantly improved (8.0 ± 1.5 vs. $7.4 \pm 0.8\%$, $p = 0.002$, and $8.0 \pm 1.6\%$ vs. $7.7 \pm 1.1\%$, $p = 0.006$, respectively), with better improvement in the SAP group (0.6% vs. 0.3%, $p = 0.005$). Insulin requirement showed a significant decrease only in SAP patients (0.88 ± 0.25 vs. 0.7 ± 0.23 U/kg/day, $p = 0.003$), without a change in body mass index during the observation period. No difference was observed in diabetic ketoacidosis episodes during the follow-up in both groups, whereas SH significantly decreased only in patients using SAP (11.9 vs. 4.1 events/100 patients/year, $p = 0.04$). No difference was found between patients using SAP who started using the insulin pump and CGM at the same time and those who started the insulin pump before using CGM.

Conclusions

In daily settings, patients using SAP can achieve better control than patients using conventional insulin pump.

COMMENT

The increasing availability of CGM is likely to have a significant impact on paediatric diabetes therapy and education in the near future. The study was designed to address the question of whether using CGM and insulin pump therapy improved glycaemic control, which it did. The main limitation of the study is that it was not a randomised controlled trial, and most probably the more motivated families choose to use the SAP. Thus, it is difficult to generalise the conclusions. However, selection of patients motivated to use SAP with proper education could be the key factors for the long-term success of these new technological advances.

Factors predictive of severe hypoglycaemia in type 1 diabetes

Juvenile Diabetes Research Foundation Continuous Glucose Monitoring Study Group, Fiallo-Scharer R[1], Cheng J[2], Beck RW[2], Buckingham BA[3], Chase HP[1], Kollman C[2], Laffel L[4], Lawrence JM[5], Mauras N[6], Tamborlane WV[7], Wilson DM[3], Wolpert H[4]

[1] *Barbara Davis Center for Childhood Diabetes, Aurora, Colorado,* [2] *Jaeb Center for Health Research, Tampa, Florida,* [3] *Stanford University, Stanford, California,* [4] *Joslin Diabetes Center, Boston, Massachusetts,* [5] *Kaiser Permanente, San Diego, California,* [6] *Nemours Children's Clinic, Jacksonville, Florida,* [7] *Yale University, New Haven, Connecticut*

*Diabetes Care 2011; **34**: 586–90*

Background

Understanding factors predictive of SH would be an obvious help in prevention and have been looked at in numerous studies. This study was unique in the large sample size (436 subjects with T1D) and a full year of close observation while using a CGM.

Methods

In this multicentre clinical study, 436 children, adolescents and adults were randomised to a treatment group that used a CGM or to a control group that continued to use standard home blood glucose monitoring for 6 months. The control group used a CGM for the second 6 months. Baseline risk factors for SH were evaluated over the 12-month period.

Results

SH in the 6 months prior to the study was the strongest predictor of SH ($p < 0.001$). Females had more frequent SH ($p = 0.05$), as did subjects with higher scores on the Hypoglycemia Fear Questionnaire ($p = 0.02$) and those with a higher percentage of baseline CGM values <70 mg/dl ($p = 0.02$). CGM-measured hypoglycaemia over the 24 h prior to an SH event was strongly associated with SH ($p < 0.001$), but the positive predictive value was low.

Conclusions

SH in the previous 6 months was the only strong predictor of SH during the study.

COMMENTS

It is unfortunate that in this large, well studied group other reliable factors predictive of SH (other than the well known previous episode) could not be found.

Effect of continuous glucose monitoring on hypoglycaemia in type 1 diabetes

Battelino T[1], Phillip M[2], Bratina N[1], Nimri R[2], Oskarsson P[3], Bolinder J[3]

[1]*Department of Pediatric Endocrinology, Diabetes and Metabolism, UMC-University Children's Hospital, Faculty of Medicine, University of Ljubljana, Ljubljana, Slovenia,* [2]*Jesse Z and Sara Lea Shafer Institute for Endocrinology and Diabetes, National Center for Childhood Diabetes, Schneider Children's Medical Center, Petah Tikva, and Sackler Faculty of Medicine, Tel-Aviv University, Israel, and* [3]*Department of Medicine, Karolinska University Hospital Huddinge, Karolinska Institutet, Stockholm, Sweden*

Diabetes Care 2011; **34***: 795–800*

Background

Frequent hypoglycaemia is associated with hypoglycaemic unawareness, impaired neurological function and impaired cognitive functions.

Aim

The aim was to evaluate the effect of using CGM on hypoglycaemia in patients with T1D.

Methods

A randomised controlled multicentre study including 120 patients (53 children and adolescents) with T1D for more than 1 year, with HbA1c < 7.5%, using intensive insulin therapy with CSII or MDI. Patients were randomly assigned to a group using the RT-CGM or to a control group performing SBGM with glucose meters and wearing a masked CGM every second week for 5 days. The study duration was 26 weeks. The primary endpoint was the time spent in hypoglycaemia (interstitial glucose level <63 mg/dl) during the study.

Results

In the study group compared with the control group the time per day spent in hypoglycaemia was significantly shorter (0.48 ± 0.57 vs. 0.97 ± 1.55 h/day, p = 0.03) and time spent in the normoglycaemic range (70–180 mg/dl) was significantly longer (17.6 vs. 16 h/day, p = 0.009). At the end of the study, HbA1c level was lower in the study group compared with the control group [difference –0.27%; 95% confidence interval (CI) –0.47 to –0.07; p = 0.008].

Conclusions

The use of CGM was associated with reduced time of hypoglycaemia and increased time of normoglycaemic levels, and with a concomitant decrease in HbA1c in paediatric and adult patients with T1D.

COMMENT

Despite the increased use of insulin analogues and CSII, only a relatively small percentage of patients with T1D attain and maintain their target HbA1c. Hypoglycaemia is considered a serious risk associated with intensive therapy (8, 9). Recurrent episodes of hypoglycaemia at a young age have been associated with neurocognitive dysfunction. The fear of hypoglycaemia prevalent in adolescents and the families of children with T1D may pose a barrier to improved glycaemic control (10).

The recent study evaluated the hypoglycaemia preventive effect of CGM, and found a significant reduction in the time spent in hypoglycaemia in relatively well controlled patients with T1D, with a parallel significant decrease in HbA1c level in patients using the device compared with standard SBGM. Thus, the improvement in metabolic control is not necessarily associated with increased risk for hypoglycaemia, contrary to the Diabetes Control and Complications Trial findings (2).

However, we have to consider some limitations of the study that may influence the interpretation of the results: more patients (41%) on MDI in the control group than in the CGM group (24%); the cohort included highly motivated (more than five blood glucose measurements a day before randomisation); well controlled (HbA1c < 7.5%) patients. Thus, in order to generalise the conclusion about the hypoglycaemia preventive effect of CGM, further studies are required in less controlled and less motivated patients, and maybe also in younger paediatric patients.

Sensor-augmented pump therapy from the diagnosis of childhood type 1 diabetes: results of the Paediatric Onset Study (ONSET) after 12 months of treatment

Kordonouri O[1], Pankowska E[2], Rami B[3], Kapellen T[4], Coutant R[5], Hartmann R[1], Lange K[6], Knip M[7,8], Danne T[1]

[1] *Bult Diabetes Centre for Children and Adolescents, Kinderkrankenhaus auf der Bult, Hannover, Germany,* [2] *Department of Paediatric Diabetology and Birth Defects, Medical University of Warsaw, Warsaw, Poland,* [3] *Department of Paediatrics, Medical University of Vienna, Vienna, Austria,* [4] *Universitätsklinik und Poliklinik für Kinder und Jugendliche, Leipzig, Germany,* [5] *Département de Pédiatrie, Centre Hospitalier Universitaire, Angers, France,* [6] *Department of Medical Psychology, Hannover Medical School, Hannover, Germany,* [7] *Hospital*

for Children and Adolescents and Folkhälsan Research Centre, University of Helsinki, Helsinki, Finland, and [8]*Department of Paediatrics, Tampere University Hospital, Tampere, Finland*

Diabetologia 2010; 53: 2487–95

Background
Intensive insulin therapy is important in avoiding diabetes-related microvascular and macrovascular complications and may also play a role in preserving residual β-cell function.

Aim
The aims of the study were to determine whether the use of SAP therapy starting from the diagnosis of T1D improves subsequent glycaemic control and preserves residual β-cell function compared with the use of conventional insulin pump combined with the use of glucose meters for SBGM.

Methods
Children and adolescents aged 1–16 years (mean 8.7 ± 4.4 years) diagnosed with T1D within 4 weeks before study entry were randomised to receive insulin pump therapy with CGM ($n = 76$) or insulin pump with conventional SBGM ($n = 78$).

Endpoints were HbA1c levels and fasting C-peptide after 12 months. Additional analysis included glucose variability, sensor usage, adverse events and a health-related quality of life questionnaire.

Results
HbA1c of both treatment groups was not significantly different throughout the total period. At 12 months, patients with regular sensor use had lower values of HbA1c compared with the combined group with no or low sensor usage (7.1% vs. 7.6%, $p = 0.032$). In the SAP group compared with the conventional SBGM group, glycaemic variability was lower (mean amplitude of glycaemic excursions 80.2 ± 26.2 vs. 92.0 ± 33.7, $p = 0.037$), and fasting C-peptide levels were higher in 12–16-year-old patients (0.25 ± 0.12 vs. 0.19 ± 0.07 nmol/l, $p = 0.033$). SH was reported only in the conventional SBGM group. No differences were observed in the tests for quality of life and disease adjustment between the groups during the study.

Conclusions
Patients who were able to use the sensor regularly with pump therapy from the diagnosis of diabetes had better glycaemic control with better preservation of C-peptide particularly in adolescents.

COMMENT

Frequent blood glucose measurements are an important factor related to improved glycaemic control (3). Thus, the use of CGM can help to better manage the diabetes treatment. Integrating CGM into the diabetes skills for treatment from the onset of the disease can give a better picture of the glucose excursions in relation to different foods and activities, and improve treatment approach in the long term.

This is the first study in the paediatric age group that examined the efficacy of SAP therapy from the time of diabetes onset. It again demonstrates as reported previously (11–13) that only patients using the CGM regularly had the benefit of better reduction in HbA1c compared with conventional SBGM, probably indicating that the sensor systems are not yet effective or user-friendly enough.

Levels of C-peptide are recognised as a primary endpoint in intervention trials in patients with newly diagnosed T1D (14). Preservation of even minor levels of β-cell function were associated with improved HbA1c (15) and a striking reduction in SH (16).

C-peptide level was also reported to be correlated with fewer chronic microvascular diabetes complications (17, 18). This study demonstrated that the use of CGM was associated with a better preservation of endogenous insulin secretion after 1 year of diabetes only among adolescents, in whom the loss of β-cell function tends to be slower than in younger children. Adolescents also tend not to adhere to the diabetes management. Thus, the early introduction of SAP may be effective from both the educational and metabolic aspects, especially in the adolescent age group.

A stimulated C-peptide level may have been more sensitive in detecting the effects of β-cell protection, but it was not evaluated in this study.

Improving epinephrine responses in hypoglycaemia unawareness with real-time continuous glucose monitoring in adolescents with type 1 diabetes

Ly TT[1], Hewitt J[1], Davey RJ[2], Lim EM[3,4], Davis E[1,5], Jones TW[1,5]

[1]Department of Endocrinology and Diabetes, Princess Margaret Hospital for Children, Perth, WA, Australia, [2]School of Sport Science, Exercise and Health, University of Western Australia, Perth, WA, Australia, [3]PathWest Laboratory Medicine, Queen Elizabeth II Medical Centre, Nedlands, WA, Australia, [4]Department of Endocrinology and Diabetes, Sir Charles Gairdner Hospital, Nedlands, WA, Australia, and [5]Telethon Institute for Child Health Research, Centre for Child Health Research, University of Western Australia, Perth, WA, Australia

Diabetes Care 2011; **34**: 50–52

Background

Both defective counter-regulatory responses (impaired epinephrine and glucagon response) and hypoglycaemia unawareness constitute the hypoglycaemia-associated autonomic failure of recurrent episodes of hypoglycaemia. This study was designed to determine whether the use of RT-CGM with preset alarms at specific glucose levels can be useful to avoid hypoglycaemia and therefore improve the counter-regulatory response to hypoglycaemia.

Methods

The study included adolescents with T1D aged 12–18 years with hypoglycaemia unawareness. All subjects underwent a hyperinsulinaemic hypoglycaemic clamp study at baseline to assess hypoglycaemic symptoms and hormonal responses. Subjects were then randomised to the use of RT-CGM ($n = 6$) or standard therapy ($n = 5$) for 4 weeks. The clamp study was repeated at the end of 4 weeks.

Results

At baseline, the epinephrine response to hypoglycaemia was blunted, without a difference between subjects randomised to CGM or standard groups. After the intervention, in the CGM group compared with the standard group a greater epinephrine response was found (change 604% ± 234% vs. 114% ± 83%, p = 0.048) and a greater peak adrenaline response during hypoglycaemia (1093 ± 221 vs. 572 ± 162 pmol/l, p = 0.048). Subjects in the CGM group compared with the standard group reported higher adrenergic symptom scores after the intervention (5.4 ± 0.4 vs. 3.4 ± 0.2, p < 0.001). Following the intervention, there was no deterioration in glycaemic control, glucagon response was absent, and no change was found in cortisol and growth hormone responses to hypoglycaemia in the two groups.

Conclusions

A greater epinephrine response during hypoglycaemia suggests that RT-CGM is a useful clinical tool to improve hypoglycaemia unawareness in adolescents with T1D.

COMMENT

The high risk of SH associated with hypoglycaemia unawareness requires that the condition will be recognised and treated. This study demonstrated that blunted counter-regulatory responses to hypoglycaemia occur in adolescents, and the use of RT-CGM is a useful tool that can improve the adrenergic response during hypoglycaemia. Although this was a small study with short duration of only 1 month its results seem to be important for their implications.

Continuous glucose monitoring in newborn babies at risk of hypoglycaemia

Harris DL[1,2], Battin MR[2,3], Weston PJ[1], Harding JE[2]

[1]*Newborn Intensive Care Unit, Waikato District Health Board, Hamilton, New Zealand,* [2]*Liggins Institute, University of Auckland, New Zealand, and* [3]*Newborn Services, Auckland City Hospital, Auckland, New Zealand*

J Pediatr 2010; **157***: 198–202.e1*

Background
Neonatal hypoglycaemia can cause brain damage. Blood glucose levels fluctuate after birth as the baby adapts to extra-uterine life. Episodes of hypoglycaemia may go undetected, and their duration and severity cannot be assessed.

Aim
The aim of this study was to determine the usefulness of CGM in babies at risk of neonatal hypoglycaemia.

Methods
Babies born at $\geq$32 weeks' gestation who were at risk of hypoglycaemia (as prematurity, infant of diabetic mother, small/large for gestational age) and were admitted to newborn intensive care ($n = 102$) received routine treatment, including intermittent blood glucose measurement using the glucose oxidase method, and blinded CGM. Mean age at entry to the study was 4.8 h. Babies remained in the study until they were no longer at risk of hypoglycaemia or for 7 days, whichever came first. Hypoglycaemia was defined as a blood glucose level <47 mg/dl.

Results
CGM was well tolerated in infants for as long as 7 days. There was good agreement between blood and interstitial glucose concentrations (mean difference 0.03 mmol/l; 95% CI, −1.02 to 1.1 mmol/l). Low glucose concentrations (<47 mg/dl) were detected in 32 babies (33%) with blood sampling and in 45 babies (44%) with CGM. There were 265 episodes of low interstitial glucose concentrations lasting between 5 and 475 min, 215 (81%) of which were not detected with blood glucose measurement.

Also, 107 episodes in 34% of the babies lasted >30 min, 78 (73%) of which were not detected with blood glucose measurement.

Conclusions

CGM detects many more episodes of low glucose concentrations than routine blood glucose measurement in newborn babies.

COMMENT

This study demonstrates the usefulness and reliability of CGM in babies at risk of neonatal hypoglycaemia. CGM in this group appears to be safe, well tolerated and easy to use. CGM detects many more episodes of low glucose concentrations than intermittent blood glucose measurement in newborn babies, even in the setting of an intensive care unit.

The physiological significance of previously undetected episodes of hypoglycaemia is unknown. The advantage of CGM is the ability to measure the duration, severity and frequency of hypoglycaemia in these neonates. However, the association between the undetected hypoglycaemic episodes and neurological outcome still needs to be evaluated to justify the routine use of CGM in the newborn intensive care unit.

NEW THERAPIES IN TYPE 1 DIABETES

Mixing insulin aspart with detemir does not affect glucose excursion in children with type 1 diabetes mellitus

Nguyen TM[1], Renukuntla VS[2], Heptulla RA[2]

[1]*Department of Pediatrics – Endocrinology Section, Nemours Children's Clinic, Jacksonville, FL, USA, and* [2]*Department of Pediatrics – Endocrinology and Metabolism Section, Baylor College of Medicine and Texas Children's Hospital, Houston, TX, USA*

Diabetes Care 2010; 33: 1750–52

Background

Mixing rapid-acting and slow-acting insulin in the same syringe can decrease the number of daily injections, and may improve adherence to therapy. The aim of the study was to evaluate whether insulin detemir mixed with aspart has equivalent effects on blood glucose as if they were given as separate injections in paediatric patients with T1D.

Methods

This was a randomised crossover, open-labelled study including 14 children with T1D aged 14.75 ± 2.69 years with HbA1c of 7.7 ± 0.7%. Patients were assigned to either study A (mixed insulins) or study B (separate insulins) for the first 10 days and crossed over for the last 10 days. Each subject underwent CGM on the last 72 h of each study arm. Sustained glucose values over time were calculated as the area under the curve (AUC), the index of blood glucose control (*M* value) and glucose excursions (the mean amplitude of glucose excursions, MAGE). The relative frequency of mild hypoglycaemic episodes was calculated as the number of glucose values of 40–60 mg/dl divided by the total number of glucose values generated during the 48 h of CGM. The study was designed to detect a 20% difference in the mean AUC for blood glucose values in the 72-h study period.

Results

The 48-h AUC, *M* value, MAGE and relative frequency of mild hypoglycaemic episodes for study A vs. study B were 457 ± 70 vs. 469 ± 112 mmol/h/l (p = 0.58), 39.67 ± 15.37 vs. 39.75 ± 9.69 mmol/l (p = 0.98), 6.35 ± 1.92 vs. 5.98 ± 0.92 (p = 0.42) and 5.3 ± 5.2% vs. 6.7 ± 11.1% (p = 0.95), respectively. There was no SH in either group.

Conclusions

Insulin detemir mixed with aspart given twice daily had equivalent effects on blood glucose compared with giving them as separate injections twice daily, in children with T1D.

COMMENT

One of the barriers to good metabolic control in children with T1D is adherence to MDI. The concerns about mixing rapid-acting and slow-acting insulin analogues in the same syringe is because it may change the action of the insulin, and therefore can change the glucose excursions and the glycaemic control.

This study demonstrated that mixing insulin detemir with aspart in the same syringe had equivalent effects on blood glucose levels and rates of hypoglycaemia compared with giving them as separate injections, similar to the findings of a previous study when insulin glargine was mixed with aspart or lispro (19).

However, the study limitations are the small number of patients included and the lack of long-term follow-up consequences such as the effect on metabolic control, evaluated by the change in HbA1c levels.

IMMUNE INTERVENTION FOR TYPE 1 DIABETES

Age of islet autoantibody appearance and mean levels of insulin, but not GAD or IA-2 autoantibodies, predict age of diagnosis of type 1 diabetes: Diabetes Autoimmunity Study in the Young

Steck AK, Johnson K, Barriga KJ, Miao D, Yu L, Hutton JC, Eisenbarth GS, Rewers MJ

Barbara Davis Center for Childhood Diabetes, University of Colorado, Denver, Aurora, CO, USA

*Diabetes Care 2011; **34**: 1397–9*

Background

Screening for autoantibodies to insulin (IAA), GAD and protein tyrosine IA-2 (ICA512) is the mainstay of risk prediction for T1D. Factors correlating and potentially predictive of age of diagnosis of children followed from birth are less well characterised.

Aim

The aim of this study was to evaluate predictors of progression to diabetes in children with high risk human leucocyte antigen (HLA) genotypes and persistent islet autoantibodies.

Methods

The Diabetes Autoimmunity Study in the Young (DAISY) has followed young children at increased risk of diabetes ($n = 2542$) including relatives and general population children screened for susceptibility HLA-DR/DQ genotypes. Autoantibodies to GAD, IA-2 and insulin (IAA) were measured in all samples at 9, 15 and 24 months of age, and annually thereafter; if positive, antibodies were measured every 3–6 months. Follow-up time was defined as the time from initial positive autoantibody test for each subject. Multiple linear regression was used to evaluate potential predictors of age of diabetes diagnosis in subjects who had their first autoantibody measurement before 1.5 years ($n = 38$).

Results

During a median follow-up of 7 years, 169 children developed persistent islet autoantibodies (one or more autoantibodies on at least two consecutive visits), and 55 of those progressed to diabetes. A total of 89% of children who progressed to diabetes expressed two or more autoantibodies. Children expressing three autoantibodies showed a linear progression to diabetes with 74% cumulative incidence by the 10-year follow-up compared with 70% with two antibodies and 15% with one antibody (p < 0.0001). The high risk DR3/4-DQB1*0302 genotype was an additional predictor of a 10-year progression to diabetes in children expressing one autoantibody (30 vs. 13%; p = 0.035) or two autoantibodies (100 vs. 54%; p = 0.029), but not among patients expressing three autoantibodies (73.6 vs. 75.1%; p = 0.91). Children with persistently positive IAA levels had a higher progression rate to diabetes (100% by 5.6 years) than children with fluctuating IAA levels (63% by the 10-year follow-up) (p < 0.0001). Both age of appearance of first autoantibody and IAA levels were major determinants of the age of diabetes diagnosis ($r = 0.79$, p < 0.0001).

Conclusions

In this prospective study of the DAISY cohort, 89% of children who progressed to diabetes expressed two or more autoantibodies, with cumulative incidence of 74% by age 10 years for individuals expressing three autoantibodies. Age of diagnosis of diabetes was strongly correlated with age of appearance of the first autoantibody and IAA levels.

COMMENT

Prevention trials of T1D in individuals during the preclinical phase of the disease (marked by the presence of persistent islet autoantibodies) have to be targeted to those patients with the highest risk to progress to diabetes. Thus, the value of identifying the most significant risk factors for progression to overt diabetes is important. However, no prevention trial in children has demonstrated a significant impact on the cessation of the immune process yet. Thus, the burden of the emotional stress experienced by parents of children with positive autoantibodies has to be assessed before implementation of routine screening.

Dietary intervention in infancy and later signs of beta-cell autoimmunity

Knip M, Virtanen SM, Seppä K, Ilonen J, Savilahti E, Vaarala O, Reunanen A, Teramo K, Hämäläinen AM, Paronen J, Dosch HM, Hakulinen T, Akerblom HK; Finnish TRIGR Study Group

Hospital for Children and Adolescents, University of Helsinki and Helsinki University Central Hospital, Helsinki, Finland

N Engl J Med 2010; 11: 1900–8

Background

The progression of T1D prior to diagnosis can manifest in emerging markers of β-cell autoimmunity. It has been suggested that β-cell autoimmunity can be induced early in life, particularly when there is early exposure to complex dietary proteins after a brief stint of breastfeeding. This study hypothesised that supplementing breast milk with highly hydrolysed milk formula vs. cow's milk formula would decrease the cumulative incidence of diabetes-associated autoantibodies in such children.

Methods

In all, 230 infants with HLA-conferred susceptibility to T1D with at least one family member with T1D were assigned to either the control group or the treatment group in this double-blind, randomised trial. The control group received conventional cow's milk formula and the treatment group received a casein hydrolysate formula. The formulas were used whenever breast milk was not available for the first 6–8 months of life. Five islet-cell autoantibodies were analysed over a mean observation period of 10 years (mean 7.5). All children were monitored for the incidence of T1D until 10 years of age.

Results

The risk for developing T1D was not significantly associated with the feeding intervention (hazard ratio with casein hydrolysate 0.80). The unadjusted hazard ratio for positivity for one or more autoantibodies in the treatment group compared with the control group was 0.54 (95% CI, 0.29–0.95), and for positivity for two or more autoantibodies was 0.52 (95% CI, 0.21–1.17). Insulin autoantibodies were the first or among the first antibodies that appeared in children in whom multiple antibodies were detectable in the first positive sample.

Conclusions

Results indicate that preventative measures, specifically dietary intervention, on high risk children can feasibly decrease the risk of developing β-cell autoimmunity. There has not yet been a significant difference in the development of T1D. This type of intervention would be necessary early in life but could be implemented relatively easily as a public health measure.

COMMENTS

This is important research in relation to the ingestion of cow's milk formula and the development of islet autoimmunity. The onset of T1D has not varied between the casein hydrolysate group and the control group. Eight of the children in the casein hydrolysate group and 17 of the children in the control group tested positive for two or more islet autoantibodies. Although more information is still needed, this paper suggests dietary casein may be one factor related to β-cell autoimmunity.

REFERENCES

1. Patterson CC, Dalquist GG, Gyurus E, Green A, Soltesz G, EURODIAB Study Group. Incidence trends for childhood type 1 diabetes in Europe during 1989–2003 and predicted new cases 2005–2020: a multicenter prospective registration study. *Lancet* 2009; **373**: 2027–33

2. The Diabetes Control and Complications Trial Research Group. The effect of intensive treatment of diabetes on the development and progression of long-term complications in insulin-dependent diabetes mellitus. *N Engl J Med* 1993; **329**: 977–86

3. Levin BS, Anderson BJ, Butler DA, Antisdel JE, Brackett J, Laffel LMB. Predictors of glycaemic control and short-term adverse outcomes in youth with type 1 diabetes. *J Pediatr* 2001; **139**: 197–203

4. Ziegler A-G, Hummel M, Schenker M, Bonifacio E. Autoantibody appearance and risk for development of childhood diabetes in offspring of parents with type 1 diabetes: the 2-year analysis of the German BABYDIAB Study. *Diabetes* 1999; **48**: 460–8

5. Knip M, Virtanen SM, Akerblom HK. Infant feeding and risk of type 1 diabetes. *Am J Clin Nutr* 2010; **91** (Suppl): 1506S–13S

6. Wilkinson J, McFann K, Chase HP. Factors affecting improved glycaemic control in youth using insulin pumps. *Diab Med* 2010; **27**: 1174–7

7. Tsalikian E, Mauras N, Beck RW, Tamborlane WV, Janz KF, Chase HP, Wysocki T, Weinzimer SA, Buckingham BA, Kollman C, Xing D, Ruedy KJ; Diabetes Research in Children Network Direcnet Study Group. Impact of exercise on overnight glycemic control in children with type 1 diabetes mellitus. *J Pediatr* 2005; **147**: 528–34

8. Shalitin S, Phillip M. Hypoglycemia in type 1 diabetes: a still unresolved problem in the area of insulin analogs and pump therapy. *Diabetes Care* 2008; **31** (Suppl 2): S121–4

9. Cryer PE. Hypoglycemia: the limiting factor in the glycaemic management of type 1 and type 2 diabetes. *Diabetologia* 2002; **45**: 937–48

10. Marrero DG, Guare JC, Vandagriff JL, Fineberg NS. Fear of hypoglycemia in the parents of children and adolescents with diabetes: maladaptive or healthy response? *Diabetes Educ* 1997; **23**: 281–6

11. Hirsch IB, Abelseth J, Bode BW, Fisher JS, Kaufman FR, Mastrototaro J, Parkin CG, Wolpert HA, Buckingham BA. Sensor-augmented insulin pump therapy: results of the first randomized treat-to-target study. *Diab Technol Ther* 2008 **10**: 377–83

12. Juvenile Diabetes Research Foundation Continuous Glucose Monitoring Study Group. Continuous glucose monitoring and intensive treatment of type 1 diabetes. *N Engl J Med* 2008; **359**: 1464–76

13. Bergenstal RM, Tamborlane WV, Ahmann A, Buse J, Dailey G, Davis SN, Joyce C, Perkins BA, Willi SM, Wood M, for the STAR 3 Study Group. Effectiveness of sensor-augmented insulin pump therapy in type 1 diabetes. *N Engl J Med* 2010; **363**: 311–20

14. Ludvigsson J. C-peptide an adequate endpoint in type 1 diabetes. *Diabetes Metab Res Rev* 2009; **25**: 691–3

15. The DCCT Research Group. Effect of intensive therapy on residual β-cell function in patients with type I diabetes in the Diabetes Control and Complications Trial. *Ann Intern Med* 1998; **128**: 517–23

16. The Diabetes Control and Complications Trial Research Group. Hypoglycemia in the Diabetes Control and Complications Trial. *Diabetes* 1997; **46**: 271–86

17. Panero F, Novelli G, Zucco C, Fornengo P, Perotto M, Segre O, Grassi G, Cavallo-Perin P, Bruno G. Fasting plasma C-peptide and micro- and macrovascular complications in a large clinic-based cohort of type 1 diabetic patients. *Diabetes Care* 2009; **32**: 301–5

18. Steffes MW, Sibley S, Jackson M, Thomas W. Beta-cell function and the development of diabetes-related complications in the Diabetes Control and Complications Trial. *Diabetes Care* 2003; **26**: 832–6

19. Fiallo-Scharer R, Horner B, McFann K, Walravens P, Chase HP. Mixing rapid-acting insulin analogues with insulin glargine in children with type 1 diabetes mellitus. *J Pediatr* 2006; **148**: 481–4

CHAPTER 12

Diabetes Technology and the Human Factor

Alon Liberman[1], Bruce Buckingham[2] and Moshe Phillip[1]

[1] *Jesse Z and Sara Lea Shafer Institute of Endocrinology and Diabetes, National Center for Childhood Diabetes, Schneider Children's Medical Center of Israel, Petah Tikva, Israel*
[2] *Stanford Medical Center, Stanford, CA, USA*

INTRODUCTION

The task of preserving the desired glucose control is challenging for both patients with type 1 diabetes mellitus (T1D) and their families. Having a chronic disease with a demanding treatment regimen means the person with diabetes must maintain a high level of motivation and adherence without having the opportunity to take a 'vacation' from their diabetes. Recent developments in diabetes technologies improved diabetes control, but were associated with the need to wear more devices and pay increased attention to the disease. At the present time using the new technologies still requires treatment decisions which remain the ultimate responsibility of the patient. In other words, the 'human factor' in diabetes technologies is still mandatory and therefore must be taken into consideration.

The 'human factor' is not a single issue; it encompasses physical and emotional and intellectual interfaces, understanding new information, as well as the 'hassle factor' of the different devices. For some patients the advantages of the new technologies such as insulin pumps, glucose sensors and self-monitoring of blood glucose (SMBG) levels are outweighed by the perceived burdens and hassles imposed by these tools. In addition, there are unique concerns for specific groups such as skin real-estate issues with young children, fear of hypoglycaemia in both parents of young children and adult patients, behavioural issues associated with identity development in adolescents (fear of being 'different') as well as the usual problems of stress, anxiety and depression which are common even in the population without diabetes. Finally, problems concerning decreased

Int J Clin Pract 2012; **66** (Suppl. 175): 68–73

adherence, lack of motivation and low quality of life can significantly affect the 'human factor'.

The present chapter will review papers published in the last year that examined some of these issues.

Poor adherence to integral daily tasks limits the efficacy of CSII in youth

O'Connell MA[1], Donath S[2], Cameron FJ[1]

[1]*Department of Endocrinology and Diabetes, Royal Children's Hospital and Murdoch Children's Research Institute, Melbourne, Australia, and* [2]*Clinical Epidemiology and Biostatistics Unit, Royal Children's Hospital and Murdoch Children's Research Institute, Melbourne, Australia*

Pediatric Diabetes 2011: 12: 556–9

Background

Utilising continuous subcutaneous insulin infusion (CSII) regimens helps many young people improve their glycaemic control; however, there is still a significant proportion of patients who do not have sustained good glycaemic control. The purpose of this study was to evaluate adherence to recommended CSII-associated tasks in a paediatric cohort (mean age 13 years) and to recognise potentially modifiable behaviours that affect their HbA1c level.

Methods

CSII data from 100 youth with T1D were uploaded and analysed using CareLink Software (Medtronic Minimed).

Results

In their study mean bolus frequency was 6.1 per day; however, 69/100 entered fewer than four blood glucose levels per day. HbA1c decreased by 0.2% for every additional blood glucose level ($p = 0.001$) and bolus event ($p < 0.001$) per day. Prandial insulin omission was frequent and related to significant increases in HbA1c. Older age and duration of CSII were associated with poorer adherence to recommended behaviours.

Conclusions

Glycaemic gain achieved by CSII regimens is closely related to the way in which CSII is utilised by the patient on a daily basis. Poor adherence to overall CSII-related tasks is frequent in adolescents and limits the efficacy of CSII in this age group.

Reasons for missed mealtime insulin boluses from the perspective of adolescents using insulin pumps: 'lost focus'

Olinder AL[1,2], Nyhlin KT[3], Smide B[2]

[1] *Sachs' Children's Hospital, Södersjukhuset, Stockholm, Sweden,* [2] *Department of Medical Sciences, Uppsala University Hospital, Uppsala, Sweden, and* [3] *School of Life Sciences, University of Skövde, Skövde, Sweden*

*Pediatric Diabetes 2011; **12**: 402–9*

Background
The aim of this study was to examine the reasons for missed bolus doses and the strategies adolescents utilise for avoiding this when using insulin pumps.

Methods
The authors choose grounded theory method as a model for the collecting and analysing of data. Data were obtained through interviews with 12 adolescents treated with CSII (five males and seven females, mean age 14.4 years) from different Swedish paediatric diabetes clinics. All interviews were tape-recorded and immediately transcribed.

Results
The core theme of 'lost focus' came up as representing the main cause for missed bolus doses. Recognised subcategories were delayed lost focus, directly lost focus and totally lost focus. There was a hazard of delayed lost focus when youth used postprandial bolusing. Focus could also be lost directly in connection with the beginning of the meal. Totally lost focus happened when the adolescent apprehended the consequence of diabetes as too high or tried to ignore that he or she had it. The category 'agreements about reminders' appeared to be the main strategy for avoiding missed bolus doses; more subcategories were personal reminders and technical reminders. An involvement of the adolescent in these agreements was necessary; otherwise, the reminding could be seen as nagging and fail to succeed.

Conclusion
The results may help diabetes care teams appreciate the circumstances in which youth miss their bolus insulin doses. This may make it easier to talk about missed doses and develop strategies for avoiding this behaviour and will enable discussions between parents and children over agreements about reminders.

COMMENT

The problem of bolus omission in CSII management among children and youth is well known and has been documented in several previous studies. Burdick *et al.* (1) reported that patients who missed less than one mealtime bolus per week had a mean of 8.0% A1c compared with 8.8% for patients that missed more than one bolus per week. They concluded that 'Missed mealtime insulin boluses seem to be the major cause of suboptimal glycaemic control in youths with diabetes receiving continuous subcutaneous insulin infusion therapy'. It is the constant, unremitting daily demands of diabetes that make adherence difficult for adolescents who have many other priorities in their daily routines. Full closed-loop or treat-to-range closed-loop therapy could provide a significant benefit to this particular age group. The same frequency of missed meal boluses may also occur in patients using multiple daily injection (MDI) therapy, but we currently do not have pens with downloadable memory to allow for collection of this data.

The two above-mentioned studies provide a complementary perspective on this subject. The first cross-sectional study has examined the problem from the quantitative aspect and has found that 'Maladaptive behaviours that correlated with higher HbA1c were alarmingly common'. The unwanted behaviour included infrequent SMBG and omission of breakfast bolus insulin and was found in 70% of the patients. The authors emphasise the importance of the influence of human behaviour on glycaemic outcomes with CSII and call for enforcing adherence in order for optimal balance.

The second qualitative study assessed the reasons adolescents gave for missing meal boluses. According to this study, many of the patients omitted insulin boluses to avoid embarrassment around their peers or to prevent hypoglycaemia by delivering the bolus after onset of the meal. In consequence some of them postpone the insulin bolus and eventually forget it. Indeed, there are a certain number of patients who find the CSII management too overwhelming and ignore many of their insulin boluses.

Missed meal boluses is a common problem that should be addressed when there are fewer than three boluses a day, or at times of the day when food is commonly consumed and there is no observed meal bolus in the pump download. Understanding the problem from the patient's point of view may help the patient feel more understood and his/her adherence to the treatment may increase. These studies also highlight the value of having good software that allows easy visualisation and documentation of insulin administration. In the CareLink software this is best observed by reviewing the 'daily details' reports with the patient. This ability to discuss daily aspects of diabetes management with concrete data is missing when patients use MDI therapy, and some pump software does not provide the same, easily assessed and visualised daily details. As we progress with additional steps to closed-loop therapy, the software should allow easy visualisation of the results to both the patient and healthcare provider.

Satisfaction with continuous glucose monitoring in adults and youths with type 1 diabetes

Tansey M[1], Laffel L[2], Cheng J[3], Beck R[3], Coffey J[1], Huang E[4], Kollman C[3], Lawrence J[5], Lee J[6], Ruedy K[3], Tamborlane W[7], Wysocki T[8], Xing D[3]; on behalf of Juvenile Diabetes Research Foundation Continuous Glucose Monitoring Study Group

[1]*Department of Pediatrics, University of Iowa, IA, USA,* [2]*Joslin Diabetes Center, Pediatrics, Harvard Medical School, Boston, MA, USA,* [3]*Jaeb Center for Health Research, Tampa, FL, USA,* [4]*University of Chicago, Medicine, Chicago, IL, USA,* [5]*Department of Research and Epidemiology, Kaiser Permanente Southern California, Anaheim, CA, USA,* [6]*University of Michigan, Child Health Evaluation and Research Unit, Ann Arbor, MI, USA,* [7]*Yale University School of Medicine, Pediatrics, New Haven, CT, USA, and* [8]*Nemours Children's Clinic, Center for Pediatric Psychology Research, Jacksonville, FL, USA*

Diabet Med 2011; **28**: 1118–22

Aim

The purpose of this study was to describe satisfaction with continuous glucose monitoring (CGM) in T1D patients; to relate CGM satisfaction scores with usage; and to identify common themes in perceived benefits and obstacles of monitoring reported by adults, adolescents and the parents of adolescents in the Juvenile Diabetes Research Foundation (JDRF) CGM trial.

Methods

The Continuous Glucose Monitoring Satisfaction Scale questionnaire was completed after 6 months of CGM use. Patients also completed open-ended queries of positive and negative attributes of CGM.

Results

A relationship was found between more frequent use of CGM and higher scores of satisfaction among adults ($n = 224$), youths ($n = 208$) and parents of youths ($n = 192$) (all $p < 0.001$). This was true for both the 'benefits' and 'hassles' subscales of the Continuous Glucose Monitoring Satisfaction Scale, but the most significant differences between the two groups involved scores on hassle factors. Common obstacles to monitoring use included sensor needle pain, system alarms and body image issues; while common benefits included glucose trend data and options to self-correct out-of-range glucose levels and to detect hypoglycaemia.

Conclusions

Although patients who use continuous glucose monitoring often have a better chance for increasing their glycaemic control without increasing hypoglycaemia, it is still important to overcome obstacles to consistent use, strengthen benefits and set realistic expectations for this technology.

Quality-of-life measures in children and adults with type 1 diabetes: Juvenile Diabetes Research Foundation Continuous Glucose Monitoring Randomised Trial

Juvenile Diabetes Research Foundation Continuous Glucose Monitoring Study Group

Diabetes Care 2010; 33: 2175–217

Background

The influence of CGM on quality of life (QOL) was examined among participants with T1D.

Methods

In this multicentre trial, 451 children and adults with T1D were assigned randomly to CGM treatment or the control group. All patients and their parents (of patients younger than 18 years) completed both generic and diabetes-specific QOL questionnaires at baseline and 26 weeks and the CGM satisfaction scale was completed by the CGM group (patients and parents) at 26 weeks.

Results

After 26 weeks of CGM use, QOL scores remained largely unchanged for both the treatment and the control group. However, a slight difference was documented in favour of the adult CGM group on several subscales ($p < 0.05$). There was substantial satisfaction with CGM technology after 26 weeks among participants and parents.

Conclusions

Baseline QOL was high, and the measures showed minor changes with CGM use, although a high level of CGM satisfaction was reported.

COMMENT

Understanding how patients perceive the benefits and barriers to CGM is important for identifying strategies to reduce barriers and enable more consistent monitoring.

Several studies have recently validated the Continuous Glucose Monitoring Satisfaction Scale as an important scale that helps in assessing directly both the benefits and hassles associated with CGM use. A large JDRF trial found that adolescents did not use the CGM as much as pre-pubertal children, were less satisfied, could not accept the hassle and burden caused by CGM use and failed to achieve the study A1c targets.

The first study presented above examined the relationship between frequency of CGM and its satisfaction by all users (adults, adolescents and their parents). They found that patients who used the CGM more frequently (6 days or more per week) reported more benefits and less hassles compared with infrequent users (4 days or more per week).

From the self-reported information, interesting discrepancies were seen when comparing the adolescents' perceived barriers with what their parents perceived as barriers. Adolescents reported that frequent alarms and the pain of insertion were the most frequent barriers to CGM usage, whereas their parents reported that the change to the adolescent's body image was a bigger barrier.

The discrepancy between the two viewpoints highlights a very common experience in the clinic. The parents as well as the diabetes team tend to seek more abstract themes as possible diabetes barriers (body image, meaning and acceptance of diabetes) while the adolescents tend to focus on more practical issues. If indeed the above conclusion is correct, there is hope for fewer complaints in this age group with improved technology.

Sensor augmented pump therapy lowers HbA1c in suboptimal controlled type 1 diabetes; a randomised controlled trial

Hermanides J[1], Nørgaard K[2], Bruttomesso D[3], Mathieu C[4], Frid A[5], Dayan CM[6], Diem P[7], Fermon C[8], Wentholt IME[1], Hoekstra JBL[1], DeVries JH[1]

[1]*Department of Internal Medicine, Academic Medical Centre, Amsterdam, The Netherlands,* [2]*Department of Endocrinology, Hvidovre University Hospital, Hvidovre, Denmark,* [3]*Department of Clinical and Experimental Medicine, Division of Metabolic Diseases, University of Padova, Padova, Italy,* [4]*Department of Endocrinology, Catholic University Leuven, Leuven, Belgium,* [5]*Division of Diabetes and Endocrinology, Malmö University Hospital, Malmö, Sweden,* [6]*Department of Medicine, University of Bristol, Bristol, UK,* [7]*Division of Endocrinology, Diabetes and Clinical Nutrition, University Hospital and*

University of Bern, Bern, Switzerland, and [8]Centre d'éducation pour le traitement de diabète et des maladies de la nutrition, Centre Hospitalier de Roubaix, Roubaix, France

Diabet Med 2011; **28**: 1158–67

Aim

The aim of this study was to examine the effectiveness of sensor augmented pump therapy vs. multiple daily injection therapy in patients with poorly controlled T1D (A1c ≥ 8.2%).

Methods

In total, 83 patients with T1D (40 women) currently treated with MDI, aged 18–65 years, were randomly assigned to 26 weeks of treatment with either a sensor-augmented insulin pump (SAP) ($n = 44$) (Paradigm® REAL-Time) or MDI ($n = 39$). Change in HbA1c between baseline and 26 weeks, sensor derived endpoints and patient reported outcomes were assessed.

Results

The mean HbA1c at baseline changed from 8.46% (SD 0.95) to 7.23% (SD 0.65) in the SAP group and from 8.59% (SD 0.82) to 8.46% (SD 1.04) in the MDI group. Mean difference in change in HbA1c after 26 weeks was −1.21% (95% confidence interval −1.52 to −0.90, p < 0.001) in favour of the SAP group. This advantage was achieved without increasing the percentage of time spent in hypoglycaemia. The SAP group showed an improvement in the Problem Areas in Diabetes and Diabetes Treatment Satisfaction Questionnaire scores.

Conclusions

SAP therapy significantly decreased HbA1c in T1D patients poorly controlled on MDI therapy.

COMMENT

This study is smaller in size but with similar study design to the Star 3 study, except in the Star 3 trial the enrolment A1c was >7.3%. In both studies SAP therapy was compared with intensive MDI therapy. In both studies there was a significant improvement in the SAP group in comparison with the MDI group. The SAP group also showed increased satisfaction scores as measured by the Problem Areas in Diabetes and Diabetes Treatment Satisfaction Questionnaire.

When comparing the quality of life scores between the two groups (measured by using the SF-36v2), there was almost no significant difference. This again demonstrates the relative insensitivity of quality of life measures to significant changes in diabetes control and diabetes related issues.

Use of continuous glucose monitoring in young children with type 1 diabetes: implications for behavioural research

Patton SR[1], Williams LB[2], Eder SJ[1], Crawford MJ[3], Dolan L[4], Powers SW[5]

[1] *Department of Pediatrics, University of Michigan/CS Mott Children's Hospital, Ann Arbor, MI, USA,* [2] *Department of Pediatrics, University of South Florida, Tampa, FL, USA,* [3] *Department of Clinical and Health Psychology, University of Florida, Gainesville, FL, USA,* [4] *Department of Pediatrics, Division of Pediatric Endocrinology, Cincinnati Children's Hospital Medical Center, Cincinnati, OH, USA, and* [5] *Department of Pediatrics, Division of Behavioral Medicine and Clinical Psychology, Cincinnati Children's Hospital Medical Center, Cincinnati, OH, USA*

*Pediatric Diabetes 2011; **12**: 18–24*

Aim

The purpose of this study was to assess the feasibility of obtaining retrospective CGM data in young children with T1D. CGM provides moment-to-moment tracking of glucose concentrations and measures of intra- and inter-day variability.

Methods

A total of 31 children (mean age 5.0 years) with T1D used a blinded Medtronic Minimed CGM for a mean of 66.8 h. The CGM was inserted in diabetes clinics and parents were instructed for 1 h on its usage.

Results

Few difficulties were reported by families in wearing the sensor for a mean of 66 h. The authors compared participants' CGM data with SMBG data and also data from older children with T1D to show differences in glucose variability existing in this population. Increased glucose variability was associated with a history of hypoglycaemic seizures.

Conclusions

CGM can be used as an acceptable research tool for obtaining glucose data in young children with T1D who frequently experience more glucose variability. Data achieved through CGM are richer and more detailed than traditional SMBG data and allow analyses of how behaviour may affect blood glucose levels.

COMMENT

This is one of a few studies that have assessed the use of CGM in young children less than 7 years of age with T1D, and once again it demonstrates increased glycaemic variability in this age group. As the authors emphasised, the reason for this study is the growing evidence suggesting that 'glucose variability is a key factor in the risk for diabetes-related complications' (i.e. microvascular complications in adults). Another variable examined in this study was diabetes-related adherence such as number of omitted insulin dosages at meals or snacks per week, daily blood glucose monitoring frequency, and number of meals or snacks per day. These young children had a mean glucose of 191 mg/dl and only 5% of readings were less than 70 mg/dl, indicating that the parents may have intentionally kept them with higher blood glucose levels. Some recent studies indicate that parental fear of hypoglycaemia may be a barrier to optimal glycaemic control. Patton et al. (2,3) examined this issue with a modified version of the fear of hypoglycaemia scale (the Hypoglycemia Fear Survey – Parents of Young Children, HFS-PYC). They found that mothers of young children who experienced a seizure were more worried and tended to have more hypoglycaemia-fear behaviour than mothers of young children who had never had a seizure. Mothers reported higher total HFS-PYC scores and higher scores on the behaviour subscale, and reported greater use of strategies that increase blood glucose levels than fathers. The authors also suggest that mothers of young children with T1D often assume the majority of care for their child's diabetes. Back to the current study, the authors suggest that CGM 'can be particularly useful for behavioural researchers examining associations between patients' psychosocial functioning, self-care behaviours, and their glycaemic control, which evidence suggests should be a target for future behavioural interventions'. According to the studies cited above, reducing parental fear of hypoglycaemia may be an important goal for this kind of intervention. The use of pumps with a low glucose suspend feature or predictive pump shut-off to prevent hypoglycaemia may be particularly appropriate in this age group where there is a high level of anxiety about hypoglycaemia.

Survey of insulin site rotation in youth with type 1 diabetes mellitus

Patton SR[1,2], Eder S[1,2], Schwab J[2,3], Sisson CM[2,3]

[1] *Division of Child Behavioral Health, C.S. Mott Children's Hospital, Ann Arbor, MI, USA,* [2] *University of Michigan Medical School, Department of Pediatrics, Ann Arbor, MI, USA,* [3] *Division of Endocrinology, C.S. Mott Children's Hospital, Ann Arbor, MI, USA*

*J Pediatr Health Care 2010; **24**: 365–71*

Background

Injection site rotation is an important constituent of insulin regimen and is helpful in preventing lipodystrophy in T1D. This study examined the number of injection/infusion sites used by youth with T1D and their perceived obstacles to using new sites in rotation for insulin administration.

Methods

A total of 201 adolescents with T1D completed a 24-item survey about site rotation practices and obstacles to site rotation during a routine diabetes appointment.

Results

Fifteen per cent of adolescents reported using at least four different sites in their rotation plan, while 22% reported using only one site. A negative association was found between number of sites used and the number of perceived obstacles reported by youth on multiple daily injections. Fear of pain was the most frequent obstacle reported by adolescents.

Conclusion

Adherence to an appropriate site rotation plan may be a problem for many adolescents with T1D. Regular evaluation of insulin sites and counselling regarding appropriate site rotation is needed when managing diabetes among adolescents. Fear of pain when rotating to new insulin sites may be reduced with the help of relaxation and distraction among adolescents.

COMMENT

One of the common issues with both multiple daily injections and pump therapy is a tendency for patients to administer their insulin in one or two 'favourite' sites. When they do, insulin stimulates lipohypertrophy, and insulin injections are less painful in this lipohypertrophied site. The lipohypertrophy and eventual scar tissue formation at these favoured sites can also alter insulin pharmacodynamics which may prevent optimal insulin absorption and may eventually cause a decline in metabolic control (4,5).

Adolescents report fear from pain in rotating to new insulin sites as the most common barrier for adherence to site rotation. Only a third of youth on CSII use the recommended site rotation. Although 61% of youth on a CSII regimen recognise that site rotation will improve their diabetes control, 67% of the same group mentioned comfort with their existing routine as a barrier to adopting new sites.

With the addition of CGM site rotation becomes a much bigger issue since, at any one time, two sites are occupied, and in young children the real estate of skin becomes an even bigger issue. The insulin causes lipohypertrophy which is not a problem with sensors; however, both pumps and sensors require adhesive tape. Every time tape is pulled off the skin it removes the top layer of the epidermis which is an important barrier to skin infections. If a site is used repeatedly, it does not allow time for the skin to heal and increases the risk for an infection where the sensor or infusion set needle penetrates the skin. The use of multiple adhesive tapes also increases the risk of tape allergy.

Fear of pain and fear of change are the main barriers to site rotation. The authors suggest that using relaxation and distraction techniques will help children cope with their fear while they become more familiar with new injection sites.

The field of relaxation and distraction has developed in recent years along with recognition of its effectiveness. Pain no longer seems a physiological phenomenon *per se* but a complicated experience containing both physiological and psychological factors, especially anxiety and the inability to relax. This field provides options such as meditation, relaxation and virtual techniques which will help the diabetes team expand their box of tools and improve patient adherence to treatment.

Fear of hypoglycaemia in type 1 diabetes managed by continuous subcutaneous insulin infusion: is it associated with poor glycaemic control?

Nixon R, Pickup JC

Diabetes Research Group, King's College London School of Medicine, Guy's Hospital, London, UK

*Diabetes Technol Ther 2011; **13**: 93–8*

Aim

The aim of this study was to examine the scope of fear of hypoglycaemia in patients with T1D using CSII and to test the hypothesis that poor glycaemic control during CSII is associated with fear of hypoglycaemia.

Methods

The authors interviewed non-pregnant T1D patients attending an insulin pump clinic with at least 6 months' duration of CSII. In 104 subjects, fear of hypoglycaemia was evaluated by questionnaire; 75 responded.

Results

The median duration of CSII was 5 years (range 1–29 years). Suboptimal glycaemic control [haemoglobin A1c (HbA1c) $\geq 8.5\%$] was present in 27%, and this group had more men than the good control group with HbA1c $< 7.0\%$ (43% vs. 11%). Significant fear of hypoglycaemia (score $> 50\%$) occurred in 27% of subjects, but fear of hypoglycaemia was not related to HbA1c. Accumulated episodes and rate of severe hypogly-caemia were the only significant correlates of fear of hypoglycaemia ($r = 0.48$, $p < 0.001$). The HbA1c on CSII was correlated with the mean HbA1c for the 6 months on MDI therapy prior to starting CSII ($p < 0.0001$).

Conclusions

Fear of hypoglycaemia is not correlated with HbA1c levels of patients using CSII therapy. Other factors (such as their previous HbA1c on MDI therapy and adherence to insulin pump procedures) are likely to be more significant. However, marked fear of hypoglycaemia exists in many CSII-treated people and may indirectly affect quality of life and psychological well-being.

Sustained efficacy of continuous subcutaneous insulin infusion in type 1 diabetes subjects with recurrent non-severe and severe hypoglycaemia and hypoglycaemia unawareness: a pilot study

Giménez M, Lara M, Conget I

Endocrinology and Diabetes Unit, Institute of Biomedical Investigations August Pi i Sunyer, CIBER of Diabetes and Associated Metabolic Diseases and Hospital Clínic i Universitari, Barcelona, Spain

*Diabetes Technol Ther 2010; **12**: 517–21*

Aim

The purpose of this study was to evaluate the effect of initiation of CSII therapy on hypoglycaemia awareness and on glucose profiles in adults with T1D followed for 2 years after CSII initiation. Patients were recruited into the study with a history of repeated non-severe (NS) or severe (SH) hypoglycaemic episodes.

Methods

The authors included in the study subjects who were older than 18 years with T1D duration of more than 5 years who were on multiple doses of insulin, without microvascular or macrovascular complications, and who had more than four NS events per week (in the last 8 weeks) and more than two SH events (in the last 2 years). NS/SH episodes and hypogly-caemia awareness were evaluated at baseline and at 6, 12 and 24 months after starting CSII therapy. A 72-h CGM was performed and subjects had a hypoglycaemic clamp to test for symptoms of hypoglycaemia at baseline and after 24 months of CSII. Quality of life was also evaluated after 6, 12 and 24 months.

Results

A total of 20 patients were included (mean age 34.0 ± 7.5 years, 12 women, mean A1c $6.7 \pm 1.1\%$, and mean 16.2 ± 6.6 years of diabetes' duration). At baseline, 19 of 20 patients had hypoglycaemia unawareness, which decreased substantially during the follow-up to three out of 20 at 24 months. NS episodes per week decreased from 5.40 ± 2.09 at baseline to 2.75 ± 1.74 at the end of the follow-up ($p < 0.001$). SH episodes fell from 1.25 ± 0.44 per subject-year to 0.05 ± 0.22 after 24 months ($p < 0.001$). There was no change in haemoglobin A1c. With CGM, the percentage of values within 70–180 mg/dl increased ($53.2 \pm 11.0\%$ to $60.3 \pm 17.1\%$, $p = 0.13$), and the percentage of values <70 mg/dl diminished ($13.7 \pm 9.4\%$ to $9.1 \pm 5.2\%$, $p = 0.07$), after 24 months. Mean amplitude of glycaemic excursions diminished after 24 months of CSII (136 ± 28 mg/dl to 115 ± 19 mg/dl; $p < 0.02$). An improvement in all the aspects of quality of life was observed. The basal alteration in symptom response to an induced hypoglycaemia improved after 24 months of initiating CSII leading to a response indistinguishable from that observed in a control group of patients with T1D without repeated NS and SH.

Conclusions

Use of CSII helps in preventing hypoglycaemic episodes, improving hypoglycaemia awareness, and achieving better glycaemic profile.

COMMENT

It is thought that fear of hypoglycaemia is a major contributor to poor glycaemic control. A cognitive-emotional model and the behavioural model have been developed to explain the effect of fear of hypoglycaemia on metabolic control. If a person with diabetes is worried and troubled about having a potential hypoglycaemic episode (perhaps even severe), he/she will develop protective behaviours oriented toward preventing a hypoglycaemic attack. These behaviours include increased food intake and/or reduced insulin doses that may eventually lead to poor glycaemic control. The Hypoglycemia Fear Survey is a measurement tool based on this model.

The first study challenges this well accepted assumption. According to the results no correlation was found between HbA1c on CSII and fear of hypoglycaemia. Patients with poorer glycaemic control did not report more fear of hypoglycaemia than patients with good glycaemic control. Taking a closer look at the results may provide some possible explanations. In this study 27% of the patients did have significant fear of hypoglycaemia which was correlated with the occurrence of episodes of SH.

In the second study by Giménez *et al.* there was a decrease in the number of hypoglycaemic episodes in a group with a history of frequent episodes of hypoglycaemia and hypoglycaemia unawareness with 2 years of CSII therapy. In this study there was a significant improvement in their diabetes quality of life, which is probably related to restoration of hypoglycaemia awareness. The study, however, did not measure fear of hypoglycaemia. In another study hypoglycaemia unawareness was reversed with 4 weeks of sensor augmented pump therapy using a high hypoglycaemic threshold of 108 mg/dl (6).

These studies show that CSII therapy, particularly when combined with a continuous glucose sensor, can have a major role in decreasing hypoglycaemia unawareness and fear of hypoglycaemia.

There is also a group that had never experienced a severe hypoglycaemia attack but still report fear of hypoglycaemia. Gonder-Frederick *et al.* (7) argue that this group may possess anxiety as a trait and not as a state. Patients that have an anxious tendency are at risk of confusing symptoms of anxiety with those of hypoglycaemia.

In conclusion, CSII and the use of CGM can have a major role in restoring hypoglycaemia awareness, but this does not necessarily translate into a lower A1c, although it can have a significant impact on the patients' quality of life. The use of these technologies can also be combined with a psychological approach to reduce anxiety and fear of hypoglycaemia.

Role of parenting style in achieving metabolic sx control in adolescents with type 1 diabetes

Shorer M[1], David R[2], Schoenberg-Taz M[1], Levavi-Lavi I[3], Phillip M[1,2], Meyerovitch J[1,2]

[1] *Jesse Z and Sara Lea Shafer Institute for Endocrinology and Diabetes, National Center for Childhood Diabetes, Schneider Children's Medical Center of Israel, Petah Tikva, Israel,* [2] *Sackler Faculty of Medicine, Tel-Aviv University, Tel-Aviv, Israel, and* [3] *Department of Medical Psychology, Schneider Children's Medical Center of Israel, Petah Tikva, Israel*

Diabetes Care 2011; 34: 1–3

Aim

The aim of this study was to examine the role of parenting style in achieving metabolic control and treatment adherence in youth with T1D.

Methods

Parents of 100 adolescents with T1D completed questionnaires on their parenting style and sense of helplessness. The patient's adherence to the treatment regimen was rated by both parents and patients. Glycaemic control was evaluated by HbA1c values.

Results

Better glycaemic control was predicted by utilising an authoritative paternal parenting style and adherence in the child; a permissive maternal parenting style predicted poor adherence. A higher sense of helplessness in both parents predicted suboptimal glycaemic control and poorer adherence to treatment. A sense of helplessness in parents was a significant predictor of diabetes control after correcting for other confounders (patient age, sex and treatment method).

Conclusions

An authoritative non-helpless parenting style is correlated with better diabetes control in youth. The authors conclude that paternal involvement is important in youth diabetes management and remark that these results have implications for psychological interventions.

COMMENT

The problem of motivation in patients with diabetes is without doubt one of the most important issues in diabetes care. Since a patient's adherence to treatment still plays a central role in glucose control, being non-cooperative to treatment regimen can cause poor glucose control. Multiple studies have shown that diabetes technology may be very successful when used by well controlled patients and parents who have high motivation and receive support of specialised diabetes care centres with expertise in diabetes technology. Nimri *et al*. (8) reported that 'Continuous subcutaneous insulin infusion improves glycemic control in children and adolescents with type 1 diabetes, especially those with a history of moderate to poor glycemic control' but the authors also mentioned that a possible explanation of the better glycaemic improvement in children compared with the adolescent group might be related to the parental supervision of the young children and their greater motivation.

It seems that there is no single solution for motivating diabetes patients. The diabetes team will have to be creative and to attack this problem from many different angles including increased parental involvement.

Adherence challenges in the management of type 1 diabetes in adolescents: prevention and intervention

Borusa JS[1], Laffel L[2]

[1] *Division of Adolescent/Young Adult Medicine, Department of Medicine, Children's Hospital Boston, Boston, MA, USA, and* [2] *Pediatric, Adolescent and Young Adult Section, Genetics and Epidemiology Section, Joslin Diabetes Center, Harvard Medical School, Boston, MA, USA*

*Curr Opin Pediatr 2010; **22**: 405–11*

Background

Although efficient therapies are available, there is still poor treatment adherence among teens with T1D compared with other children. The purpose of this paper was to review the obstacles that influence adherence and discuss interventions that have shown promise in improving results for this age group.

Results

Adolescents face many barriers to adherence, including developmental behaviours, changes in family dynamics, and the adolescent's own perception of social stress, as well as the physiological insulin resistance brought on by pubertal physiology. Some successful treatments have been based on encouraging non-judgmental family support in the daily tasks of blood glucose monitoring and insulin regimen. Other interventions have utilised motivational interviewing and problem-solving techniques, flexibility in nutrition recommendations, and extending provider outreach and support with technology.

Summary

Effective treatments build upon adolescents internal and external supports (family, technology and internal motivation) in order to make their management of diabetes simpler and provide opportunities for the adolescents to share the burden of care. Although such strategies help reduce the demands placed upon adolescents with diabetes, poor glycaemic control will probably persist for the majority of adolescents until technological breakthroughs allow for automated insulin delivery in closed-loop systems.

COMMENT

The problem of compliance and adherence is one of the central issues that medical and rehabilitation psychology deals with. Increased adherence to diabetes management favourably impacts glycaemic control and lower haemoglobin A1c (HbA1c) levels reduce the risk for diabetes complications. It is therefore accepted that psychological treatment should focus on increasing adherence to diabetes treatment. In their discussion the authors point out that adherence is not necessarily an independent factor. Rather, 'there is a constellation of factors that impacts adherence in adolescents with type 1 diabetes'. These factors include both modifiable and unmodifiable factors. One of these factors is implementation of technologies for diabetes management (alongside diabetes-specific family conflict, increased family involvement with diabetes management and gender- and age-specific issues).

Diabetes technology in general and continuous glucose monitors in particular may become an obstacle for teens rather than a useful instrument.

Adolescents tend to overemphasise the demands and personal intrusions caused by the CGM use and ignore its benefits. The authors suggest that 'strategies to increase treatment adherence for teens must require minimal distraction from the teen's routine tasks of daily living'. We indeed agree and suggest that people who develop new technologies for patients with diabetes should remember that any new technology should reduce the burden imposed on the patients especially in the adolescent age group.

REFERENCES

1. Burdick J, Chase HP, Slover RH, Knievel K, Scrimgeour L, Maniatis AK, Klingensmith GJ. Missed insulin meal boluses and elevated hemoglobin A1c levels in children receiving insulin pump therapy. *Pediatrics* 2004; **113** (3 Pt 1): e221–4

2. Patton SR, Dolan LM, Henry R, Powers SW. Parental fear of hypoglycemia: young children treated with continuous subcutaneous insulin infusion. *Pediatr Diabetes* 2007; **8**: 362–8

3. Patton SR, Dolan LM, Henry R, Powers SW. Fear of hypoglycemia in parents of young children with type 1 diabetes mellitus. *J Clin Psychol Med Settings* 2008; **15**: 252–9

4. Hofman PL, Lawton SA, Peart JM, Holt JA, Jefferies CA, Robinson E, Cutfield WS. An angled insertion technique using 6-mm needles markedly reduces the risk of intramuscular injections in children and adolescents. *Diabet Med* 2007; **24**: 1400–5

5. Johansson UB, Amsberg S, Hannerz L, Wredling R, Adamson U, Arnqvist HJ, Lins PE. Impaired absorption of insulin aspart from lipohypertrophic injection sites. *Diabetes Care* 2005; **28**: 2025–7

6. Ly TT, Hewitt J, Davey RJ, Lim EM, Davis EA, Jones TW. Improving epinephrine responses in hypoglycemia unawareness with real-time continuous glucose monitoring in adolescents with type 1 diabetes. *Diabetes Care* 2011; **34**: 50–2

7. Gonder-Frederick L, Fisher CD, Ritterband LM, Cox DJ, Hou, L, DasGupta AA, Clarke WL. Predictors of fear of hypoglycemia in adolescents with type 1 diabetes and their parents. *Pediatr Diabetes* 2006; **7**: 215–22

8. Nimri R, Weintrob N, Benzaquen H, Ofan R, Fayman G, Phillip M. Insulin pump therapy in youth with type 1 diabetes: a retrospective paired study. *Pediatrics* 2006; **117**: 2126–31

CHAPTER 13

New Medications for the Treatment of Diabetes

Satish K. Garg[1] and Jay S. Skyler[2]

[1] University of Colorado Health Sciences Center, Aurora, CO, USA
[2] Division of Endocrinology, Diabetes and Metabolism and Diabetes Research Institute, University of Miami Miller School of Medicine, Miami, FL, USA

INTRODUCTION

A number of new medications are being developed for the treatment of diabetes. In this chapter, we review recent papers describing some of these. We begin with insulins – an overview paper, two papers about insulin degludec (one each for type 2 and type 1 diabetes), one paper about a pre-mixed insulin combining insulin degludec with insulin aspart, one paper about very early development of a possible method to prolong the action of insulin glargine, and two papers about ultra-rapid-acting insulins – one that uses an inhaled insulin formulation in which insulin is adsorbed onto fumaryl diketopiperazine powder, and one in which action is accelerated by mixture with hyaluronidase.

Next we cover a new weekly formulation of the glucagon-like peptide 1 (GLP-1) receptor agonist exenatide; the development of two new classes of antidiabetic drugs, sodium glucose cotransporter 2 (SGLT-2) inhibitors and glucokinase activators; a potential new indication for the GLP-1 receptor agonists and dipeptidyl peptidase 4 (DPP-4) inhibitors – use in type 1 diabetes; and finally we look at new studies trying to prevent type 2 diabetes.

The future of basal insulin supplementation

Simon AC, DeVries JH

Department of Internal Medicine, Academic Medical Centre, Amsterdam, The Netherlands

*Diabetes Technol Ther 2011; **13** (Suppl 1): S103–8*

Int J Clin Pract 2012; **66** (Suppl. 175): 74–83

Background

Both patients and physicians are often reluctant to start or intensify insulin therapy because of perceived fear of painful injections, hypoglycaemia, weight gain, complexity of insulin regimens, and drug costs. Optimising basal insulin therapy and addressing these barriers can facilitate the achievement of optimal glycaemic control in patients with type 2 diabetes. The currently available long-acting basal insulin analogues (detemir and glargine) show advantages compared with the NPH insulin. The aim of this review is to present an overview of the candidates for improved basal insulin in the pharmaceutical pipeline.

Results

The first new basal insulin to enter the market is most probably insulin degludec (IDeg), currently reporting in phase 3 of development, from Novo Nordisk (Bagsvaerd, Denmark), which has a longer duration of action than currently available analogues. Phase 2 studies show comparable efficacy and safety outcomes compared with insulin glargine once daily with less hypoglycaemia in type 1 diabetes. The final results of phase 3 studies seem to confirm this, also in type 2 diabetes. Biodel (Danbury, CT, USA) has two long-acting basal insulin formulations in the pipeline, both in the pre-clinical phase of development: BIOD-Adjustable Basal, a modified formulation of insulin glargine, is being developed in long-, medium- and short-acting forms and could be mixed, and BIOD-Smart Basal releases insulin proportional to the subcutaneous glucose concentration. Clinical trials with the new patch pump from CeQur (Montreux, Switzerland) have recently started in Europe. This pump delivers subcutaneously both basal and bolus doses and is intended for people with type 2 diabetes who need multiple daily injection insulin therapy.

COMMENT

Simon and DeVries project the future of basal insulin supplementation in this paper. They highlight some new information on insulin degludec (not yet approved in any part of the world). Phase 2 studies on insulin degludec show significantly lower hypoglycaemia in subjects with type 1 diabetes. The authors also report on Biodel-adjustable basal, a modified formulation of insulin glargine that could possibly be mixed with ultra-fast-acting insulin for a single injection treatment. The ideal way to deliver basal insulin might be the use of patch pumps using rapid-acting or ultra-fast-acting insulin to replicate what happens in healthy individuals. Below are some of the studies with new basal insulins and their development.

Insulin degludec, an ultra-long-acting basal insulin, once a day or three times a week versus insulin glargine once a day in patients with type 2 diabetes: a 16-week, randomised, open-label, phase 2 trial

Zinman B[1], Fulcher G[2], Rao PV[3], Thomas N[4,] Endahl LA[5], Johansen T[5], Lindh R[5], Lewin A[6], Rosenstock J[7], Pinget M[8], Mathieu C[9]

[1] *Samuel Lunenfeld Research Institute, Mount Sinai Hospital, University of Toronto, Toronto, ON, Canada,* [2] *Royal North Shore Hospital and University of Sydney, Sydney, NSW, Australia,* [3] *Nizam's Institute of Medical Sciences University, Hyderabad, India,* [4] *Christian Medical College, Vellore, India,* [5] *Novo Nordisk, Soeborg, Denmark,* [6] *National Research Institute, Los Angeles, CA, USA,* [7] *Dallas Diabetes and Endocrine Center at Medical City, Dallas, TX, USA,* [8] *University Hospital Strasbourg, Strasbourg, France, and* [9] *UZ Gasthuisberg Katholieke Universiteit Leuven, Leuven, Belgium*

*Lancet 2011; **377**: 924–31*

Background

Insulin degludec is an ultra-long-acting insulin in clinical development, and its action profile is mainly attributable to formation of soluble multihexamers at the injection site, from which monomers gradually separate and are absorbed into the circulation, resulting in a flat and stable pharmacokinetic profile at steady state. This clinical proof-of-concept trial aimed to assess efficacy and safety of insulin degludec once a day or three times a week compared with insulin glargine once a day, in combination with metformin, in insulin-naive patients with type 2 diabetes who were inadequately controlled on oral antidiabetic medications.

Methods

This was a multicentre (28 clinical sites in Canada, India, South Africa and the USA) randomised open-label, parallel-group phase 2 trial of 16 weeks in which participants with type 2 diabetes (age 18–75 years, HbA1c 7%–11%) were enrolled and treated. Participants were randomly allocated in a 1:1:1:1 ratio to receive insulin degludec either once a day or three times a week or insulin glargine once a day, all in combination with metformin. Investigators were masked to data until database release. The primary outcome was HbA1c after 16 weeks of treatment.

Results

Of 367 patients screened, 245 were eligible for inclusion. Of these, 62 participants were randomly allocated to receive insulin degludec three times a week [starting dose 20 U per injection (1 U = 9 nmol)], 60 to receive insulin degludec once a day [starting dose 10 U (1 U = 6 nmol); group A], 61 to receive insulin degludec once a day [starting dose 10 U (1 U = 9 nmol); group B] and 62 to receive insulin glargine [starting dose 10 U (1 U = 6 nmol)] once a day. At study end, mean HbA1c levels were the same across treatment groups. Estimated mean HbA1c treatment differences from insulin degludec, by comparison with insulin glargine, were 0.08% [95% confidence interval (CI) –0.23 to 0.40] for the three dose per week schedule, 0.17% (–0.15 to 0.48) for group A and 0.28% (–0.04 to 0.59) for group B. Few participants had hypoglycaemia and the number of adverse events was the same across groups, with no apparent treatment-specific pattern.

Conclusions

Findings from this trial show that insulin degludec can provide equivalent glycaemic control to insulin glargine without new or increased rates of adverse events in insulin-naive people with type 2 diabetes. The safety, efficacy and optimum use of treatment regimens for insulin degludec need to be established.

COMMENT

Zinman *et al.* report phase 2 results on insulin degludec in patients with type 2 diabetes. There was comparable glycaemic control and the rates of hypoglycaemia did not differ between groups. This study also explored whether insulin degludec given in higher dose could possibly be given three times a week, thus limiting the number of injections per week. Although it is interesting to see the development of a new basal insulin, it should be noted that insulin degludec was similar to insulin glargine in terms of glycaemic control.

Insulin degludec in type 1 diabetes: a randomised controlled trial of a new-generation ultra-long-acting insulin compared with insulin glargine

Birkeland KI[1], Home PD[2], Wendisch U[3], Ratner RE[4], Johansen T[5], Endahl LA[5], Lyby K[5], Jendle JH[6], Roberts AP[7], DeVries JH[8], Meneghini LF[9]

[1]*Oslo University Hospital and Faculty of Medicine, Oslo, Norway,* [2]*Newcastle University, Newcastle upon Tyne, UK,* [3]*Group Practice in Internal Medicine and Diabetology, Hamburg, Germany,* [4]*MedStar Research Institute, Washington, DC, USA,* [5]*Novo Nordisk A/S, Soeborg, Denmark,* [6]*Örebro University Hospital,*

Örebro, Sweden, [7]Royal Adelaide Hospital, Adelaide, SA, Australia, [8]University of Amsterdam, Amsterdam, The Netherlands, and [9]University of Miami Miller School of Medicine, Miami, FL, USA

*Diabetes Care 2011; **34**: 661–5*

Background

Despite the advantages offered by current basal insulin analogues, hypoglycaemia remains a treatment limitation. Insulin degludec (IDeg) is a new-generation ultra-long-acting basal insulin that forms soluble multi-hexamers after subcutaneous injection, resulting in an ultra-long-action profile and a smooth and stable pharmacokinetic profile at steady state. These attributes are expected to provide improved glycaemic control and to lower the risk of hypoglycaemia. The aim of this trial was to compare the efficacy, safety and tolerability of two different IDeg formulations (IDeg(A) and IDeg(B)) with insulin glargine (IGlar), all in combination with insulin aspart (IAsp) as mealtime insulin, in people with type 1 diabetes.

Methods

A 16-week, randomised, open-label trial, in which patients (mean age 45.8 years, A1c 8.4%, fasting plasma glucose 9.9 mmol/l, body mass index 26.9 kg/m^2) received subcutaneous injections of IDeg(A) (600 μmol/l; $n = 59$), IDeg(B) (900 μmol/l; $n = 60$) or insulin glargine (IGlar; $n = 59$), all given once daily in the evening, and insulin aspart was administered at mealtimes.

Results

At 16 weeks, mean A1c was comparable for IDeg(A) (7.8 ± 0.8%), IDeg(B) (8.0 ± 1.0%) and IGlar (7.6 ± 0.8%), as was fasting plasma glucose (8.3 ± 4.0, 8.3 ± 2.8 and 8.9 ± 3.5 mmol/l, respectively). Estimated mean rates of confirmed hypoglycaemia were 28% lower for IDeg(A) compared with IGlar [rate ratio (RR) 0.72 (95% CI 0.52–1.00)] and 10% lower for IDeg(B) compared with IGlar [RR 0.90 (0.65–1.24)]; rates of nocturnal hypoglycaemia were 58% lower for IDeg(A) [RR 0.42 (0.25–0.69)] and 29% lower for IDeg(B) [RR 0.71 (0.44–1.16)]. Mean total daily insulin dose was similar to baseline. The frequency and pattern of adverse events was similar between insulin treatments.

Conclusions

This clinical trial showed that IDeg, used in combination with mealtime IAsp, is a well tolerated and efficacious treatment when used in patients with type 1 diabetes, providing comparable glycaemic control to insulin glargine at comparable doses but with lower rates of hypoglycaemia.

> **COMMENT**
>
> Similar to the trial reported above, IDeg used in type 1 diabetes for 4 months had an apparent, but not statistically significant, reduction in hypoglycaemia, with similar glucose control. This study investigated two different formulations of IDeg and concluded that it is safe and well tolerated in patients with type 1 diabetes compared with IGlar. The real question that still needs to be answered is whether there are meaningful differences between IDeg and IGlar.

A new-generation ultra-long-acting basal insulin with a bolus boost compared with insulin glargine in insulin-naive people with type 2 diabetes: a randomised, controlled trial

Heise T[1], Tack CJ[2], Cuddihy R[3], Davidson J[4], Gouet D[5], Liebl A[6], Romero E[7], Mersebach H[8], Dykiel P[8], Jorde R[9]

[1]*Profil Institut für Stoffwechselforschung, Neuss, Germany,* [2]*Radboud University, Nijmegen Medical Centre, Nijmegen, The Netherlands,* [3]*International Diabetes Center, Park Nicollet, Minneapolis, MN, USA,* [4]*Department of Medicine, Division of Endocrinology, University of Texas, Southwestern Medical School, Dallas, TX, USA,* [5]*Hôpital Saint Louis, Centre Hospitalier de La Rochelle, La Rochelle, France,* [6]*Center for Diabetes and Metabolism, Fachklinik, Bad Heilbrunn, Germany,* [7]*University of Valladolid, Instituto de Endocrinología y Nutrición, Valladolid, Spain,* [8]*Novo Nordisk A/S, Søborg, Denmark, and* [9]*Institute of Clinical Medicine, University of Tromsø, Tromsø, Norway*

*Diabetes Care 2011; **34**: 669–74*

Background

Insulin degludec (IDeg) can be co-formulated with insulin aspart (IAsp) resulting in a soluble preparation comprising two different insulin analogues (IDegAsp: 70% v/v IDeg as basal insulin and 30% v/v IAsp as prandial insulin). By providing both basal and rapid-acting insulin analogues in one injection, IDegAsp could be an attractive alternative to the common strategy of initiating insulin therapy with basal insulin only on top of oral antidiabetic drugs. In this clinical proof-of concept trial, the safety and efficacy of IDegAsp was compared with insulin glargine (IGlar), both given once daily in combination with metformin in insulin-naive subjects with type 2 diabetes inadequately controlled on oral antidiabetic therapy. To establish the optimal ratio of IDeg to IAsp, an alternative formulation of IDegAsp (AF) containing a higher percentage of IAsp (45%) was also evaluated.

Methods

In this 16-week, open-label trial, subjects (mean age 59.1 years, A1c 8.5%, body mass index 30.3 kg/m^2) were randomised to once-daily IDegAsp ($n = 59$), AF ($n = 59$) or IGlar ($n = 60$), all in combination with metformin. Insulin was administered before the evening meal and dose-titrated to a fasting plasma glucose target of 4.0–6.0 mmol/l.

Results

After 16 weeks, mean A1c decreased in all groups to comparable levels (IDegAsp 7.0%; AF 7.2%; IGlar 7.1%). A similar proportion of subjects achieved A1c < 7.0% without confirmed hypoglycaemia in the last 4 weeks of treatment (IDegAsp 51%; AF 47%; IGlar 50%). Mean 2-h post-dinner plasma glucose increase was lower for IDegAsp (0.13 mmol/l) and AF (0.24 mmol/l) than for IGlar (1.63 mmol/l), whereas mean fasting plasma glucose was similar (IDegAsp 6.8 mmol/l; AF 7.4 mmol/l; IGlar 7.0 mmol/l). Hypoglycaemia rates were lower for IDegAsp and IGlar than for AF (1.2, 0.7 and 2.4 events per patient-year). Nocturnal hypoglycaemic events occurred rarely for IDegAsp and IGlar compared with AF (27 events).

Conclusions

Despite the limitations of this proof-of-concept study with a small sample size, a relatively short treatment duration and an open study design, it did show IDegAsp to be a promising treatment option for initiating insulin therapy in subjects with type 2 diabetes inadequately controlled with oral antidiabetic drugs. IDegAsp was safe and well tolerated, providing comparable overall glycaemic control to IGlar with lower doses and with the additional benefit of post-dinner plasma glucose control that did not result in an increased risk of nocturnal hypoglycaemia.

COMMENT

This is a proof-of-concept study using a new pre-mixed insulin – a combination of insulin degludec and insulin aspart (IDegAsp) as a 'basal plus' concept for managing diabetes. This 4-month trial documented lower hypoglycaemic events with IDegAsp with similar glucose control (A1c) compared with IGlar. As should be expected, there was a significant decrease in post-dinner glucose levels since IDegAsp has a rapid-acting insulin component. However, there was no rapid-acting component with IGlar. A better comparator would have been a currently available pre-mixed insulin. Such preparations, with a combination of rapid and basal insulin, in the future might allow uncontrolled patients with type 2 diabetes to achieve both lower fasting glucose and a reduction in the rise in blood glucose after eating their major meal.

Effect of sulfobutyl ether-β-cyclodextrin on bioavailability of insulin glargine and blood glucose level after subcutaneous injection to rats

Uehata K[1], Anno T[1], Hayashida K[1], Motoyama K[1], Hirayama F[2], Ono N[3], Pipkin JD[3], Uekama K[2], Arima H[1]

[1]*Graduate School of Pharmaceutical Sciences, Kumamoto University, Kumamoto, Japan,* [2]*Faculty of Pharmaceutical Sciences, Sojo University, Kumamoto, Japan, and* [3]*CyDex Pharmaceuticals Inc., Lenexa, KS, USA*

Int J Pharm 2011; **419**: 71–6

Background

Insulin glargine is the first long-acting basal insulin analogue used for subcutaneous administration once daily in patients with type 1 or type 2 diabetes mellitus. The aim of the study was to evaluate the potential use of sulfobutyl ether-β-cyclodextrin (SBE4-β-CyD), with the degree of substitution of the sulfobutyl ether group 3.9, on bioavailability of insulin glargine, the sustained-glucose lowering effect, the effects on physico-chemical properties and pharmacokinetics/pharmacodynamics of insulin glargine and the release of insulin glargine after subcutaneous injection into rats.

Methods

Serum insulin glargine and glucose levels of rats were measured. The solution of the insulin glargine in phosphate buffer in the absence and presence of SBE4-β-CyD was subcutaneously injected into male rats, and at appropriate intervals blood samples were taken.

Results

SBE4-β-CyD increased the solubility and suppressed aggregation of insulin glargine in phosphate buffer at pH 9.5, probably due to the interaction of SBE4-β-CyD with aromatic amino acid residues such as tyrosine of insulin glargine. In addition, SBE4-β-CyD accelerated the dissolution rate of insulin glargine from its precipitates, compared with that of insulin glargine alone. Furthermore, subcutaneous administration of an insulin glargine solution with SBE4-β-CyD enhanced the bioavailability of insulin glargine and sustained the glucose lowering effect, possibly due to the inhibitory effects of SBE4-β-CyD on the enzymatic degradation at the injection site.

Conclusions

SBE4-β-CyD enhanced both bioavailability and a persistence of the blood-glucose lowering effect of insulin glargine after subcutaneous injection to rats, probably due to the inhibitory effects of SBE4-β-CyD on the enzymatic degradation at the injection site, resulting from interaction with the insulin glargine molecule. These findings indicate that SBE4-β-CyD can be a useful excipient for sustained release of insulin glargine.

COMMENT

Since basal insulin treatment is becoming more popular in patients with type 2 diabetes, especially when they start to fail on oral hypoglycaemic agents and/or incretin therapies, there is an ongoing effort to improve the qualities of insulin glargine or to develop a better basal insulin. In this study, the authors investigated SBE4-β-CyD on the properties of insulin glargine. Their results conclude that SBE4-β-CyD can be a useful excipient for sustained release of insulin glargine. To achieve the same effect, there are also studies being pursued with higher concentrations of insulin glargine (U-200 or U-500) to see if these result in better basal insulin effect than insulin glargine in U-100 formulations.

Prandial inhaled insulin plus basal insulin glargine versus twice daily biaspart insulin for type 2 diabetes: a multicentre randomised trial

Rosenstock J[1], Lorber DL[2], Gnudi L[3], Howard CP[4], Bilheimer DW[4], Chang PC[4], Petrucci RE[4], Boss AH[4], Richardson PC[4]

[1] *Dallas Diabetes and Endocrine Center at Medical City, Dallas, TX, USA,*
[2] *Diabetes Control Foundation, Diabetes Care and Information Center, Flushing, NY, USA,* [3] *Unit for Metabolic Medicine, Cardiovascular Division, King's College London, London, UK, and* [4] *MannKind Corporation, Valencia, CA, USA*

Lancet 2010; **375**: *2244–53*

Background

Insulin therapy is often a delayed strategy in patients with type 2 diabetes mellitus because it is associated with weight gain, hypoglycaemia and the need for subcutaneous injections. The aim of this study was to compare the efficacy and safety of prandial Technosphere inhaled insulin plus bedtime insulin glargine vs. twice daily biaspart insulin for treatment of type 2 diabetes in patients previously treated with insulin, with or without oral agents.

Methods

This was a multicentre multinational randomised, open-label, parallel-group study of adult patients with type 2 diabetes and poor glycaemic control despite insulin therapy, with or without oral antidiabetic drugs. Patients were randomly allocated in a 1:1 ratio to receive 52 weeks' treatment with prandial Technosphere inhaled insulin powder plus bedtime insulin glargine, or twice daily pre-mixed biaspart insulin (70% insulin aspart protamine suspension and 30% insulin aspart of rDNA origin). The primary endpoint was a comparison of change in HbA1c from baseline to week 52 between treatment groups; the non-inferiority margin was 0.4%. Analysis was by per protocol for non-inferiority testing of the primary endpoint.

Results

Patients were allocated to inhaled insulin plus insulin glargine (n = 334) and to biaspart insulin (n = 343); 107 patients on inhaled insulin plus insulin glargine and 85 on biaspart insulin discontinued the trial. A total of 211 patients on inhaled insulin plus insulin glargine and 237 on biaspart insulin were included in per-protocol analyses. Change in HbA1c with inhaled insulin plus insulin glargine (–0.68%, SE 0.077, 95% CI –0.83 to –0.53) was similar and non-inferior to that with biaspart insulin (–0.76%, 0.071, –0.90 to –0.62). The between-group difference was 0.07% (SE 0.102, 95% CI –0.13 to 0.27). Patients had significantly lower weight gain and fewer mild-to-moderate and severe hypoglycaemic events on inhaled insulin plus insulin glargine than on biaspart insulin. The safety and tolerability profile was similar for both treatments, apart from increased occurrence of cough and change in pulmonary function in the group receiving inhaled insulin plus insulin glargine.

Conclusions

Inhaled insulin plus insulin glargine, alone or in combination with an oral antidiabetic drug (e.g. metformin), is an effective alternative to conventional insulin therapy (biaspart insulin) in uncontrolled type 2 diabetes.

COMMENT

Ultra-rapid-acting insulin has the theoretical advantage of matching the timing of exogenous insulin availability with that which would occur in healthy individuals. Prandial Technosphere inhaled insulin powder is one formulation that offers that potential. Its current development programme uses a small inhaler the size of a thumb. These two features are in sharp contrast to the previously marketed inhaled insulin Exubera which offered no unique pharmacokinetic advantage vs. injected prandial insulin preparations and had a rather large and cumbersome inhalation device. In the current study, there was less weight gain and less hypoglycaemia with the inhaled insulin plus insulin glargine programme, probably related to the rapid preprandial action and rapid dissipation of effect, so that there was no continuing postprandial hyperinsulinaemia which increases the risk of hypoglycaemia and results in weight gain.

Accelerated insulin pharmacokinetics and improved postprandial glycaemic control in patients with type 1 diabetes after co-administration of prandial insulins with hyaluronidase

Hompesch M[1], Muchmore DB[2], Morrow L[1], Vaughn DE[2]

[1] *Profil Institute for Clinical Research, Chula Vista, CA, USA, and* [2] *Halozyme Therapeutics, San Diego, CA, USA*

Diabetes Care 2011; **34**: 666–8

Background

Many patients with diabetes fail to meet target blood glucose levels, suggesting that the pharmacokinetic and efficacy profiles of available prandial insulin products should be improved. A previous study demonstrated that recombinant human hyaluronidase (rHuPH20) accelerates the pharmacokinetics of the insulin analogue lispro and regular human insulin (RHI) in healthy volunteers. The aim of this study was to confirm these findings in patients with type 1 diabetes using patient-specific, optimised doses of insulin and to explore the impact of these pharmacokinetic effects on glycaemic response to a standardised meal.

Methods

This was a four-way, crossover study including patients with type 1 diabetes ($n = 22$) who received injections of individually optimised doses of lispro or RHI with and without rHuPH20 before a liquid meal.

Results

With rHuPH20 co-administration, early insulin exposure (0–60 min) increased by 54% ($p = 0.0011$) for lispro and 206% ($p < 0.0001$) for RHI compared with the respective insulin alone. Peak blood glucose decreased 26 mg/dl for lispro ($p = 0.002$) and 24 mg/dl for RHI ($p = 0.017$), reducing hyperglycaemic excursions (area under the curve for blood glucose >140 mg/dl) by 79% ($p = 0.09$) and 85% ($p = 0.049$), respectively. Rates of hypoglycaemia were comparable for lispro with or without rHuPH20, whereas co-administration of RHI and rHuPH20 reduced hypoglycaemia.

Conclusions

The results of this study suggest that a co-formulation of prandial insulins with rHuPH20 may provide benefits for treating patients with diabetes by decreasing postprandial hyperglycaemic excursions without increasing the risk for late postprandial hypoglycaemic events.

COMMENT

Adding rHuPH20 to insulin results in more rapid absorption and is another strategy for accelerating the action of insulin resulting in an ultra-rapid-acting time course of action. The current study demonstrates that the concept is viable and that both regular insulin and current rapid acting insulin analogues can have their time course accelerated. Studies are under way testing this insulin in full-scale clinical trials.

Efficacy and safety of exenatide once weekly versus sitagliptin or pioglitazone as an adjunct to metformin for treatment of type 2 diabetes (DURATION-2): a randomised trial

Bergenstal RM[1], Wysham C[2], Macconell L[3], Malloy J[3], Walsh B[3], Yan P[3], Wilhelm K[3], Malone J[4], Porter LE[3]; DURATION-2 Study Group

[1] *International Diabetes Center at Park Nicollet, Minneapolis, MN, USA,* [2] *Rockwood Clinic, Spokane, WA, USA,* [3] *Amylin Pharmaceuticals, San Diego, CA, USA, and* [4] *Eli Lilly, Indianapolis, IN, USA*

Lancet 2010; **376***: 431–9*

Background

Most patients with type 2 diabetes begin pharmacotherapy with metformin but eventually need additional treatment. In this DURATION-2 study (Diabetes Therapy Utilization: Researching Changes in A1c, Weight and Other Factors Through Intervention with Exenatide Once Weekly), a comparison of the efficacy, safety and tolerability of three recommended therapies for patients not sufficiently controlled on metformin was assessed: exenatide once weekly (GLP-1 receptor agonist), and maximum approved doses of sitagliptin (DPP-4 inhibitor) and pioglitazone (thiazolidinedione).

Methods

In this multicentre (72 sites) randomised, double-blind, double-dummy, superiority trial of 26 weeks, patients with type 2 diabetes who had been treated with metformin (baseline mean HbA1c of 8.5%, fasting plasma glucose of 9.1 mmol/l, weight of 88.0 kg) were enrolled. Patients were randomly assigned to receive 2 mg injected exenatide once weekly plus oral placebo once daily; or 100 mg oral sitagliptin once daily plus injected placebo once weekly; or 45 mg oral pioglitazone once daily plus injected placebo once weekly. The primary endpoint was change in HbA1c between baseline and week 26. Analysis was by intention to treat, for all patients who received at least one dose of study drug.

Results

A total of 170 patients were assigned to receive once-weekly exenatide, 172 to receive sitagliptin and 172 to receive pioglitazone. In all, 491 patients received at least one dose of study drug and were included in the intention-to-treat analysis (160 on exenatide, 166 on sitagliptin and 165 on pioglitazone). Treatment with exenatide reduced HbA1c (least squares mean –1.5%, 95% CI –1.7 to –1.4) significantly more than did sitagliptin (–0.9%, –1.1 to –0.7) or pioglitazone (–1.2%, –1.4 to –1.0). Treatment differences were –0.6% (95% CI –0.9 to –0.4, p < 0.0001) for exenatide vs. sitagliptin, and –0.3% (–0.6 to –0.1, p = 0.0165) for exenatide vs. pioglitazone. Weight loss with exenatide (–2.3 kg, 95% CI –2.9 to –1.7) was significantly greater than with sitagliptin (difference –1.5 kg, 95% CI –2.4 to –0.7, p = 0.0002) or pioglitazone (difference –5.1 kg, –5.9 to –4.3, p < 0.0001). No episodes of severe hypoglycaemia occurred. The most frequent adverse events with exenatide and sitagliptin were nausea and diarrhoea; upper respiratory tract infection and peripheral oedema were the most frequent events with pioglitazone.

Conclusions

This study provides one of the most comprehensive direct comparisons of key intermediate outcome markers with adjunctive treatments to metformin. The improvements in HbA1c and bodyweight with once-weekly exenatide with a minimum number of hypoglycaemic episodes suggest that this drug should be considered as an adjunct to metformin in patients who need improvements in glucose control and bodyweight and in whom the risk of hypoglycaemia needs to be kept to a minimum.

DURATION-2: efficacy and safety of switching from maximum daily sitagliptin or pioglitazone to once-weekly exenatide

Wysham C[1], Bergenstal R[2], Malloy J[3], Yan P[3], Walsh B[3], Malone J[4], Taylor K[3]

[1] *Rockwood Clinic, Spokane, WA, USA,* [2] *International Diabetes Center at Park Nicollet, Minneapolis, MN, USA,* [3] *Amylin Pharmaceuticals Inc., San Diego, CA, USA, and* [4] *Eli Lilly and Company, Indianapolis, IN, USA*

*Diabetic Medicine 2011; **28**: 705–14*

Background

In the initial 26-week, double-blind, double-dummy assessment period of the DURATION-2 trial in patients with type 2 diabetes on metformin, the once-weekly GLP-1 receptor agonist exenatide once weekly resulted in greater HbA1c improvement and weight reduction compared with maximum approved daily doses of sitagliptin or pioglitazone. This trial was designed to evaluate the glycaemic and non-glycaemic (bodyweight, blood pressure, fasting lipids, markers of cardiovascular risk) changes in patients (i) treated with exenatide once weekly for 52 weeks; (ii) who switched from daily inhibition of DPP-4 (sitagliptin) to a therapy that results in continuous exposure to greater concentrations of the GLP-1 receptor agonist exenatide; and (iii) who switched from daily peroxisome proliferator activated receptor gamma (PPAR-γ) stimulation with pioglitazone, which increases insulin sensitivity to a therapy that augments glucose-dependent insulin secretion and is associated with weight loss.

Methods

In a 26-week, open-label, uncontrolled assessment period oral medications were discontinued and all patients received exenatide once weekly. Of the 364 patients (baseline HbA1c 8.5 ± 1.1%, fasting plasma glucose 9.0 ± 2.5 mmol/l, weight 88 ± 20 kg) who continued into the open-label period, 319 patients (88%) completed 52 weeks.

Results

Patients who received only exenatide once weekly demonstrated significant 52-week improvements in HbA1c (−1.6 ± 0.1%), fasting plasma glucose (−1.8 ± 0.3 mmol/l) and weight (−1.8 ± 0.5 kg). Patients who switched from sitagliptin to exenatide once weekly demonstrated significant incremental improvements in HbA1c (−0.3 ± 0.1%), fasting plasma glucose (−0.7 ± 0.2 mmol/l) and weight (−1.1 ± 0.3 kg). Patients who switched from pioglitazone to exenatide once weekly maintained HbA1c and fasting plasma glucose improvements (−1.6 ± 0.1%, −1.7 ± 0.3 mmol/l), with significant weight reduction (−3.0 ± 0.3 kg). Exenatide once weekly was generally well tolerated and adverse events were predominantly mild or moderate in intensity. Nausea was the most frequent adverse event in this assessment period. No severe hypoglycaemia was observed.

Conclusions

Exenatide once weekly has been demonstrated to elicit greater HbA1c improvement when directly compared with three agents that are commonly used after metformin (sitagliptin, pioglitazone, insulin glargine). The current findings suggest that exenatide once weekly may also be a suitable treatment alternative in patients with type 2 diabetes on a background of metformin who are not currently achieving adequate glycaemic control with a DPP-4 inhibitor or in whom thiazolidinedione-related bodyweight gain is a concern.

COMMENT

Exenatide once weekly is a long-acting formulation of a GLP-1 receptor agonist, the first diabetes drug that can be given on a weekly basis. The DURATION studies are a series of trials that compare exenatide once weekly with other diabetes drugs. In DURATION-2, the comparison is with the DPP-4 inhibitor sitagliptin and the thiazolidinedione pioglitazone in patients treated with metformin. During the first 26 weeks, in the *Lancet* paper, there was both greater lowering of HbA1c and greater weight loss with exenatide once weekly than with sitagliptin or pioglitazone. During the next 26 weeks, in the *Diabetic Medicine* paper, patients who had been on sitagliptin or pioglitazone were switched to exenatide once weekly. Those previously on sitagliptin had incremental improvements in both HbA1c and weight loss; those previously on pioglitazone maintained HbA1c and had significant weight loss. Together with the other DURATION studies, this indicates that exenatide once weekly offers the potential to reduce the frequency of injections to once weekly while attaining both excellent glycaemic control and better weight control.

Effect of dapagliflozin in patients with type 2 diabetes who have inadequate glycaemic control with metformin: a randomised, double-blind, placebo-controlled trial

Bailey CJ[1], Gross JL[2], Pieters A[3], Bastien A[4], List JF[4]

[1]*Life and Health Sciences, Aston University, Birmingham, UK,* [2]*Endocrine Division, Universidade Federal do Rio Grande do Sul, Porto Alegre, Brazil,* [3]*Global Biometric Sciences, Bristol-Myers Squibb, Brainel'Alleud, Belgium, and* [4]*Global Clinical Research, Bristol-Myers Squibb, Princeton, NJ, USA*

Lancet 2010; **375**: *2223–33*

Background

Correction of hyperglycaemia and prevention of glucotoxicity are important objectives in the management of type 2 diabetes. Dapagliflozin, a selective sodium glucose cotransporter-2 (SGLT-2) inhibitor, reduces renal glucose reabsorption in an insulin-independent manner. This study assessed the efficacy and safety of dapagliflozin when added to metformin in adult patients with type 2 diabetes who are not adequately controlled with metformin alone.

Methods

In this phase 3, multicentre, double-blind, parallel-group, placebo-controlled trial, adults with type 2 diabetes ($n = 546$) who were receiving daily metformin ($\geq$1500 mg per day) and had inadequate glycaemic control were randomly assigned to receive one of three doses of dapagliflozin (2.5 mg, $n = 137$; 5 mg, $n = 137$; or 10 mg, $n = 135$) or placebo ($n = 137$) orally once daily. Patients continued to receive their pre-study metformin dosing. The primary outcome was change from baseline in HbA1c at 24 weeks. All randomised patients who received at least one dose of double-blind study medication and who had both a baseline and at least one post-baseline measurement were included in the analysis.

Results

In total, 534 patients were included in the analysis of the primary endpoint (dapagliflozin 2.5 mg, $n = 135$; dapagliflozin 5 mg, $n = 133$; dapagliflozin 10 mg, $n = 132$; placebo, $n = 134$). At week 24, mean HbA1c had decreased by –0.30% (95% CI –0.44 to –0.16) in the placebo group, compared with –0.67% (–0.81 to –0.53, p $= 0.0002$) in the dapagliflozin 2.5 mg group, –0.70% (–0.85 to –0.56, p < 0.0001) in the dapagliflozin 5 mg group, and –0.84% (–0.98 to –0.70, p < 0.0001) in the dapagliflozin 10 mg group. Symptoms of hypoglycaemia occurred in similar proportions of patients in the dapagliflozin and placebo groups. Signs, symptoms and other reports suggestive of genital infections were more frequent in the dapagliflozin groups [2.5 mg, 11 patients (8%); 5 mg, 18 (13%); 10 mg, 12 (9%)] than in the placebo group [seven (5%)]. Seventeen patients had serious adverse events (four in each of the dapagliflozin groups and five in the placebo group).

Conclusions

This trial shows that dapagliflozin can improve glycaemic control in patients who have inadequate control with metformin. The drug acts independently of insulin, lowers weight, and is not associated with risk of hypoglycaemia. Safety and tolerability of the drug were also confirmed. Therefore, addition of dapagliflozin to metformin provides a new therapeutic option for the treatment of type 2 diabetes.

COMMENT

There are many SGLT-2 inhibitors currently under development. Dapagliflozin is the first of these to come to regulatory review, having been a subject of a US Food and Drug Administration advisory committee in 2011. The SGLT-2 inhibitors block reabsorption of glucose in the kidney, resulting in loss of glucose in the urine and consequent lowering of plasma glucose. In rodent models, this mechanism of reducing glycaemia corrects glucose toxicity, resulting in improved insulin secretion and decreased insulin resistance. If such mechanisms are confirmed in human beings, this class of therapeutic agent might have great potential in the management of diabetes. On the other hand, the increased glycosuria may increase the risk of urinary tract infections and genital fungal infections. The issue will be balancing benefits with risks. The current study gives some insight into this balance.

A novel approach to control hyperglycaemia in type 2 diabetes: sodium glucose cotransport (SGLT) inhibitors. Systematic review and meta-analysis of randomised trials

Musso G[1], Gambino R[2], Cassader M[2], Pagano G[2]

[1]Gradenigo Hospital, Turin, Italy, and [2]Department of Internal Medicine, University of Turin, Italy

Ann Med 2011 Apr 15 [Epub ahead of print]

Aim

To assess the efficacy and safety of the new antidiabetic drugs SGLT-2 inhibitors in type 2 diabetes.

Methods

Among 151 papers published on Medline, Cochrane Library, EMBASE, PubMed and international meeting abstracts through December 2010, 13 randomised placebo-controlled trials were included. Two reviewers retrieved papers and evaluated study quality by appropriate scores. Main outcomes were pooled using random- or fixed-effects models.

Results

Dapagliflozin significantly reduced HbA1c (–0.52%; 95% CI –0.46 to –0.57%; $p < 0.00001$), fasting plasma glucose (–18.28 mg/dl; 95% CI –20.66 to –15.89; $p < 0.00001$), body mass index (–1.17%; –1.41 to –0.92%; $p < 0.00001$), systolic (–4.08 mmHg; –4.91 to –3.24) and diastolic (–1.16 mmHg; –1.67 to –0.66) blood pressure, and serum uric acid (–41.50 μmol/l; –47.22 to –35.79). Other SGLT-2 inhibitors showed similar results. Dapagliflozin treatment increased the risk of urinary tract (odds ratio 1.34; 1.05–1.71) and genital tract (odds ratio 3.57; 2.59–4.93) infection; it also mildly increased the risk of hypoglycaemia (odds ratio 1.27; 1.05–1.53) when co-administered with insulin.

Conclusions

Pending confirmation from larger randomised controlled trials, this analysis shows that SGLT-2 inhibitors are safe and effective for hyperglycaemia treatment in type 2 diabetes.

COMMENT

The authors report a meta-analysis of randomised clinical trials of SGLT-2 inhibitors. Based on the statistical analysis there was significant reduction in HbA1c in patients randomised to dapagliflozin compared with other antidiabetic treatment. As indicated above, this study also noted a significant increase in genital and urinary tract infections along with a small increase in hypoglycaemic episodes when dapagliflozin was co-administered with insulin. In this rapidly evolving field, it is probably too early to evaluate the long-term efficacy and safety of SGLT-2 inhibitors.

Piragliatin, a novel glucokinase activator, lowers plasma glucose both in the post-absorptive state and after a glucose challenge in patients with type 2 diabetes mellitus: a mechanistic study

Bonadonna RC[1], Heise T[2], Arbet-Engels C[3], Kapitza C[2], Avogaro A[4], Grimsby J[3], Zhi J[3], Grippo JF[3], Balena R[5]

[1] *Division of Endocrinology and Metabolism, Department of Medicine, University of Verona School of Medicine, Verona, Italy,* [2] *Profil Institute, Neuss, Germany,* [3] *Hoffmann La-Roche, Nutley, New Jersey, USA,* [4] *Department of Clinical and Experimental Medicine and Metabolic Diseases, University of Padova, Padova, Italy, and* [5] *Hoffmann-La Roche, Basel, Switzerland*

J Clin Endocrinol Metab 2010; **95**: 5028–36

Background

Glucokinase plays a key role in glucose homeostasis. Glucokinase activators can lower glucose levels in both animal and human type 2 diabetes. The present study was undertaken to elucidate the mechanisms of the acute glucose-lowering action of glucokinase activator piragliatin in patients with type 2 diabetes in both fasting and fed (oral glucose tolerance test) states.

Methods

This was a phase Ib randomised, double-blind, placebo-controlled crossover trial of two (25 and 100 mg) doses of piragliatin, using a double-tracer glucose technique and mathematical modelling of the glucose-stimulated insulin secretion system to assess glucose fluxes and β-cell function. A single administration of piragliatin was chosen to avoid the potentially confounding influences of the metabolic changes associated with chronic drug treatment. The primary measure was plasma glucose concentration. The secondary measure was model assessed β-cell function and tracer-determined glucose fluxes.

Results
Piragliatin caused a dose-dependent reduction of glucose levels in both fasting and fed states ($p < 0.01$). In the fasting state, piragliatin caused a dose-dependent increase in β-cell function, a fall in endogenous glucose output and a rise in glucose use (all $p < 0.01$). In the fed state, the primary effects of piragliatin were on β-cell function ($p < 0.01$).

Conclusions
The glucokinase activator piragliatin has shown net glucose-lowering effects both in the post-absorptive state and after a glucose challenge. The mechanisms underlying these piragliatin glucose-lowering effects include a unique capability to improve all measured facets of β-cell function, with a consequent restraint of endogenous glucose output in the post-absorptive state and a remodelling in time of the homeostatic response after the glucose challenge. Furthermore, there is potential evidence of non-insulin-mediated improvements in glucose use, which await further experimental elucidations. Some concerns regarding hypoglycaemic risk at later times after a glucose challenge should be investigated more thoroughly. Altogether, this study supports that piragliatin may be a promising antidiabetic agent, with a primary target in human β-cell function.

COMMENT

Glucokinase is an important enzyme, serving in the pancreatic β-cell as a glucose sensor, a veritable 'glucose receptor' in β-cells, because the rate of conversion of glucose to glucose-6-phosphate is the rate-limiting step in glucose-stimulated insulin secretion. In the liver, glucokinase determines the rate of glucose disposal and of glycogen synthesis. Thus, activation of glucokinase would be expected to result in major improvements in glucose metabolism. Consequently, a number of glucokinase activators are under development as potential therapeutic agents for diabetes. Piragliatin is one such agent. Although there have been many reports using glucokinase activators in animal models, this is one of the first studies in human beings. We await additional studies both with piragliatin and other glucokinase activators.

Liraglutide as additional treatment for type 1 diabetes

Varanasi A, Bellini N, Rawal D, Vora M, Makdissi A, Dhindsa S, Chaudhuri A, Dandona P

Division of Endocrinology, Diabetes and Metabolism, State University of New York at Buffalo, and Kaleida Health, Buffalo, NY, USA

Eur J Endocrinol 2011; 165: 77–84

Background

The use of a GLP-1 analogue, liraglutide, may help in controlling hyperglycaemia and the oscillations in glucose concentrations in type 1 diabetes. The aim of the present trial was to determine whether the addition of liraglutide to insulin to treat patients with type 1 diabetes leads to an improvement in glycaemic control and diminishes glycaemic variability.

Methods

In this study, patients with well controlled type 1 diabetes ($n = 14$) on continuous glucose monitoring and intensive insulin therapy were treated with liraglutide for 1 week. Of the 14 patients, eight continued therapy for 24 weeks.

Results

In all the 14 patients, mean fasting and mean weekly glucose concentrations significantly decreased after 1 week from 130 ± 10 to 110 ± 8 mg/dl ($p < 0.01$) and from 137.5 ± 20 to 115 ± 12 mg/dl ($p < 0.01$) respectively. Glycaemic excursions significantly improved at 1 week. The glucose concentrations decreased from 56 ± 10 to 26 ± 6 mg/dl ($p < 0.01$) and the coefficient of variation decreased from 39.6 ± 10 to 22.6 ± 7 ($p < 0.01$). There was a concomitant fall in basal insulin from 24.5 ± 6 to 16.5 ± 6 units ($p < 0.01$) and bolus insulin from 22.5 ± 4 to 15.5 ± 4 units ($p < 0.01$). In patients who continued therapy with liraglutide for 24 weeks, mean fasting, mean weekly glucose concentrations, glycaemic excursions, and basal and bolus insulin dose also significantly decreased ($p < 0.01$). HbA1c decreased significantly at 24 weeks from 6.5% to 6.1% ($p = 0.02$), as did the bodyweight by 4.5 ± 1.5 kg ($p = 0.02$).

Conclusion

The addition of liraglutide to insulin therapy in well controlled type 1 diabetes patients resulted in a significant and rapid reduction in glycaemic excursions with a concomitant reduction in insulin dose and a reduction in appetite and food intake. The glycaemic effects were rapidly reversed after the cessation of liraglutide treatment. Bodyweight fell significantly in the group followed up for 24 weeks.

Effect of sitagliptin on glucose control in adult patients with type 1 diabetes: a pilot, double-blind, randomised, crossover trial

Ellis SL[1,2], Moser EG[1], Snell-Bergeon JK[1], Rodionova AS[1], Hazenfield RM[1], Garg SK[1,3]

[1] *Barbara Davis Center for Childhood Diabetes, Aurora, CO, USA,* [2] *Department of Clinical Pharmacy, University of Colorado Denver, Aurora, CO, USA, and* [3] *Department of Internal Medicine and Pediatrics, University of Colorado Denver, Aurora, CO, USA*

Diabetic Medicine 2011; 28: 1176–81

Background

Patients with type 1 diabetes have significantly elevated postprandial glucagon secretion. DPP-4 inhibitors improve HbA1c by several mechanisms, including increasing GLP-1 and glucose-dependent insulinotropic peptide concentrations, which decreases postprandial rises in glucagon in both type 1 and type 2 diabetes. The purpose of this pilot study was to assess the clinical benefit of sitagliptin in adult patients with type 1 diabetes.

Methods

This double-blind, randomised, crossover, 8-week, pilot study enrolled adult subjects with type 1 diabetes ($n = 20$). Subjects received sitagliptin 100 mg/day or placebo for 4 weeks and then crossed over. Outcomes included 2-h postprandial blood glucose and 24-h area under the curve changes in glucose measurements from continuous glucose monitoring, HbA1c, fructosamine and insulin dose.

Results

Sitagliptin significantly reduced blood glucose (2-h postprandial and 24-h area under the curve) despite reduced total and prandial insulin dose. Based on continuous glucose monitor findings, sitagliptin improved measures of glycaemic control, including mean blood glucose (-0.6 mmol/l; $p = 0.012$) and time in euglycaemic range 4.4–7.8 mmol/l (0.4 ± 0.2 h; $p = 0.046$). After controlling for period, treatment and insulin dose, the HbA1c was also significantly reduced ($-0.27 \pm 0.11\%$; $p = 0.025$) when patients were taking sitagliptin.

Conclusions

This study demonstrated that sitagliptin significantly reduced blood glucose, both the 2-h and 24-h area under the curve, in patients with type 1 diabetes. Sitagliptin also significantly reduced total daily insulin dose and HbA1c values while improving mean glucose from continuous glucose monitor downloads and time spent in the euglycaemic range. Further investigation is warranted in patients with type 1 diabetes in a larger cohort designed to assess both clinical outcomes and mechanism of action.

COMMENT

These two reports are small pilot studies assessing the potential role of the GLP-1 receptor agonist liraglutide and the DPP-4 inhibitor sitagliptin in type 1 diabetes. Both studies suggest that there is a beneficial effect. It is intriguing that patients with long-standing type 1 diabetes benefited from these interventions, suggesting that their mechanism of action in this circumstance is independent of stimulation of insulin secretion and is perhaps related to inhibition of glucagon secretion. Moreover, there has been an emerging interest in insulin resistance in type 1 diabetes and the fact that some patients with type 1 diabetes become overweight and really have the pathophysiological features of type 1 diabetes plus type 2 diabetes. Here, the potential role of GLP-1 receptor agonists or DPP-4 inhibitors promoting weight loss or limiting weight gain may also prove beneficial. These pilot studies demonstrate significant improvement in glucose control in patients with type 1 diabetes treated with liraglutide or sitagliptin. Additional studies with these agents are ongoing, and we await more to appear.

Low-dose combination therapy with rosiglitazone and metformin to prevent type 2 diabetes mellitus (CANOE trial): a double-blind randomised controlled study

Zinman B[1,2], Harris SB[3], Neuman J[1], Gerstein HC[4], Retnakaran RR[1], Raboud J[5,6], Qi Y[1], Hanley AJ[1,6]

[1] *Leadership Sinai Centre for Diabetes, Department of Medicine, Mount Sinai Hospital, and University of Toronto, Toronto, ON, Canada,* [2] *Samuel Lunenfeld Research Institute, Mount Sinai Hospital, Toronto, ON, Canada,* [3] *Centre for Studies in Family Medicine, University of Western Ontario, London, ON, Canada,* [4] *Division of Endocrinology and Metabolism and the Population Health Research Institute, Department of Medicine, McMaster University, and Hamilton Health Sciences, Hamilton, ON, Canada,* [5] *Division of Infectious Diseases,*

University Health Network, Toronto, ON, Canada, [6]Dalla Lana School of Public Health and Department of Nutrition and Public Health Sciences, University of Toronto, Toronto, ON, Canada

Lancet 2010; **376**: 103–11

Background
The evolving epidemic of type 2 diabetes has challenged healthcare providers to assess the safety and efficacy of various diabetes prevention strategies. Thiazolidinediones and metformin have different mechanisms of action (increasing insulin sensitivity and reducing hepatic glucose production, respectively) and have both been shown to reduce the development of diabetes in patients with impaired glucose tolerance. The Canadian Normoglycaemia Outcomes Evaluation (CANOE) trial assessed whether combination therapy with half the maximum dose of rosiglitazone and metformin on a background of a structured lifestyle intervention would prevent type 2 diabetes in individuals with impaired glucose tolerance.

Methods
In a double-blind, randomised controlled trial undertaken in clinics in Canadian centres, patients with impaired glucose tolerance ($n = 207$) were randomly assigned to receive combination rosiglitazone (2 mg) and metformin (500 mg) twice daily or matching placebo for a median of 3.9 years (interquartile range 3.0–4.6). The primary outcome was time to development of diabetes, measured by an oral glucose tolerance test or two fasting plasma glucose values of 7.0 mmol/l or greater.

Results
In all, 103 participants were assigned to rosiglitazone and metformin, and 104 to placebo; all were analysed. Vital status was obtained in 198 (96%) participants, and medication compliance (taking at least 80% of assigned medication) was 78% ($n = 77$) in the metformin and rosiglitazone group and 81% ($n = 80$) in the placebo group. Incident diabetes occurred in significantly fewer individuals in the active treatment group [$n = 14$ (14%)] than in the placebo group [$n = 41$ (39%); p < 0.0001]. The relative risk reduction was 66% (95% CI 41–80) and the absolute risk reduction was 26% (14–37). In total 70 (80%) patients in the treatment group regressed to normal glucose tolerance compared with 52 (53%) in the placebo group (p = 0.0002). Insulin sensitivity decreased by study end in the placebo group (median –1.24, interquartile range –2.38 to –0.08) and remained unchanged with rosiglitazone and metformin treatment (–0.39, –1.30 to 0.84; p = 0.0006 between groups). The change in β-cell

function, as measured by the insulin secretion sensitivity index 2, did not differ between groups (placebo −252.3, −382.2 to −58.0, vs. rosiglitazone and metformin −221.8, −330.4 to −87.8; p = 0.28). Diarrhoea was more often observed among participants in the active treatment group compared with the placebo group [16 (16%) vs. 6 (6%); p = 0.0253).

Conclusions

Findings from the CANOE trial have shown that the combination of the thiazolidinedione rosiglitazone with metformin at half the maximum dose was highly effective in prevention of diabetes and in normalization of glucose tolerance in individuals with impaired glucose tolerance, with little effect on the well known clinically relevant adverse events of these two drugs. These results lend support to the notion of the use of low dose combination therapies as an effective means to manage complex metabolic disorders.

Pioglitazone for diabetes prevention in impaired glucose tolerance

DeFronzo RA[1], Tripathy D[1], Schwenke DC[3,4], Banerji M[5], Bray GA[6], Buchanan TA[7], Clement SC[8], Henry RR[9], Hodis HN[7], Kitabchi AE[9], Mack WJ[7], Mudaliar S[9], Ratner RE[9,10], Williams K[2], Stentz FB[9], Musi N[1], Reaven PD[3]; ACT NOW Study

[1] Texas Diabetes Institute and University of Texas Health Science Center, San Antonio, TX, USA, [2] KenAnCo Biostatistics, San Antonio, TX, USA, [3] Phoenix Veterans Affairs Health Care System, Phoenix, AZ, USA, [4] College of Nursing and Health Innovation, Arizona State University, Phoenix, AZ, USA, [5] SUNY Health Science Center at Brooklyn, Brooklyn, NY, USA, [6] Pennington Biomedical Research Center, Louisiana State University, Baton Rouge, LA, USA, [7] University of Southern California Keck School of Medicine, Los Angeles, CA, USA, [8] Division of Endocrinology and Metabolism, Georgetown University, Washington, DC, USA, [9] VA San Diego Healthcare System and University of California at San Diego, San Diego, CA, and University of Tennessee, Division of Endocrinology, Diabetes and Metabolism, Memphis, TN, USA, and [10] Medstar Research Institute, Hyattsville, MD, USA

New Engl J Med 2011; 364: 1104–15

Background

Impaired glucose tolerance is associated with increased rates of cardiovascular disease and conversion to type 2 diabetes mellitus. Interventions that may prevent or delay such occurrences are of great clinical importance. The aim of the present study was to examine the effect of pioglitazone on diabetes risk factors and cardiovascular risk factors in adults with impaired glucose tolerance.

Methods

A randomised, double-blind, placebo-controlled study included 602 patients that were randomly assigned to receive pioglitazone or placebo. Fasting glucose was measured quarterly, and oral glucose tolerance tests were performed annually. Conversion to diabetes was confirmed on the basis of the results of repeat testing. The median follow-up period was 2.4 years.

Results

Annual incidence rates for type 2 diabetes mellitus were 2.1% in the pioglitazone group and 7.6% in the placebo group, and the hazard ratio for conversion to diabetes in the pioglitazone group was 0.28 (95% CI 0.16–0.49; $p < 0.001$). Conversion to normal glucose tolerance occurred in 48% of the patients in the pioglitazone group and 28% of those in the placebo group ($p < 0.001$). Treatment with pioglitazone compared with placebo was associated with significantly reduced levels of fasting glucose (a decrease of 11.7 mg/dl vs. 8.1 mg/dl, $p < 0.001$), 2-h glucose (a decrease of 30.5 mg/dl vs. 15.6 mg/dl) and HbA1c (a decrease of 0.04% vs. an increase of 0.20%, $p < 0.001$). Pioglitazone therapy was also associated with a decrease in diastolic blood pressure (by 2.0 mmHg vs. 0.0 mmHg, $p = 0.03$), a reduced rate of carotid intima-media thickening (31.5%, $p = 0.047$) and a greater increase in the level of high-density lipoprotein cholesterol (by 7.35 mg/dl vs. 4.5 mg/dl, $p = 0.008$). Weight gain was greater with pioglitazone than with placebo (3.9 kg vs. 0.77 kg, $p < 0.001$) and oedema was more frequent (12.9% vs. 6.4%, $p = 0.007$).

Conclusions

Treatment with pioglitazone in patients with impaired glucose tolerance reduced the risk of diabetes, although pioglitazone was associated with significant weight gain and oedema. Use of pioglitazone improved diastolic blood pressure, high-density lipoprotein cholesterol levels and serum levels of alanine aminotransferase and aspartate aminotransferase, and it slowed progression of carotid intima-media thickening.

Long-term effect of rosiglitazone and/or ramipril on the incidence of diabetes

DREAM-On (Diabetes Reduction Assessment with Ramipril and Rosiglitazone Medication Ongoing Follow-up) investigators, Gerstein HC[1], Mohan V[2], Avezum A[3], Bergenstal RM[4], Chiasson JL[5], Garrido M[6], MacKinnon I[7],

*Rao PV[8], Zinman B[9], Jung H[10], Joldersma L[10], Bosch J[1], Yusuf S[1];
DREAM-On Writing Group*

[1] *McMaster University and Hamilton Health Sciences and Population Health
Research Institute, Hamilton, ON, Canada,* [2] *Dr Mohan's Diabetes Specialities
Centre, Chennai, India,* [3] *Research Division, Dante Pazzanese Institute of
Cardiology, São Paulo, Brazil,* [4] *International Diabetes Center at Park Nicollet,
Minneapolis, MN, USA,* [5] *CHUM, University of Montreal, Montreal, QC, Canada,*
[6] *Clínica Privada Provincial, Buenos Aires, Argentina,* [7] *Instituto de
Investigaciones Clinicas, Mar del Plata, Argentina,* [8] *Nizam's Institute of Medical
Sciences University, Hyderabad, India,* [9] *Samuel Lunenfeld Research Institute,
Mount Sinai Hospital, University of Toronto, Toronto, ON, Canada,* [10] *Population
Health Research Institute, Hamilton, ON, Canada*

Diabetologia 2011; **54***: 487–95*

Background

The Diabetes Reduction Assessment with Rosiglitazone and Ramipril
Medication (DREAM) trial was a multicentre, randomised, placebo-
controlled trial of rosiglitazone and/or ramipril in people aged 30 and
over with impaired fasting glucose and/or impaired glucose tolerance. It
showed that, during the active treatment phase, rosiglitazone reduced the
incidence of the primary composite outcome of diabetes or death by 60%,
reduced diabetes alone by 62% and increased the likelihood of regression
to normoglycaemia by 83%. A subset of sites participating in the DREAM
trial followed DREAM participants after the active treatment phase of the
study was completed. The aim of this study was to investigate whether an
effect on diabetes prevention persists more than 1.5 years after therapy
has been discontinued.

Methods

The DREAM-On passive follow-up study was conducted at 49 of the 191
DREAM sites. Consenting participants were invited to have a repeat oral
glucose tolerance test 1–2 years after active therapy ended. A diagnosis
of diabetes at that time was based on either a fasting or 2-h plasma glucose level of $\geq$7.0 mmol/l or $\geq$11.1 mmol/l, respectively, or a confirmed
diagnosis by a non-study physician. Regression to normoglycaemia was
defined as a fasting and 2-h plasma glucose level of <6.1 mmol/l and
<7.8 mmol/l, respectively.

Results

After a median of 1.6 years after the end of the trial and 4.3 years after randomisation, rosiglitazone participants had a 39% lower incidence

of the primary outcome [hazard ratio (HR) 0.61, 95% CI 0.53–0.70; $p < 0.0001$] and 17% more regression to normoglycaemia (95% CI 1.01–1.34; $p = 0.034$). When the analysis was restricted to the passive follow-up period, a similar incidence of both the primary outcome and regression was observed in people from both treatment groups (HR 1.00, 95% CI 0.81–1.24, and HR 1.14, 95% CI 0.97–1.32, respectively). Similar effects were noted when new diabetes was analysed separately from death. Ramipril did not have any significant long-term effect.

Conclusions

These findings indicate that 3 years of treatment have a legacy effect on incident diabetes, suggesting that rosiglitazone preserves β-cell function while it is being taken without harming the β-cell.

COMMENT

These three studies further explore the potential use of thiazolidinediones in the prevention or delay of type 2 diabetes. One, CANOE, used low dose rosiglitazone in combination with metformin. One, ACT-NOW, used pioglitazone at full dosage. The third, DREAM-On, was a post-treatment follow-up of a subset of subjects in the earlier DREAM study (1). As with previous studies, all of these demonstrated significant reductions in progression to type 2 diabetes and increased the likelihood of reversal to normoglycaemia with active treatment compared with placebo. In DREAM-On, however, during follow-up after cessation of active therapy, rates of progression to diabetes and of regression were similar in both treatment groups. This is a highly important observation, in that it suggests that treatment must be maintained to achieve the beneficial effect. The lack of evident side effects in CANOE suggests that this may be feasible with low doses of drugs. The development of weight gain and oedema in ACT-NOW may prove limiting at the high doses used. A trial with low dose pioglitazone, which generally avoids these adverse effects, would seem warranted. The real question is whether it is time to revise the glycaemic criteria for diagnosis of diabetes to include those who have impairments of glycaemia but not yet diabetes by the current criteria.

OVERALL COMMENTARY

Current therapies for diabetes are imperfect, with complications still developing at distressing rates. Coupled with the exploding worldwide epidemic of diabetes, new treatment strategies are warranted. Here we have discussed new medications, modification of existing medications to offer improvement, new uses of existing medications, and earlier intervention to try to halt the course of the disease process. We anticipate that this wave of development will continue until such time as we are able to eradicate this disease.

REFERENCE

1. Effect of rosiglitazone on the frequency of diabetes in patients with impaired glucose tolerance or impaired fasting glucose: a randomised controlled trial. The DREAM (Diabetes REduction Assessment with ramipril and rosiglitazone Medication) Trial Investigators. *Lancet* 2006; **68**: 1096–1105

Index

Printed and bound by CPI Group (UK) Ltd, Croydon, CR0 4YY

27/10/2024

14580219-0002